MRCPsych:
Passing the CASC Exam
SECOND EDITION

MRCPsych:
Passing the CASC Exam
SECOND EDITION

Edited by

Justin Sauer
Maudsley Hospital, London, UK

Malarvizhi Babu Sandilyan
Prospect Park Hospital, Reading, UK

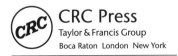

CRC Press
Taylor & Francis Group
Boca Raton London New York

CRC Press is an imprint of the
Taylor & Francis Group, an **informa** business

Whilst the advice and information in this book are believed to be true and accurate at

the date of going to press, neither the author[s] nor the publisher can accept any legal

responsibility or liability for any errors or omissions that may be made. In particular,

(but without limiting the generality of the preceding disclaimer) every effort has been

made to check drug dosages; however it is still possible that errors have been missed.

Furthermore, dosage schedules are constantly being revised and new side-effects

recognized. For these reasons the reader is strongly urged to consult the drug

companies' printed instructions before administering any of the drugs recommended

in this book.

CRC Press
Taylor & Francis Group
6000 Broken Sound Parkway NW, Suite 300
Boca Raton, FL 33487-2742

© 2017 by Taylor & Francis Group, LLC
CRC Press is an imprint of Taylor & Francis Group, an Informa business

No claim to original U.S. Government works

Printed in Great Britain by Ashford Colour Press Ltd
Version Date: 20160826

International Standard Book Number-13: 978-1-4987-2218-6 (Paperback)

Library of Congress Cataloging-in-Publication Data

Names: Sauer, Justin, editor. | Babu Sandilyan, Malarvizhi, editor.
Title: MRCPsych : passing the CASC exam / [edited by] Justin Sauer and
Malarvizhi Babu Sandilyan.
Description: Second edition. | Boca Raton : Taylor & Francis, 2017. |
Includes bibliographical references and index.
Identifiers: LCCN 2016019550 | ISBN 9781498722186 (alk. paper)
Subjects: | MESH: Psychiatry | Mental Disorders | Examination Questions
Classification: LCC RC457 | NLM WM 18.2 | DDC 616.890076--dc23
LC record available at https://lccn.loc.gov/2016019550

Visit the Taylor & Francis Web site at
http://www.taylorandfrancis.com

and the CRC Press Web site at
http://www.crcpress.com

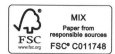

Contents

Preface

The importance of unhurried, comprehensive assessments of real patients in psychiatric training is key in terms of skill acquisition and development, something that is quite distinct from the time-limited scenarios with role-players as part of the CASC or 'Clinical Assessment of Skills and Competencies'. However, this examination is now a firmly established component of the Royal College membership examinations, and there are decent arguments that underpin its inclusion, despite the limitations.

Learning the mechanics of the process and the CASC 'tricks of the trade' are key to success. Passing an examination of this type can never be guaranteed, but as with everything, the more you practice, the 'luckier you will be'.

We hope the examination guidance and breadth of scenarios in this updated edition will help you in your examination success and future careers.

Justin Sauer and Malarvizhi Babu Sandilyan

Acknowledgements

We are grateful to the chapter authors for their time, effort and wisdom. We would like to thank Lance Wobus and the rest of the team at Taylor & Francis for their support and patience.

Editors

Justin Sauer is a consultant psychiatrist at the Maudsley Hospital in London. He has been involved in teaching trainees for Royal College examinations for many years, including running courses.

Malarvizhi Babu Sandilyan is a consultant psychiatrist at Berkshire Healthcare NHS Foundation Trust. She won the Alexander Mezey Prize and the Laughlin Prize in 2010 for best overall performance in the MRCPsych written and CASC examinations.

Contributors

Sangita Agarwal MBBS BSc MSc MRCPsych
Consultant Rheumatologist
Department of Rheumatology
Guy's Hospital
London, UK

Oliver Bashford BSc (Hons) MBChB DGM MRCPsych
Consultant Old Age Psychiatrist
Surrey and Borders Partnership NHS Foundation Trust
England, UK

Sharada Deepak MBBS MD MRCPsych
Consultant Psychiatrist
Berkshire Healthcare NHS Foundation Trust
Berkshire, UK

Matthew Fernando MBBS BSc (Hons) MRCPsych
Specialist Registrar in Child and Adolescent Psychiatry
South London and Maudsley NHS Foundation Trust
Fellow in Medical Education
NELFT NHS Foundation Trust
London, UK

Russell Foster BSc BA CandMag MSc PhD MBBS MRCPsych
Honorary Consultant Psychiatrist
Institute of Liver Studies
King's College Hospital
London, UK

Thomas Gilberthorpe MBChB MRCPsych
Specialist Registrar in Liaison Psychiatry
South London and Maudsley NHS Foundation Trust
London, UK

Marc Lyall MBBS BSc MRCPsych LLM
Consultant Forensic Psychiatrist
Centre for Forensic Mental Health
John Howard Centre
London, UK

James Main BM BCh MA MRCPsych
Lishman Unit
South London and Maudlsey NHS Foundation Trust
London, UK

Babu Mani MBBS DMH MRCPsych
Consultant Psychiatrist
Berkshire Healthcare NHS Foundation Trust
Berkshire, UK

Ruaidhri McCormack MRCPsych
Section of Cognitive Neuropsychiatry
Institute of Psychiatry, Psychology and Neuroscience
London, UK

Priyadarshini Natarajan MBBS PGDipPsych (Cardiff) MRCPsych
Consultant Psychiatrist
Berkshire Healthcare NHS Foundation Trust
Berkshire, UK

David Okai MD (Res) MBBS BMedSci (Hons) MRCPsych DipCBT
Consultant in Psychological Medicine and Neuropsychiatry
Psychological Medicine Service
Oxford University Hospitals NHS Foundation Trust
Oxford, UK

Dennis Ougrin MBBS MRCPsych PGDip (Oxon) PhD
Consultant Child and Adolescent Psychiatrist
Clinical Senior Lecturer
Course Leader, MSc in Child and Adolescent Mental Health
Child and Adolescent Psychiatry
Institute of Psychiatry
London, UK

Mark Parry MBChB MRCPsych
Consultant Psychiatrist
Berkshire Healthcare NHS Foundation Trust
Berkshire, UK

Pranathi Ramachandra MBBS DPM MRCPsych
Consultant Psychiatrist
Cambridgeshire and Peterborough NHS Foundation Trust
Cambridge, UK

Justin Sauer MBBS BSc FRCPsych
Consultant Psychiatrist
South London and Maudsley NHS Foundation Trust
London, UK

Dinesh Sinha MBBS MSc MBA MRCPsych
Consultant Psychiatrist in Psychotherapy
East London NHS Foundation Trust
London, UK

Derek Tracy MB BCh BAO MSc FHEA MRCPsych
Consultant Psychiatrist and Associate Clinical Director
Oxleas NHS Foundation Trust
The Memorial Hospital
London, UK

Exam guidance

Use the stations in this book for practice with colleagues and for individual rehearsal. Refer to the Royal College website for any CASC updates. Currently, you need to pass 12 out of 16 stations. All stations have equal weighting towards the total number required to pass. Half of the stations (8 in total) are single stations lasting 7 minutes, with 90 seconds to read the scenario. The other half are linked stations lasting 10 minutes each, with 90 seconds to read (4 linked scenarios, 8 stations in total). Linked stations are designed so the task in the first station is followed by a related task in the second. Single stations are run in the same way as the old part 1 OSCE. Some of the scenarios may be similar to the OSCE, but a higher performance standard will be required. Don't be surprised to find two examiners in the station, one marking and one playing a medical role (who will not contribute to the marking).

The CASC standards are high and as a more senior trainee you will be expected to show competence in management issues. However, you will still need to demonstrate ability in history taking, assessment and formulation of cases. Diagnosis, aetiology and prognosis will similarly be assessed. Without doubt, the most important skill is clear and effective communication and it is here that candidates usually fall down, rather than lack of knowledge. Clarity when communicating in lay terms or when dealing with a colleague is crucial. Showing genuine empathy where appropriate is similarly important. If communication is a weakness, you must rehearse intensely to change your style – which is difficult a few weeks before the exam. It can take time and hard work. If English is not your first language ask colleagues how they might 'phrase' questions or demonstrate empathy. If you are able to 'act', like the actors in the scenarios, you will also be at an advantage. Treat the scenarios as real, and you will perform better.

The marks given for each station are as follows:

- Good Pass
- Pass
- Borderline
- Fail
- Clear Fail

The chances are that a poor performance in one station does not mean complete failure. You are unlikely to be in a good position to judge your own performance, so do not dwell on this. Concentrate on the job at hand and carry on!

A list of some top tips

In your preparation consider how you would manage disorders using the matrix on the next page or something similar. It is important to have a structure in your mind for the common scenarios.

Management	Short term	Medium term	Long term
Biological			
Psychological			
Social			

In aetiological scenarios, consider the predisposing, precipitating and perpetuating factors.

Examiners are looking for:

- Competence in your assessment and management
- Structure
- Logic
- Safety
- Emotional intelligence

Examiners do not like:

- Repetition
- Waffling
- Poor communication skills
- Poor listening skills
- Disorganisation
- Arrogance
- Arguments

The examiners do not want to fail you. They sit as a group before the CASC to consider what areas need to be covered to pass a station – so they have all agreed on this. If you are borderline in a performance but have been a great communicator with evidence of emotional intelligence you may just pass the station.

Consider your own

Appearance and behaviour

- Confident, professional, but not arrogant
- Don't panic – rehearse opening phrases for different scenarios to build initial confidence
- If you are anxious, the examiners become anxious too
- Dress smart, formal – like a future colleague!
- Body language – stop any habits – ask colleagues to comment – your non-verbal communication should be of someone who is calm, interested and supportive

Speech

- Should be clear, confident and unrushed – many of us have a tendency to speak faster when anxious
- Verbal habits – again ask colleagues or record your interview – addressing your 'ums' or similar utterances can make a huge difference in how you come across
- Where possible start with an open question
- Avoid swing questions

- Avoid leading questions
- Speak in lay terms to patients – avoid psychobabble
- The use of silence, where appropriate, can be very valuable

Interview technique

- Read the scenario carefully
- Answer the tasks that have been set for you and not what you want to talk about (a common error)
- Clarification is important if you are unsure – there will be a copy of the scenario in the examination cubicle if you need to refer to this (but hopefully this will not be necessary)
- Introduce yourself to the patient
- Ask if it would be alright to 'talk to them/ask some questions etc.'
- Reassure/empathise where appropriate
- Use normalisation where appropriate
- Learn stock phrases in case you run dry e.g. 'Do you have any questions for me at this point?' 'So to summarise...'
- Don't end the station until you are told to end – if you get the timing wrong it can feel very awkward
- If running short on time, explain this to the patient/relative
- Better to say you don't know, than to get it very wrong
- Always be polite and courteous throughout – even if you've had a hard time – and thank the actor at the end
- Don't take the actors' behaviour personally
- Smiling can put everyone at ease
- Know the ICD-10 or DSM 5 diagnostic criteria for the main conditions as these will instruct your assessments
- Do not ignore non-verbal cues – e.g. EPSE, agitation
- Listen to what the patient or relative is saying. It is a common mistake to ignore valuable information and to talk 'at' people rather than enter into a dialogue
- Always consider risk
- Practise with a stopwatch and Dictaphone

O LINKED STATIONS

STATION 1(a): TREATMENT-RESISTANT DEPRESSION

INSTRUCTION TO CANDIDATE

Mr Jones is a 74-year-old depressed patient. He has not responded to therapeutic doses of lofepramine and sertraline and, more recently, a combination of venlafaxine and mirtazapine. A worsening of mood and the emergence of psychotic features led to a compulsory admission to hospital under the Mental Health Act. He has been seen by the ward psychologist but is too depressed currently to engage with cognitive behavioural therapy (CBT). The nursing staff are concerned with his dietary intake, which has declined since his admission. Over the last week, fluid intake has reduced and blood tests show abnormal urea and electrolytes consistent with dehydration. His wife wonders if he should be transferred to a medical ward. In the absence of the consultant, you see this gentleman on the ward.

Explain to Mr Jones how you wish to manage him further and what this is likely to involve.

DO NOT INCLUDE A RISK ASSESSMENT.

ACTOR (ROLE-PLAYER) INSTRUCTIONS

You are withdrawn and relatively unforthcoming.

You do not recall the details of current or past treatments.

You are somewhat fearful and upset by the prospect of electro-convulsive therapy (ECT), but want to know more about it.

You recognise that you have not been eating or drinking well, but you are not delirious.

You do not actively want to end your life, but do not care if you die.

You would quite like to be left alone (halfway through the station), but you allow the candidate to continue if they are polite.

SUGGESTED APPROACH

Setting the scene

Begin the task by addressing the patient by name and introducing yourself. Acknowledge his current circumstances and explain the purpose of your meeting: 'Hello Mr Jones, I am Dr_____, a psychiatrist. I am sorry that things have been difficult for you lately; I understand your depression hasn't improved despite treatment with several antidepressants…'

Allow the patient to respond to your introduction and maintain a flow in your conversation.

Then explain your concerns: 'I can see that you haven't been able to eat and drink well lately; is something stopping you from eating or drinking?' 'Do you remember you had some recent blood tests? Well, the results are concerning because they are abnormal, probably because you aren't drinking very much.'

Explain the purpose of your discussion and offer him any clarifications: 'I would like to discuss with you the various treatment options available to help you recover from this depression. Please do interrupt me if you want to ask me anything in-between.'

Medical treatment

Here, you have to explain your concerns about his physical health and how you are planning to manage this: 'Mr Jones, it is very important that we talk about your physical health. Your recent blood tests were abnormal (deranged kidney function and salt levels in the blood), indicating that you are dehydrated. We will need to closely monitor this as, unless you are drinking, we might need to transfer you to the general hospital so they can rehydrate you with fluids. So we will be keeping a very close eye on your daily food and fluid intake over the next 24 hours to make sure your general health is satisfactory. We will need to take further blood tests and check your blood pressure and pulse rate frequently on the ward and I will be asking the nursing staff to encourage you to eat and drink at frequent intervals. Though all of this may seem like we are disturbing you quite often, these are important measures to support your general wellbeing.'

Psychological treatment

Here, you can briefly explore the outcome of the psychological assessment: 'I understand that you met with the psychologist to work out ways of overcoming your depression. Can you tell me how it went?' Then you can briefly explain the rationale of CBT and why it may not be suitable for him right now: 'Cognitive behavioural therapy aims at modifying your thoughts and behaviours which contribute to depression. However, it may take up to several weeks to achieve this, and given the severe nature of your depression, we may have to leave it for the future and not consider it as an option right now.'

Pharmacological treatment

Here, briefly explain the options available for treatment-resistant depression. You will have to familiarise yourself with the literature evidence for the various drugs (see 'Further Reading').

You should explain that changes to medication will depend on him being physically well and appropriately hydrated. If the patient is somewhat unresponsive, it might seem inappropriate to discuss the detail of particular drugs; but you can talk in broad terms: 'Mr Jones, there are further changes to your medication that might help you. Adding medication can have a positive effect on mood; however, this often takes some time to see a positive effect.'

Possibilities here for discussion include lithium, tri-iodothyronine or quetiapine.

ECT

ECT should be considered as an option when the effects of depression are potentially life threatening, such as through poor fluid or dietary intake. It will be important to demonstrate to the examiner that you recognise the severity of the depression and the risks faced by the patient and that ECT may be an appropriate treatment option. You should be familiar with the mental health law surrounding the administration of ECT in a consenting/non-consenting patient in principle, but are unlikely to be asked specifics in relation to the Mental Health Act law in a CASC station.

'Mr Jones, unfortunately, you remain very depressed despite treatment and it is seriously affecting your general health now. We are concerned that your physical health will deteriorate further without appropriate treatment. Taking all of this into consideration, one option that we need to discuss is ECT.' At this point, you should ask if he has heard about ECT or knows anyone who has been treated with ECT. This will help to address any preconceptions that he may have about ECT.

How does ECT work?

'The treatment is well established and its role has been well recognised in treating depression for many years. Because of the advances in medicine, it has become safer over the years. ECT involves passing a mild electric current through the brain whilst you are asleep under anaesthesia. This will artificially create a fit, and during this fit, there is a release of natural brain chemicals or neurotransmitters which help improve the symptoms of depression.'

What is the process like?

'Before we begin ECT, we have to check your physical health. This involves a thorough clinical examination, further blood tests, a tracing of your heart (ECG) and a chest x-ray if necessary. The anaesthetist will want to examine you and will also be at your bedside monitoring you throughout the procedure itself. I will go through all of this with you again in detail if you decide to proceed with ECT. You will have to sign a form to indicate that you are happy to go ahead with ECT. But of course, you can change your mind at any time before the procedure itself. The treatment is usually given twice a week and may last up to 12 sessions.'

What are the side effects?

'There are some short-term side effects following ECT; the common ones are headache, muscular pain, nausea and confusion. The risk of serious harm such as death is 1 in 100,000, which is very rare and is related to anaesthetic complications. This risk is reduced by having a proper anaesthetic fitness check prior to the procedure. In the longer term, about a third of people complain of loss of memory for life events often surrounding the period of depression. This is something we would have to monitor in the future.'

Rapport and communication

The patient will show a degree of psychomotor retardation, being somewhat withdrawn and slow to talk. It is important not to rush the patient, to give him enough time to absorb all the information you give and to check he understands what you say. Give him opportunities to ask questions and for there to be a dialogue. Addressing the patient by name personalises the interview and makes him feel valued. Whilst explaining all the risks, it is important to simultaneously explain how you are going to manage the risks so as to not alarm the patient. It is very important to give realistic and honest hope and reassurances, which will instil confidence in him (and the examiner).

Conclusion

Here, you can summarise what you have discussed, any further information you want to give and what the next steps will be: 'Mr Jones, we have had a discussion about your depression and how we can help you get better. I know there's been a lot of information for you to take in, but I am going to leave a written summary with your key nurse about what we've discussed. We can then meet again tomorrow, after you have had a chance to discuss this with your family. Does that sound OK? It's been very nice talking to you.'

FURTHER READING

Cleare, A., Pariante, C.M., Young, A.H. et al. (2015) Evidence-based guidelines for treating depressive disorders with antidepressants: A revision of the 2008 British Association for Psychopharmacology guidelines. *Journal of Psychopharmacology*, 29(5), 459–525.

Depression in adults: Recognition and Management. Clinical Guideline 90 (CG90) by National Institute for Health and Clinical Excellence. Published in October 2009 and updated in April 2016.

Taylor, D., Paton, C. & Kapur, S. (2015) *The Maudsley Prescribing Guidelines in Psychiatry*, 12th edition, London: Wiley-Blackwell.

www.nice.org.uk/guidance/ta59 – National Institute for Health and Care Excellence (NICE) guidance on the use of electroconvulsive therapy.

www.rcpsych.ac.uk/healthadvice/treatmentswellbeing/ect.aspx

The examiner's mark sheet

Domain/ percentage of marks	Essential points to pass	✓	Extra marks/comments (make notes here)
1. Rapport and communication 25% of marks	Clear communication Open and closed questions Empathy Demonstrating patience		
2. Pharmacological treatment for depression 20% of marks	Demonstrates options in treatment-resistant depression		
3. ECT option 20% of marks	Discusses of ECT as an option Addresses concerns Provides reassurances		
4. Medical treatment for dehydration and malnutrition 25% of marks	Highlights the importance of physical health Need for medical treatment in the first instance		
5. Psychological treatment for depression 10% of marks	Basic enquiries (we know he is too impaired)		

STATION 1(b): ECT

INSTRUCTION TO CANDIDATE

You meet with his wife, Mrs Jones, who is concerned about her husband's further deterioration since admission to hospital. You inform her that the team believe that ECT should now be considered in view of his worsening condition.

Mrs Jones has heard only negative things about ECT. Discuss the ECT with Mrs Jones and answer any questions.

ACTOR (ROLE-PLAYER) INSTRUCTIONS

You are very concerned about your husband and want him to get the best treatment.

You have heard bad things about 'electric shock therapy'.

You have seen it portrayed in films and are worried that it could turn your husband into a 'zombie' or might 'wipe out his memory'.

You want to ask questions about side effects, risks of memory loss and why it is being suggested.

You are initially anxious but are willing to listen to the candidate's explanation.

SUGGESTED APPROACH

Setting the scene

Introduce yourself and explain your reason for wanting to speak with her: 'Hello, Mrs Jones, my name is Dr_____, a psychiatrist. Thank you for meeting with me today. I would like to discuss your husband's treatment with you and answer any questions you may have.' Mention that you have just met with her husband and have discussed the treatment options, which include ECT. Acknowledge that ECT does have bad press, but that it is extremely effective in depression and that you would be happy to discuss any concerns she may have. It is useful to start by asking what she already knows about ECT.

Rationale

It is important to explain why ECT is being suggested, and to convey to Mrs Jones the seriousness of the situation and why alternative treatment options are less suitable. 'Mrs Jones, your husband has been treated with several different antidepressants and is now taking a combination of medications without any improvement. Psychological therapy can be helpful, but at the present time, your husband is not able to engage with this. There are other medications that we could add, but these would take a while to work, and because he is now not eating and drinking adequately, we need to intervene more quickly. ECT is often used for cases such as this because it is known to work quickly and is very effective.'

Procedure

An explanation of the procedure, if pitched at the appropriate level, can allay patients' and relatives' anxieties. Remember to invite questions and check that you have been understood.

'Would it help if I explain what happens during the treatment? Please feel free to interrupt and ask questions at any time. ECT involves the use of electricity to induce a very brief "fit" or "seizure" that usually lasts no more than 30 seconds. It takes place in a special treatment room. An anaesthetist gives a general anaesthetic, so that the person is asleep during the procedure, and a muscle relaxant to reduce the body movements that happen during a fit. The patient is not aware of what is happening and it is not painful. A brief electric current is given by the psychiatrist using two pads that are placed on the head for just a few moments. At all times, the anaesthetist, psychiatrist and ECT nurses will be present. After the fit has finished, the patient wakes up a short while later and then remains in a recovery area supervised by staff until ready to return to the ward.'

A usual course of treatment is between 6 and 12 sessions and given twice a week.

Benefits and adverse effects

It is important to give a balanced account of the intended benefits and possible side effects, without understating the adverse effects. Explain that the likelihood of a good response increases from two-thirds with antidepressants alone to four-fifths with ECT. It is one of the most effective treatments for depression. It is generally considered safe and there is no evidence base to date showing that ECT harms the brain.

Short-term adverse effects
- Common side effects include headache and drowsiness immediately after ECT, which usually settle within a few hours.
- Sometimes people complain of short-term memory loss, but this is usually temporary and only involves recent memories; for example, what the patient had done just before the treatment.
- Unilateral treatment can reduce the effects on memory.

Long-term adverse effects
- Some individuals describe longer-term memory problems.

How it works

A detailed account is unlikely to be required here. It is sufficient to describe in lay terms an alteration to the brain's chemistry: 'We are not sure exactly how ECT works, but believe that the treatment causes a release of neurotransmitters or "natural brain chemicals," whose imbalance is thought to underlie depression. This artificially induced release of "feel-good chemicals" may be how it works.'

Risk

It is important to emphasise that whilst ECT is associated with some risks, there are also risks of not having treatment, which include further delay in recovery from depression and deterioration in physical health, which could lead to death if not eating or drinking sufficiently. Mention that the risk of death following ECT is approximately 1 in 100,000 treatments, due to the anaesthetic risk.

Rapport and communication

There are those that consider ECT to be ineffective, inhumane and degrading and that it belongs to a different era. It has often been portrayed in a very negative light in the media. The character in this station may hold similar views and for this reason it is very important that she is given the opportunity to express her ideas and concerns, that she is listened to attentively and that her concerns are taken seriously. It is helpful to check her understanding and invite questions throughout the interview.

Conclusion

As the interview is nearing its end, you should summarise the content of the discussion and comment on anything else that you might like to do. This can provide a neat ending to the station: 'Mrs Jones, just to summarise what we have discussed: I have tried to explain the rationale for recommending ECT for your husband and hopefully have given you some idea of what it involves and what the main side effects are. I am happy to provide you with written information to have a read through and if you have any further questions or concerns, please don't hesitate to ask.'

ADDITIONAL POINTS

1. Some of the neurochemical changes following ECT include increased noradrenaline, dopamine and serotonin and reduced acetylcholine.

2. ECT can also be used in prolonged mania and catatonia, and has been used in Parkinson's disease and neuroleptic malignant syndrome.

3. Medical investigations are routinely checked beforehand including full blood count, urea and electrolytes, ECG and chest x-ray when indicated and sickle-cell screening is important for Afro-Caribbean and Mediterranean people.

FURTHER READING

https://www.nice.org.uk/guidance/ta59 – NICE guidance on the use of ECT.

http://www.rcpsych.ac.uk/healthadvice/treatmentswellbeing/ect.aspx – information from the Royal College of Psychiatrists.

The examiner's mark sheet

Domain/ percentage of marks	Essential points to pass	✓	Extra marks/comments (make notes here)
1. Rapport and communication 25% of marks	Clear communication Avoids medical jargon Empathy Elicits concerns		
2. Rationale 20% of marks	Mentions that other treatments have failed and emphasises urgency of the situation		

⇧ 3. ECT procedure
    20% of marks

Accurate and clear description of the procedure

4. Benefits and
    adverse effects
    20% of marks

Covers the most common and the more serious adverse effects. Gives a balanced account

5. Risk
    15% of marks

Mentions risk of not treating as well as of treating

% SCORE _____

OVERALL IMPRESSION

5   (CIRCLE ONE)

Good Pass

Pass

Borderline

Fail

Clear Fail

NOTES/Areas to improve

STATION 2(a): MEMORY LOSS

INSTRUCTION TO CANDIDATE

You are about to see a patient in your clinic. Below is the referral letter.

Dear Doctor,

Re: Prof. Michael Baugh – 15.06.32. Weston Hill Rise, Southwark, London

Thank you for seeing this retired sociologist who lives alone. He has reported worsening of his memory and I wonder if he has a dementing illness. He has a history of hypertension. No major surgical procedures. I have given him an antibiotic for a recent UTI.

Current medication: Trimethoprim 200 mg b.d.
                      Simvastatin 20 mg
                      Aspirin 75 mg
                      Enalapril 20 mg

He has one daughter, Mrs Carol Davies. She works but is happy to speak to you.

Sincerely,
Dr Byron Moore

Take a history of memory loss and explain your management plan.

Do not perform a cognitive assessment.

ACTOR (ROLE-PLAYER) INSTRUCTIONS

Over a period of 1 year, you have noticed that you have become forgetful and you think it has been getting gradually worse.

You keep losing your keys and on one occasion left them in your front door when you went out.

You have forgotten to attend a number of appointments.

Your family have commented on your declining memory.

Over the last week, you have been particularly muddled and on one occasion got lost.

SUGGESTED APPROACH

Setting the scene

'Hello, Professor Baugh. My name is Dr_____, and I am a psychiatrist. I have received a letter from your GP saying that you have been concerned about your memory. Is this correct? Can you tell me what's been happening?'

Start with open questions and then move on to closed questions as appropriate.

The interview will involve taking the patient through the development of the memory impairment, any associated features and how this impairment has affected different facets of his life. The impact on social and occupational functioning is very important in the assessment of the severity and in making a diagnosis. The medical history is also essential.

History of the presenting complaint

Note that he is on treatment for a urinary tract infection (UTI), so the history should include questions regarding delirium. It should also incorporate some of the other common causes of memory loss. It is helpful to ask about what other people have noticed and it is important to establish the premorbid level of functioning, such as with regards to education and employment, as this can give an indication of the extent of decline.

Questions might include: 'What kind of problems have you noticed? What sort of things do you forget? How long has this been going on? Since it started, has it been getting any better, worse or stayed the same? Have you noticed any other symptoms? Have other people commented on this? In what way is this affecting your life? Are there things you used to do that you can no longer do because of forgetfulness?'

Differential

Dementia in Alzheimer's disease has a slow, insidious course and usually affects recent memory first and the learning of new information, with relative preservation of longer-term memory.

Vascular dementia may have a sudden onset or a stepwise decline, may be associated with a known stroke and there may be relative preservation of insight. The pattern of cognitive deficits depends upon the extent and location of cerebrovascular disease.

Dementia with Lewy bodies (DLB) may present with marked fluctuations in cognition and level of alertness, visual hallucinations, rapid eye movement (REM) sleep behaviour disorder or spontaneous features of Parkinsonism.

Personality changes with early loss of insight may indicate a fronto-temporal dementia.

Delirium usually has a rapid onset, presents with fluctuating consciousness and marked inattention, there may be visual hallucinations or other psychotic features and is associated with acute physical illness. There may be an increase or decrease in motor activity.

Depression can present with poor attention, concentration and bradyphrenia and may occur following life events and physical ill health. Often there are subjective complaints of memory loss in depression, unlike in dementia, where people will frequently hide or compensate for deficits.

It is important to differentiate isolated memory impairment from multiple or global cognitive deficits. Enquire about aphasia (e.g. nominal), agnosia, apraxia (e.g. dressing) and executive functioning (planning, organising, sequencing and abstract ability). In amnestic disorders, there is memory impairment rather than global cognitive decline.

Also consider alcohol and substance misuse, schizophrenia and malingering.

Medical history

Currently, he has a UTI. Has this caused an acute confusional state?

Ask broadly about his medical history, and specifically enquire about cardiovascular risk factors: 'I see that you are on treatment for cholesterol and high blood pressure. How long have you been on treatment for these? Do you know why you are prescribed aspirin? Do you smoke? Have you ever had a heart attack, angina or an irregular heart beat? Do you have diabetes?'

Also ask about neurological conditions: 'Have you ever had a stroke or a mini-stroke, or a head injury that knocked you unconscious? Have you had a tremor?'

Ask about alcohol consumption: 'How much alcohol do you typically drink in a week?' (and enquire about harmful use and dependence if appropriate).

Ask if he has ever had a brain scan and whether the GP has arranged blood tests or an ECG. If these have not been done, they should be included in your management plan.

Social functioning

It is essential to establish how the symptoms affect his day-to-day functioning. Remember that functional impairment is needed in order to make a clinical diagnosis of dementia. Mild memory impairment without significant functional decline is termed mild cognitive impairment and does not always lead to dementia.

Domains to ask about include basic self-care, domestic tasks around the home and more complex tasks like driving, finances, shopping and using public transport: 'How are these problems affecting your day to day life? Do you get any help from family or friends, or have professional carers visiting? (If so, ask what tasks they perform.) Do you have any difficulties with washing, getting dressed or eating dinner? How are you with tasks around the house, like cooking, cleaning and washing up? How do you manage your finances? Are you still driving? Do you do your own shopping or does someone help you with that?'

Risk

'Have you ever forgotten to turn off the gas, left the taps running by accident or left your keys in the door when you've gone out? How often does this happen? Have you found any ways to manage this? Are you still driving (and if so, have you had any problems with this)? Have you got lost at all?' Establish whether he has gotten into any risky or vulnerable situations and how often this has happened.

Management

This will depend on the diagnosis, which is based on your clinical assessment, physical examination and investigations that include memory tests, blood tests and brain imaging.

The actor may ask you what you think is wrong with him and what you will do should he have dementia. You should explain that further investigations/test results are required, but you believe there is a memory problem.

Most likely diagnoses in this scenario are Alzheimer's or vascular dementia, and recent worsening due to a delirium, secondary to urinary tract infection.

Consider management under biological, psychological and social headings. Management will depend on the degree of cognitive and functional impairment, so not all of the suggestions below will be relevant in every case.

Biological
- Optimising vascular risk factors (e.g. hypertension, dyslipidaemia, diabetes, atrial fibrillation and smoking cessation [if present])
- Additional medication for untreated physical risk factors; ensure current UTI is treated adequately
- Possible role for acetylcholinesterase inhibitors or memantine in Alzheimer's disease (AD) – be aware of recent NICE guidelines
- Treat any psychiatric comorbidity (e.g. antidepressants)
- Advice about alcohol if drinking heavily
- Encourage exercise for its wide range of physical and psychological benefits

Psychological
- Cognitive stimulation, memory groups and CBT for depression
- Reality orientation, validation therapy and reminiscence therapy

Social
- Ensuring adequate social support (e.g. carer/home help/meals-on-wheels/day centres)
- Compliance aids for medication (if still self-medicating; e.g. pill-box or blister pack)
- Occupational therapy (OT) assessment and adaptations for the home environment (e.g. memory prompts, Telecare devices and Keysafe)
- Alzheimer's Society – information resources, support groups and carer's assessment
- Support for daughter (e.g. carer's group)
- Advice about finances and lasting power of attorney

Rapport and communication

Some patients are very anxious about seeing a doctor regarding their memory and worry about the possibility of dementia. It is important to identify this and respond appropriately in order to put the patient at ease as much as possible. The patient might not be able to give a very clear history or might be slow in answering questions; in this case, you must demonstrate patience.

Conclusion

A good way to finish the station is to thank the patient and comment on further action you will take: 'Thank you for coming today, Professor Baugh. If you would like, I will write to you to summarise our discussion and send you some information leaflets that will be of interest. Also, if you are in agreement, I would like to speak to your daughter about the matters we have discussed today. Is that OK? I look forward to seeing you again next time.'

ADDITIONAL POINTS

1. When considering anti-dementia treatment, remember to take into account the NICE guidelines, any arrhythmias and a history of dyspepsia or gastric ulceration. It is important to explain that the drugs are not a cure and that benefits are modest, but they can help with cognitive symptoms for some people.

2. Three acetylcholinesterase inhibitors (donepezil, galantamine and rivastigmine) are currently recommended by NICE for Alzheimer's disease. They are all similar in their clinical effect on memory and improved attention and motivation. Common side effects include headache, nausea, vomiting, anorexia, weight loss and diarrhoea.

3. Memantine is now recommended for managing severe Alzheimer's disease and for moderately severe disease if acetylcholinesterase inhibitors cannot be taken. Memantine is an N-methyl-D-aspartate (NMDA) receptor antagonist that affects glutamate transmission. The dose is reduced in renal impairment.

FURTHER READING

http://pathways.nice.org.uk/pathways/dementia – NICE guidance on dementia.

http://www.alzheimers.org.uk/ – Alzheimer's Society website.

The examiner's mark sheet

Domain/ percentage of marks	Essential points to pass	✓	Extra marks/comments (make notes here)
1. Rapport and communication 15% of marks	Clear communication Open and closed questions Empathy Demonstrating patience		
2. History of presenting complaint 20% of marks	Explores the course of the symptoms Includes features of common causes of memory loss Includes risk incidents and behaviours		
3. Medical history 15% of marks	Elicits relevant history and excludes relevant negatives		
4. Social functioning 20% of marks	Establishes the impact of the symptoms on a range of basic and extended activities of daily living (ADLs) and current level of functioning		
5. Management 30% of marks	Appropriate suggestions for bio-psycho-social approach to management		

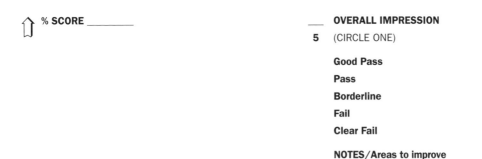

STATION 2(b): FRONTAL/TEMPORAL/PARIETAL LOBES

INSTRUCTION TO CANDIDATE

You meet with Prof. Baugh again in your clinic. Following a full initial assessment and the results of investigations, you diagnosed this gentleman with Alzheimer's type dementia and initiated acetylcholinesterase inhibitor treatment. A letter from his daughter tells you in confidence that his personality has changed significantly. She finds him to be difficult, embarrassing and on several occasions he has exposed himself. This is completely out of character and predates the new medication.

Assess his frontal, temporal and parietal lobe function.

ACTOR (ROLE-PLAYER) INSTRUCTIONS

You are fed up with all of the questions, but agree to cooperate.

You are somewhat disinhibited in manner, but not to the extent that it interferes significantly with the tasks.

SUGGESTED APPROACH

Setting the scene

'Hello, Professor Baugh, it's very nice to see you again. Do you remember our last meeting?' Asking him how he has been getting on with the new medication would be a good way to lead in to the station. Explain that you would like to do some more tests to see how the different parts of his brain are working. Inform him that you ask these questions of many people you see and not to worry if it makes a few mistakes, as some of the questions are more difficult than others.

Managing your time is important in this station, and you will lose marks if you do not cover all three sections. The examiners will not expect to see every single test for each lobe squeezed into 10 minutes, but rather a sensible, broad selection of tests that are performed properly.

Frontal lobes

Personality	'Have you changed in yourself in any way? In what way?'
Motor sequencing (Luria's test)	Demonstrate the hand sequence 'fist, edge, palm' five times, and then ask the patient to repeat with both hands. Perform for 30 seconds on each side.
Verbal fluency	Ask the patient to generate as many words as possible (not names or places) for the letters F, A or S. Perform for 1 minute and record all responses (there will not be sufficient time to test all three letters).
Category fluency	Ask the patient to name, for example, as many animals with four legs as they can in 1 minute. Record all responses.
Abstract reasoning (proverb interpretation)	Ask the patient to interpret what a proverb might mean: 'too many cooks spoil the broth' (or similar; bear in mind cultural differences here).
Cognitive estimates	'How many camels are there in Holland?' 'How tall is the Post Office Tower?'
Abstract similarities	Ask the patient in what way the following are similar: an apple and a banana; a table and chair; and/or a wall and a fence.
Primitive reflexes	Grasp reflex/rooting reflex/palmomental reflex.

Temporal lobes

Dominant lobe
Receptive dysphasia

Alexia	Ask to read something
Agraphia	Ask to write something

Impaired learning and retention of verbal material

Ask to repeat an address – 42 West Register Street – and to recall this after 5 minutes

Non-dominant lobe
Visuospatial difficulties

Anomia	Ask to name a wrist watch, strap and buckle
Prosopagnosia	Ask if he recognises the Queen on a £5 note
Hemisomatopagnosia	Belief that a limb is absent when it is not

Impaired learning and retention of non-verbal material such as music or drawings

Ask to copy a simple drawing and to repeat it from memory 5 minutes later

Bilateral lesions
Amnesic syndromes (Korsakoff's amnesia and Kluver–Bucy syndrome): assess short- and long-term memories.

Parietal lobes

	Function	Task
Dominant lobe		
Dysphasia	Receptive dysphasia	Obvious from conversation
Gerstmann's syndrome	Finger agnosia	'Point to left ring finger with right index finger'
	Dyscalculia	Simple arithmetic
	Right–left disorientation	'Touch left ear with right hand'
	Agraphia	Ask to draw something
Non-dominant lobe		
Neglect (inattention)	Neglects one side	Ask to draw clock face with dials and numbers
Prosopagnosia	Failure to recognise faces (as above)	
Anosognosia	Failure to recognise disabled body part	
Constructional apraxia	Unable to copy visually presented drawing	Copy interlocking pentagons
Topographical disorientation	Difficulty finding way, especially in new environment	Ask if he gets lost or confused in new places
Bilateral parietal lobe function		
Astereognosia	Inability to identify object through touch alone	Ask to identify key/coin with his eyes closed
Agraphagnosia	Failure to identify letters drawn on the palm	Ask him to identify H or W drawn with top of pen on his palm, with his eyes closed

Rapport and communication

It would be prudent to sensitively mention the reports of his having exposed himself and briefly assess risk issues. The patient might be offended by your mentioning this, and so this is a potential source of conflict. The style in which you ask your questions makes all the difference. For example: 'You exposed yourself in front of other people. Why did you do this?' is clumsier and less considerate than 'Some people I see who have had problems with their memory do things out of character, such as exposing themselves. Has anything like this happened to you?' Also be mindful that he might become fed up with all of the tasks being asked of him in this station, so good communication skills are essential.

ADDITIONAL POINTS

Features of frontal lobe dysfunction

Disinhibition, distractibility

Lack of drive

Errors of judgement

Failure to anticipate

Perseveration

Poor adaptation to change

Overfamiliarity

Sexual indiscretion

Consequences of neurological damage to temporal lobe structures

Changes in behaviour/personality

Increased aggression, agitation or instability (limbic system)

Contralateral homonymous upper quadrantanopia (assess visual fields)

Depersonalisation

Disturbance of sexual function

Epileptic phenomena

Psychotic disturbances akin to schizophrenia

Potential neurological consequences of parietal lobe damage

Homonymous lower quadrantanopia (optic radiation)

Astereognosis, reduced discrimination (sensory cortex)

FURTHER READING

Hodges, J.R. (2007) *Cognitive Assessment for Clinicians*, 2nd edn. New York, NY: Oxford University Press.

Lishman, W.A. (1998) *Organic Psychiatry*, 3rd edn. Oxford: Blackwell Science.

The examiner's mark sheet

Domain/ percentage of marks	Essential points to pass	✓	Extra marks/comments (make notes here)
1. Rapport and communication 25% of marks	Clear instructions Empathy		
2. Frontal lobes 25% of marks	Correct use of a range of frontal lobe tests		
3. Temporal lobes 25% of marks	Correct use of a range of temporal lobe tests		
4. Parietal lobes 25% of marks	Correct use of a range of parietal lobe tests		

⇧ % SCORE _____

___ **OVERALL IMPRESSION**

4 (CIRCLE ONE)

Good Pass

Pass

Borderline

Fail

Clear Fail

NOTES/Areas to improve

O SINGLE STATIONS

STATION 3: WANDERING

INSTRUCTION TO CANDIDATE

This elderly woman with vascular dementia was taken to hospital by the police after she was found wandering the streets in the early hours of the morning barefoot and dressed only in her nightclothes. She was confused and afraid.

She has been assessed in accident and emergency (A&E) and they have ruled out a physical aetiology. The casualty doctor informs you that she was seen in hospital a year ago by the neurologists after she had a transient ischaemic attack. She denies drinking alcohol, but is a smoker. She scored 7 out of 10 on an abbreviated mental test score today and is now asking to return home.

Assess if this patient is safe to go home. Do not carry out a cognitive assessment.

ACTOR (ROLE-PLAYER) INSTRUCTIONS

You cannot remember many details about what happened, but you are able to answer general questions about your accommodation and social circumstances.

You deny having any memory impairment.

SUGGESTED APPROACH

This woman has put herself in an extremely vulnerable situation and management will involve an assessment of risk and of her current mental state. It will also depend on her current social circumstances and whether there are any family members or close friends who will be able to provide support should she return home today.

Setting the scene

'Good morning, I'm Dr_____, a psychiatrist. I'd like to talk to you about what led to you coming into hospital today. Could you tell me what happened?' If she cannot remember what happened, take her through events in order to prompt her memory.

Taking a history

Can she remember what happened?

Why did she leave the property?

Can she remember her home address?

Has anything like this happened before? (You would want to corroborate this from A&E, police and a family doctor.)

Does she live alone? (You would want to speak to anyone living at home with her, her neighbours or her warden. If in a supported accommodation, how has she been managing?)

Does she have any next of kin or friends who you would be able to talk to?

Are there any healthcare professionals (or allied professionals) involved? (community mental health team [CMHT] for older adults, community psychiatric nurse [CPN], social worker, occupational therapist or day centre.)

It is important to find out about her living conditions (food, hygiene and gas/electricity).

Is she looking after herself appropriately?

It is important to note her current level of personal care (unkempt/undernourished).

History of alcohol or substance misuse?

History of falling?

Likelihood of repeating episodes? (Any old medical records in A&E.)

History of harming self or others?

History of behavioural disturbances? (Public or at home.)

Is she prescribed any regular medication? (Psychotropic medication; is she taking them appropriately?)

Has she been started on any new medication (e.g. diuretics or digoxin)?

Risk assessment

Consider the following:

In the household: gas, appliance use, smoking, fire, flooding or poor heating in winter

Financial: managing bills, access to money and pension

Diet: doing the shopping, preparing meals and malnutrition

Falls: at home and outside. What adaptations might be needed?

Abuse: financial (family, friends, tradesmen and opportunists) and emotional

Security: wandering and locking up (theft and burglary)

Current mental state

Excluding functional illness is important and will affect your management. Ask relevant questions in order to rule out:

- Psychosis (presence of abnormal perceptions/delusions paranoid/persecutory/command hallucinations)

- Affective illness (mania/severe depression)
- Neurotic, stress-related and somatoform disorder (dissociative fugue)
- Behavioural syndromes (somnambulism)

Capacity

Demonstrating capacity with regards to the event and associated risks would be somewhat reassuring if considering a return home. Capacity is defined as follows: the person must be able to understand and retain information long enough to make a judgement. They should be able to weigh up the pros and cons of his or her choice. The person should be able to communicate the decision made.

Further management

Respite or hospital admission
Admitting the patient would depend upon the information gathered during the interview. Even if cognitively impaired, the patient should be part of the process and continually updated. Admitting an elderly patient with dementia can be extremely distressing and you would want to provide them with appropriate reassurance. Rather than hospital admission, it might be that a period of respite in a residential or nursing home would be more appropriate.

CMHT follow-up
If not already known to mental health services, she would benefit from an assessment and follow-up. The multi-disciplinary team (MDT) will almost certainly play a role in looking at her medication, considering her cardiovascular risk factors, nursing input to monitor her mental state and OT to look at her accommodation and any modifications, particularly in view of her wandering behaviour.

Care package
She might benefit from more support depending on her social circumstances and ability to care for herself and her home environment. The social worker or care manager will be able to advise on financial matters and moving to more supported accommodation where appropriate.

Rapport and communication

The actor will put you under pressure to make a decision to let her go home. If you have performed a full risk assessment and key aspects of the mental state examination, you would still need to talk to family members and professionals that might be involved before arriving at a decision. If she has capacity and no evidence of mental illness, then she would be within her rights to leave, but you should try to persuade her to stay a little longer until you have spoken to the relevant people who are involved in her care.

ADDITIONAL POINTS

1. Assistive technology: devices can be installed in the home that alert a centre to an individual's activities. These can, for example, alert one to the fact that the front door has been opened at night. Similarly, the use of mobile phones or other devices attached to coats can allow people to be tracked if they put themselves at risk from wandering.

2. Further medical assessment: she has been cleared medically and for the purposes of the exam you would assume that to be the case. However,

in reality, you want to know the details of what examinations and tests have been performed. Is there any evidence of a fall or head injury? She should have had a full neurological assessment, and if not, you would want to do this. What were the results of blood tests and urinalysis? Does her presentation represent an acute confusional state (delirium)? Ideally, she should have had brain imaging (computed tomography/magnetic resonance imaging) in view of the history of transient ischemic attack (TIA).

FURTHER READING

Kales, H.C., Gitlin, L.N. & Lyketsos, C.G. (2015) Assessment and management of behavioural and psychological symptoms of dementia. *BMJ, 350*, h369.

The examiner's mark sheet

Domain/ percentage of marks	Essential points to pass	✓	Extra marks/comments (make notes here)
1. Rapport and communication 20% of marks	Clear communication Open and closed questions Empathy		
2. Taking the history 20% of marks	Elicits relevant aspects of the presenting event and social circumstances and level of functioning		
3. Risk 20% of marks	Enquires specifically about a range of risk behaviours (e.g. fire risk, flooding and finance)		
4. Mental state 20% of marks	Explores psychopathology and considers functional causes		
5. Further management 20% of marks	Appropriate suggestions for her ongoing management		

% SCORE _____

___

5

OVERALL IMPRESSION

(CIRCLE ONE)

Good Pass

Pass

Borderline

Fail

Clear Fail

NOTES/Areas to improve

STATION 4: TESTAMENTARY CAPACITY

INSTRUCTION TO CANDIDATE

You have been asked by a solicitor to assess this elderly woman. Her son has concerns that his mother has suddenly changed her will. He believes that his sister is plotting to exclude him from any inheritance.

Assess this woman to see if she has testamentary capacity (TC).

ACTOR (ROLE-PLAYER) INSTRUCTIONS

You are a 77-year-old lady with mild dementia.

You are carrying a notebook that you refer to at times to prompt your memory.

You know the approximate value of your house and savings and you know you have an ISA, but you do not know which bank it is in.

You have a son and daughter and three or four grandchildren. Your daughter has recently asked you to change your will, saying that she is in far greater need of financial help than her brother, but you do not know the details of this.

Your old will divided your estate equally between your two children, but your new one leaves your property and most of your savings to your daughter.

You are widowed and live alone. In the past, you ran a small cleaning company.

SUGGESTED APPROACH

Setting the scene

'Hello, my name is Dr_____, a psychiatrist. I have been contacted by a solicitor, on behalf of your son, to talk to you about your will. As I'm sure you understand, it is very important when we make a will that we fully understand what it means and what the consequences are. When we have finished today, I will write a report to the solicitor based upon our meeting today. Is that OK? Do you have any questions?'

Assessment of testamentary capacity

Testamentary capacity is the ability to make a valid will. When there is doubt as to TC, doctors are often asked for an opinion, usually a psychiatrist. Mental impairment can be grounds for a legal challenge, as can undue influence on the individual in making or changing a will.

The specific components of TC can be assessed by asking about their understanding of a will and its purpose. A general estimate of their property and its value is essential. Ask about the potential heirs and their wishes with respect to each. Reasons to include or exclude individuals should be explored. Ask about previous wills and whether they have a copy to show you.

Requirements for testamentary capacity:

1. The person must understand the nature of the act and its effects. The individual understands that they are giving their property to one or more objects of their regard.
2. The person must know the extent of his/her property. An exact knowledge is not expected, rather an idea of what property they have and its extent.

3. The person must know the legal heirs – those included and excluded – and how the will distributes the property.
4. The person has no mental disorder affecting 1–3 above. If a mental disorder is present, any legal challenge will depend upon demonstrating its impact on the ability to complete a will as set out in the criteria for TC as shown above.
5. The person must not be subject to undue influence by one or more third parties.

In assessing TC, it should be determined:

- Whether there is/was a major psychiatric disorder
- Whether this psychiatric disorder impairs the ability to know she was making a will
- Whether delusions are present that involve the estate or heirs
- Whether this disorder impairs her ability to know the nature and value of the estate
- Whether this disorder impairs her ability to identify the heirs that would usually be considered
- Whether the individual is vulnerable to undue influence

Clinical assessment is very important, as a number of conditions can interfere with valid will completion. Major psychiatric illnesses such as schizophrenia and organic diseases such as dementia are common examples. Their presence, however, does not always mean that the individual lacks TC. Someone with a psychotic illness who believes the FBI has bugged their apartment, for example, may know very well the size of their estate, their children and how it should be divided between them. Psychosis/delusions that would invalidate a person's capacity to make a will often involve their heirs in a negative way. If dementia is suspected, you would need to perform a test of cognitive function (e.g. mini-mental state examination [MMSE]).

Risk

As in all scenarios in the exam, where there is an opportunity to demonstrate that you are a safe trainee, do so. A screening question as part of your mental state examination (MSE) on suicide/self-harm would do.

Rapport and communication

The patient may be offended by the suggestion that she might not fully understand the act of making her will. To minimise this, good rapport and a sensitive explanation of why you have been asked to see her are required.

ADDITIONAL POINTS

1. Elderly people are often advised by lawyers to have an evaluation of testamentary capacity at the time a will is executed. Videotaping is increasingly used at the time of will execution, which can later be used in court.
2. Ordinarily, all relevant medical and psychiatric records would be available, as well as an estimate of the value and nature of the estate. This information would be sent to you by the solicitor. The criteria for testamentary capacity (TC) date back to 1870 and the case of *Banks v. Goodfellow*.

FURTHER READING

Banks v. Goodfellow (1870) LR 5 QB 549.

The examiner's mark sheet

Domain/ percentage of marks	Essential points to pass	✓	Extra marks/comments (make notes here)
1. Rapport and communication 20% of marks	Clear communication Open and closed questions Empathy		
2. Assessment of testamentary capacity 60% of marks	Covers the legal requirements for testamentary capacity		
3. Mental state 20% of marks	Elicits relevant psychopathology and enquires about risk		

% SCORE _____

___ **OVERALL IMPRESSION**

3 (CIRCLE ONE)

Good Pass

Pass

Borderline

Fail

Clear Fail

NOTES/Areas to improve

STATION 5: COGNITIVE ASSESSMENT

INSTRUCTION TO CANDIDATE

This 67-year-old civil engineer has noticed that his memory has deteriorated. He has felt less 'sharp' at work and, although he has no concerns about his ability to do the job, has found grasping new information quite difficult. He has a history of dyslipidaemia and hypertension, for which he is prescribed medication. He has seen his GP and the clinical examination is reported as unremarkable. There is no past psychiatric history. The GP has concerns that the presentation represents a likely dementing process, although this has not been discussed with the patient.

Carry out a cognitive assessment.

ACTOR (ROLE-PLAYER) INSTRUCTIONS

You have been more forgetful for the past one year.

You forget appointments frequently and generally slower at work than before.

The IT system has recently been updated at work and you are struggling to learn the new system.

You are required to do some memory tests and you struggle to recall information but otherwise fine.

Your mother had Alzheimer's disease and so does your sister. You are worried if you may have developed it too, and express your concerns to the doctor.

SUGGESTED APPROACH

Setting the scene

'Hello, I'm Dr_____. I've had a letter from your GP who says you've had some concerns about your memory. Is that correct? Would you tell me what's been happening?' Take a very brief history of the symptoms before moving on to the cognitive assessment.

'I'd like to run through some questions with you to test your memory. Some you may find very easy, others more difficult, but the most important thing is not to worry, just try your best. Is that OK?' Try to put him at ease.

The examination

You will be expected to use a brief memory test such as the mini-mental state examination or The Montreal Cognitive Assessment and should memorise it. You should be able to complete this assessment with time to spare. We are unable to reproduce the MMSE here due to copyright.

You should produce a score at the end. Writing the results down as you go along is therefore important. You will then be able to explain any areas of concern and what these mean. Giving feedback to the patient is important, as is reassurance.

If appropriate and if time allows, other cognitive tests may be used in addition to the MMSE. Clock-drawing is a quick and simple general test of cognition. In some cases, frontal lobe assessment is needed. It is also useful to ask questions relating to remote memory, both personal (wedding date and children's birthdays – although you will not be able to validate this) and impersonal (historical events).

Discussion about dementia risk

A discussion concerning the risk of developing dementia might ensue regarding:

- Older age
- Strong family history
- Cardiovascular disease
- Hypertension, diabetes, hypercholesterolaemia and atrial fibrillation
- Head trauma

In such scenarios, people often also express a concern about the risks to their children. Explain that we are all at risk of developing AD if we live long enough. The risk can only be approximated in the broadest terms. On balance, the risk to first-degree relatives of patients with AD who develop the disorder at any time up to the age of 85 years is slightly increased. The risk to the children of an affected individual is in the region of 1 in 5 to 1 in 6.

Conclusion

A neat way to end can be to state any further action you would take: 'Thank you for completing these tests. I think it would be helpful for us to gather more information. If you are in agreement, I would like to arrange for you to have a brain scan and for you to meet a psychologist to do more detailed testing. Is that OK?'

ADDITIONAL POINTS

Clock-drawing is increasingly used in cognitive assessment. It is easy to do and is a useful way of demonstrating disease progression with time. 'This is a clock face. Please fill the numbers and then set the time to 10 past 11.'

a. Sensitive to deterioration

b. Repeat three to six monthly

It assesses:

a. Comprehension

b. Abstract thinking

c. Planning

d. Visual memory

e. Visuospatial abilities

f. Motivation

g. Concentration

FURTHER READING

Folstein, M.F., Folstein, S.E. & McHugh, P.R. (1975) 'Mini-mental state': A practical method for grading the cognitive state of patients for the clinician. *Journal of Psychiatric Research*, *12*, 189–98.

The examiner's mark sheet

Domain/ percentage of marks	Essential points to pass	✓	Extra marks/comments (make notes here)
1. Rapport and communication 20% of marks	Clear communication Empathy		
2. Cognitive examination 60% of marks	MMSE Additional tests if relevant		
3. Discussion 20% of marks	Responds appropriately to the patient's concerns		
% SCORE _____		___ **3**	**OVERALL IMPRESSION** (CIRCLE ONE) **Good Pass** **Pass** **Borderline** **Fail** **Clear Fail** **NOTES/Areas to improve**

STATION 6: BEHAVIOURAL AND PSYCHOLOGICAL SYMPTOMS OF DEMENTIA

INSTRUCTION TO CANDIDATE

This is Mr Shaw. Your team have been seeing his mother at a nursing home since her admission there 2 months ago. She has Alzheimer's disease and had been irritable, aggressive and wandering whilst living in her own home. At that time, she was assessed and prescribed olanzapine. She settled initially, but has since become irritable again and the GP increased the dose.

Today, the son has asked to see you. He is angry and upset that his mother has been prescribed an anti-psychotic and thinks she is over-sedated. He also read an article about the 'dangers' of these medications in dementia.

Manage this situation and advise him on alternative approaches to behavioural changes in dementia.

ACTOR (ROLE-PLAYER) INSTRUCTIONS

You have read that anti-psychotics are dangerous drugs that can cause stroke, diabetes and even sudden death.

From your point of view, your mother was only aggressive once and that was with provocation, and this does not constitute 'severely' agitated behaviour.

You are very angry and demand that the drug be stopped and you do not settle down unless the doctor agrees.

SUGGESTED APPROACH

Setting the scene

'Hello, my name is Dr_____, I'm one of the psychiatrists. Thanks for coming to see me today. We've been involved in your mother's care for the last few months and I understand you have some questions about her treatment. Please tell me your concerns and I'll try my best to help.'

Rapport and communication

A major part of this station is managing the son's anger. To do this requires a calm approach, a clear explanation of the rationale for the treatment and suggestions of alternatives. If your impression is that the level of risk or the side effects do not justify the ongoing use of an anti-psychotic, then it may be appropriate to agree to discontinue it in favour of an alternative management plan. Avoid entering into an argument with the son, but allow him to voice his concerns.

'I am very concerned to hear about your mother being over-sedated, and I am glad that you have brought this to my attention. I will review her medication immediately after our discussion, and I agree that if she is suffering from significant side effects, then we should think about stopping this medication.' Answer his questions about the use of medication in dementia and the rationale. Demonstrating some knowledge in this area and providing options should help diffuse his anger.

Rationale for using an anti-psychotic

NICE guidelines state that anti-psychotics should be used for challenging behaviour in dementia only if there is severe distress or an immediate risk of harm to the person with dementia or others. There should be a full discussion of the risks and benefits and it should be time limited and reviewed at a minimum of every 3 months.

A Cochrane Review (Ballard et al., 2012) reported that evidence suggests that risperidone and olanzapine are useful in reducing aggression and risperidone reduces psychosis, but both are associated with serious adverse cerebrovascular events and extrapyramidal symptoms. Despite their modest efficacy, the significant increase in adverse events confirms that neither risperidone nor olanzapine should be used routinely to treat dementia patients with aggression or psychosis, unless there is severe distress or risk of physical harm to those living and working with the patient.

Some recommendations are that risperidone and olanzapine should not be used for behavioural symptoms of dementia. Certainly, the possibility of cerebrovascular events should be considered carefully before treating any patient with a history of stroke or transient ischaemic attack; risk factors for cerebrovascular disease (CVD) (hypertension [HT], diabetes mellitus [DM], smoking and atrial fibrillation [AF]) should also be considered.

Other atypical anti-psychotics, such as quetiapine and amisulpride, are sometimes used in place of risperidone or olanzapine, but cardiovascular events are possibly a class effect.

Explanation of the behavioural and psychological symptoms of dementia

The behavioural and psychological symptoms of dementia (BPSD) can be extremely difficult for carers to handle. In nursing homes, staff should be trained to manage these with simple non-pharmacological approaches in the first instance. However, medication is often needed when such approaches have failed, particularly where carers are subjected to ongoing physical and verbal aggression, night-time disturbance and sexual disinhibition.

Explain that BPSD are often due to our inability to understand the needs of the person with dementia. Many patients respond well to sensory stimulation, activities and social interaction. Simple interventions such as frequent toileting, good lighting, quality communication, fresh air and time in the open can make a difference. Hearing aids and analgesia for pain can make significant differences, where appropriate. A historical account of their likes and dislikes can assist the nursing home (e.g. their dietary preferences). Making the environment more homely (e.g. by putting up old family photographs) can be helpful.

Alternative management plan

First-line treatment should always be non-pharmacological, and may include:

- Aromatherapy and massage.
- Animal-assisted therapy.
- Multi-sensory stimulation.
- Music and dance-assisted therapy.
- Bright light therapy (related to melatonin).
- Psychology – looking for triggers or management advice to carers or staff.
- Structured interventions: using prompts (e.g. encouraging them to reminisce about important or enjoyable events) can help the person maintain an activity.
- Simulated presence therapy: where a video or audio recording is made by friends or family recalling events in the life. This can help to calm people or encourage their participation.

In some cases, other pharmacological approaches should be considered:

- Treating an affective component (antidepressants).
- Acetylcholinesterase inhibitors in severe cases if anti-psychotics cannot be taken.
- Memantine (some evidence for efficacy, but not in the NICE guidance for this indication).
- Mood stabilisers (anticonvulsants) can also be used for agitation.
- Benzodiazepines should be avoided other than in urgent situations, when lorazepam can be given for rapid tranquilisation.

ADDITIONAL POINTS

BPSD include:

- Motor behaviour: agitation, aggression and restlessness
- Social interactions: withdrawal, inappropriateness and disinhibition
- Speech: increased or reduced, mumbling and shouting
- Mood/anxiety: anger, lability, anxiety and fear
- Thoughts: delusions, paranoia and depression
- Perceptions: visual and auditory hallucinations
- Biological: sleep disturbance, incontinence and reduced appetite

FURTHER READING

Ballard C.G., Waite J. & Birks J. (2012) Atypical antipsychotics for aggression and psychosis in Alzheimer's disease. *Cochrane Database of Systematic Reviews* (1), CD003476.

http://pathways.nice.org.uk/pathways/dementia/dementia-interventions

The examiner's mark sheet

Domain/ percentage of marks	Essential points to pass	✓	Extra marks/comments (make notes here)
1. Rapport and communication 25% of marks	Clear communication Listens to concerns Remains calm		
2. Explanation of rationale 25% of marks	Mentions severe distress and risk to self or others Balance of benefits and risks		
3. Explanation of BPSD 25% of marks	Gives an appropriate overview of BPSD that is relevant to the case		
4. Alternative management plan 25% of marks	Mentions a range of non-pharmacological methods Suggests alternative medication options		

⇧ **% SCORE** _____

STATION 7: PSYCHOTIC DEPRESSION IN THE ELDERLY

INSTRUCTION TO CANDIDATE

You are about to meet Mrs Mary Evans, a 69-year-old lady who has been brought into hospital after neighbours reported that she was behaving strangely and was seen starting a bonfire in her front garden. When the police arrived, she told them that she wanted to kill herself and asked to be left alone.

Take a history to establish whether there are delusions, and if so whether these are primary or secondary. Also perform a risk assessment.

ACTOR (ROLE-PLAYER) INSTRUCTIONS

Earlier today, you were burning your possessions because 'they are all worthless.'

Around 3 weeks ago, you came to believe that you are impoverished, and even though there is money in the bank, you feel that this is 'just numbers.'

You have been feeling increasingly depressed for around 3 months since your husband died; you have very low energy levels, you have lost all enjoyment in life, your appetite has gone, you have lost some weight and you have no hope for the future.

You live alone, you are a widow and you stopped going to bingo 3 months ago.

You were planning to take your own life after you had destroyed your possessions.

SUGGESTED APPROACH

Setting the scene

'Hello, Mrs Evans, my name is Dr_____, a psychiatrist. I understand you've been brought to hospital today after people noticed you making a bonfire in your garden, could you tell me what's been happening?'

Taking the history

The task here is to take a history and mental state examination that guides you to a diagnosis. In this version of the station, the lady has delusions of poverty, but there are alternative versions in which she has nihilistic delusions believing herself to be dead, and one in which she believes herself to be guilty of an awful crime.

Explore what exactly has been happening that led to the police being called by her neighbours, and enquire into the build-up to this; ask how she has been for the last few weeks and months. Ask about any significant life events or psycho-social stressors that may have triggered the episode.

Ask about past psychiatric history to see if there have been any previous similar episodes, past admissions, previous self-harm or any previous psychiatric diagnoses. Screen for substance misuse, including alcohol. Ask about current social circumstances.

Assessment of mental state

You should demonstrate to the examiner that you know the diagnostic features of depression, and check for features of other causes of delusions, such as schizophrenia and delirium: 'How would you describe your mood or emotional state? How long have you felt like this? Do you still get enjoyment from things? How are your energy levels?'

The core features of depression are persistent sadness or low mood, anhedonia and anergia. It makes sense to ask about these before exploring other symptoms such as disturbed sleep, diurnal variation of mood, reduced appetite and weight loss, impaired concentration, feelings of guilt or self-blame, low self-esteem, thoughts of self-harm and hopelessness about the future.

Once you have established the presence of delusions, ask about other features of psychosis; examples include: 'Have you had the experience of hearing voices that others can't hear? Have you ever had a sensation that thoughts are being taken out of or inserted into your mind? Have you ever had a strange feeling that somehow your thoughts, feelings or movements don't belong to you?'

Assessment of the delusions

In this station, you are not only asked to establish the presence of delusions, but also to show the examiner that you can differentiate primary from secondary delusions.

Ask in detail about the patient's beliefs and follow up any cues that she gives you: 'You mentioned that you have no money; have you checked in your account? How much does it say is in there? What makes you think your possessions are worthless?'

A delusion is described as primary if it does not arise in response to another form of psychopathology, such as a mood disturbance. Primary delusions can be thought of as *un-understandable*. In contrast, secondary delusions arise as a symptom of other psychopathology, such as a mood disorder, or can be understood in light of the patient's cultural setting. The defining feature of both primary and secondary delusions is that the reason the patient gives for holding the belief is false or unacceptable.

In this station, it is not necessary to explicitly state whether you think the delusion is primary or secondary, but you should make it clear to the examiner that you know the difference: 'So let me check I have understood: you were feeling increasingly depressed for several months, and spending more and more time in bed feeling hopeless, and then you started to have the thought that you are impoverished and that all your possessions are worthless, is that right? It sounds like these ideas didn't just come out of the blue, but came to you when you were feeling very down?'

The key is to elicit a history of depression that clearly preceded the delusions.

Risk

In addition to finding out exactly what she was doing in setting the bonfire, you will need to ask some specific questions in order to form an impression of the level of risk that she poses both to herself and others.

'You were setting up a bonfire at home, could the fire have spread to the house or neighbouring properties? Now that you are here and the fire has stopped, how do you feel about that? Do you still want to burn your possessions? Do you think you would do the same again? You mentioned earlier that you had thoughts about taking your own life, could you tell me more about that? Have you thought about how you may end your life? Is there anything you can tell yourself that stops you doing that? Have you found yourself having thoughts about harming anyone else? Do you have any plans to do this?'

If you think the patient is high risk, you could indicate this to the examiner by saying something like: 'What you have told me is very concerning, and I think it is very important that you get the right help and treatment to get you through this.'

Rapport and communication

When exploring the phenomenology of a patient's beliefs, it is important to be sensitive in phrasing questions and to avoid being confrontational when testing the intensity of the belief. 'Is it possible that you could be mistaken in thinking that the money in your bank account is not really there? If someone was to say that actually your furniture is valuable, what would you think of that?'

Conclusion

It can be helpful to summarise your conversation at the end in order to check that you have understood what she has told you, and to thank her for talking to you. 'Before we finish, let me check that I have understood. Is there anything I've missed? Thank you for being so open with me today.'

FURTHER READING

Oyebode, F. (2008) Sim's *Symptoms in the Mind. An Introduction to Descriptive Psychopathology*, 4th edn. Philadelphia, PA: Saunders Elsevier.

The examiner's mark sheet

Domain/ percentage of marks	Essential points to pass	✓	Extra marks/comments (make notes here)
1. Rapport and communication 20% of marks	Clear communication Empathy Sensitive wording of questions		
2. Taking the history 20% of marks	Thorough history of presenting complaint Includes substance misuse and past psychiatric history		

⇧	3. Assessment of mental state 20% of marks	Thorough exploration of depressive symptoms and checks for other causes of delusions
	4. Assessment of the delusions 20% of marks	Establishes that the delusions are secondary to low mood rather than arising *de novo*
	5. Risk 20% of marks	Includes risk to self and others

% SCORE _____

___

5

OVERALL IMPRESSION

(CIRCLE ONE)

Good Pass

Pass

Borderline

Fail

Clear Fail

NOTES/Areas to improve

STATION 8: LEWY BODY DEMENTIA

INSTRUCTION TO CANDIDATE

You are about to meet the daughter of Mrs Dorothy Groves. Mrs Groves is a 75-year-old lady with a history of progressive memory impairment, and more recently has developed signs of Parkinsonism. You have just received the report of the dopamine transporter (DAT) scan, which shows degeneration of the dopaminergic system of the striatum. This confirms your suspicion of DLB.

Meet with Mrs Groves' daughter to explain the diagnosis, prognosis and management, and address her concerns.

ACTOR (ROLE-PLAYER) INSTRUCTIONS

You are worried that your mother has been talking about seeing little animals crawling around the sofa and you think she has been hallucinating.

You have noticed that she seems to be very stiff in her movements and has had a number of falls.

You have never heard of DLB, but last week saw a documentary about Alzheimer's and you want to know if it is similar.

You are especially worried that she will 'end up in a care home'.

SUGGESTED APPROACH

Setting the scene

'Thank you for coming to speak to me today. I'm Dr_____, a psychiatrist. I'd like to discuss with you your mother's diagnosis and care plan, and answer any questions you may have. Is that alright? Can I start by asking how much you know already about her diagnosis?'

Explanation of diagnosis and prognosis

'Your mother has a type of dementia called Lewy body dementia. Have you ever heard of this? It can cause problems with memory and other mental faculties, similar to other types of dementia, but it also causes difficulties with movements similar to those seen in Parkinson's disease. This can include stiffness, tremors, slowness and a shuffling sort of gait. Other symptoms include visual hallucinations and moving and vocalising during sleep, and some people get other physical symptoms, like a drop in blood pressure, constipation or bladder problems. It affects everyone differently and it's not possible to predict exactly how the illness will progress for a given individual, but in general, over time, the symptoms tend to get more severe and the level of support needed gradually increases.'

The DLB Consortium provide diagnostic criteria as follows:

Probable DLB:

1. The presence of dementia
2. At least two of three core features:
   a. Fluctuating cognition with pronounced variations in attention and alertness
   b. Recurrent visual hallucinations that are typically well formed and detailed
   c. Spontaneous features of Parkinsonism

Suggestive clinical features include:

- REM sleep behaviour disorder
- Severe neuroleptic sensitivity
- Low dopamine transporter uptake in basal ganglia demonstrated by single-photon emission computed tomography or positron emission tomography imaging

In the absence of two core features, the diagnosis of probable DLB *can also be made if dementia plus at least* one suggestive feature *is present* with one core feature.

Supportive clinical features include repeated falls and syncope, transient loss of consciousness, marked autonomic dysfunction, hallucinations in other modalities, depression and systematised delusions.

Management

It is helpful to present discussions of management using the bio-psycho-social framework. Treatment in DLB can be complex and it can be helpful to think about the different symptom clusters separately: cognitive, neuropsychiatric, motor, autonomic and sleep.

'There is no cure for Lewy body dementia, but we can help with some of the symptoms and we can help your mother remain as independent as possible, for as long as possible.'

Pharmacological

Rivastigmine and donepezil have both been shown to be effective for cognition and psychiatric symptoms. Donepezil is well tolerated, but rivastigmine is licenced for the treatment of Parkinson's disease dementia.

Anti-psychotics should be avoided due to the risk of hypersensitivity and neuroleptic malignant syndrome (NMS), but where needed, it is preferable to use quetiapine or clozapine, and to start with very low doses.

In cases where there is marked Parkinsonism, dopaminergic treatments can be used, but they carry a risk of neuropsychiatric side effects and would usually be given under the guidance of a neurologist or geriatrician.

Autonomic dysfunction including constipation, urinary incontinence and postural hypotension should be addressed with standard treatments.

Antidepressants can be used if there is comorbid depression, which is common.

REM sleep behaviour disorder can be treated with clonazepam, but this should be tried cautiously because of the risks associated with benzodiazepines, including cognitive impairment and sedation.

Social

Refer to OT for functional assessment and home adaptations, which may include Telecare devices. Physiotherapy may be able to help with mobility. In some cases, it may be appropriate to think about moving into more supported housing, such as sheltered accommodation. Refer to social services for assessment for a package of care to help with ADLs. Suggest that attendance at a day centre may be beneficial in order to address social isolation and boredom. Refer for assistance with finances and accessing benefits if appropriate. Give advice regarding lasting power of attorney.

Psychological

Cognitive stimulation groups, memory groups and music and dance therapy are recommended.

Do not forget to mention interventions for carers, which includes support groups and access to respite services.

The Alzheimer's Society can be a valuable support to people with all types of dementia, so consider offering a referral to them.

Addressing concerns

DLB is not well recognised by the general public and it is unlikely that the patient's daughter will be familiar with it. She may, however, have concerns based upon reports in the media about the care of people with dementia; she may be worried about her mother ending up in a care home or putting herself at risk by wandering at night or leaving gas hobs on. The way to approach this is to give a realistic impression of the kinds of problems that may arise, but also to reassure her that there are a lot of things that can be done to help her mother be as safe and independent as possible, and that there is support available for carers as well.

Allow her to voice her concerns and repeatedly check her understanding of your explanation.

Conclusion

'Thank you for coming to see me today. I know it is a lot to take in, so before you go, I will get some written information leaflets for you to take away. I also recommend the Alzheimer's Society website, as they have information about all types of dementia, not just Alzheimer's, and the website of the Lewy Body Dementia Association. I'll also give you our phone number so you can call at any time if you have any questions or concerns.'

FURTHER READING

McKeith, I.G., Dickson, D.W. & Lowe, J. et al. (2005) Diagnosis and management of dementia with Lewy bodies: A third report of the DLB Consortium. *Neurology, 65*, 1863–72.

http://www.alzheimers.org.uk/ – website of the Alzheimer's Society.

http://www.lbda.org/ – website of the Lewy Body Dementia Association.

The examiner's mark sheet

Domain/ percentage of marks	Essential points to pass	✓	Extra marks/comments (make notes here)
1. Rapport and communication 20% of marks	Clear communication Empathy Listens to concerns Checks understanding		
2. Diagnosis and prognosis 20% of marks	Clear explanation of the diagnosis Realistic account of what to expect		
3. Management – pharmacological 20% of marks	Mentions acetylcholinesterase inhibitors (AChEIs) and considers treatment of symptoms other than dementia		
4. Management – non-pharmacological 20% of marks	Suggests a range of appropriate interventions for psychological and social care		
5. Addressing concerns 20% of marks	Elicits concerns well Gives sensible suggestions and reassurance where appropriate		

% SCORE _____

OVERALL IMPRESSION

____

5   (CIRCLE ONE)

Good Pass

Pass

Borderline

Fail

Clear Fail

NOTES/Areas to improve

Chapter 2

Anxiety disorders
Priyadarshini Natarajan

O LINKED STATIONS

STATION 1(a): SOMATISATION DISORDER

INSTRUCTION TO CANDIDATE

Mrs Christine Ward is a 44-year-old woman and a mother of three children. She has been referred to the Community Mental Health Team by her GP, Dr Thomas, who had recently joined as a partner at the surgery. Dr Thomas is wary of Mrs Ward presenting to his clinic again and again with various physical symptoms, mainly pain, and requesting referrals to specialist clinics. It seems that her old GP, retired Dr Jones, knew what to say to Mrs Ward to reassure her. In her recent review with Dr Thomas, Mrs Ward is alleged to have threatened to complain against him for negligence. He has now requested an urgent psychiatric assessment.

You are a core trainee in the Community Mental Health Team. Take a history from the patient, including a brief risk assessment.

You will be asked to discuss your findings and management plan with a consultant psychiatrist in the next station (or) discuss diagnosis and management with the patient in the next station.

ACTOR (ROLE-PLAYER) INSTRUCTIONS

You are angry with your GP for referring you to the psychiatric services.

You do not want to see a psychiatrist.

You respond to appropriate reassurance from the candidate (and allow the candidate to continue).

You are somewhat tearful when asked about your ailments.

You fear you will die of cancer like your mother.

You are anxious all the time and sometimes wish you were dead.

SUGGESTED APPROACH

Setting the scene

Begin the task by addressing the patient by name and introduce yourself. Acknowledge that they might have had some reservation in attending this appointment and explain the purpose of your assessment: 'Hello, Mrs Ward, I am Dr_____, a trainee psychiatrist. It sounds like the past few months have been stressful for you. I am here to understand your difficulties and see if we can help you manage them.'

Allow the patient to respond. If they get angry, reassure them by making it clear that you accept that their symptoms are real and that you will try and help as best as you can. You may want to add that most people would be apprehensive of seeing a psychiatrist.

Then take a history of somatisation disorder, including the presenting complaints, duration of illness, differential diagnosis (which would include hypochondriasis), comorbid condition such as depression and a brief risk assessment.

Completing the task

Elaborate on history
Start the assessment interview by giving the patient the information that you have been given by her GP. Then elicit the somatic symptoms and their effects on daily life. Elaborate on the history by taking a chronological account of their symptoms: 'Mrs Ward, you seem to be suffering from pain for a long time. Could you tell me how it started? Have the symptoms changed? Are there other symptoms? How have they affected your daily life?'

Symptoms may be referred to any part or system of the body:

- Gastrointestinal: pain, belching, vomiting, nausea, etc.
- Skin: itching, burning, tingling, numbness, etc.
- Cardiovascular: breathlessness and chest pain
- Genitourinary: dysuria, frequent urination, unpleasant sensation around genitals, vaginal discharge, etc.
- Other sexual or menstrual complaints

Understand what the patient wants
Include a history of various contacts with the GP and other doctors. Elicit a history of previous referrals and treatments. This is the part of the assessment in which a patient's experience with professionals is disclosed. Give an opportunity for the patient to talk, and make appropriate empathic statements: 'I can see you have seen a few specialists over the time for your problems, but still you seem frustrated that there is no solution. I can imagine this could be hard on you.'

Elicit fears and beliefs about illness
Enquire about past illnesses in the patient which may or may not be linked to their current symptoms. Include a similar history of their family. Also ask about attitudes towards illness during their upbringing. 'Thinking back to your childhood days, what do you recollect? Were there any health-related worries in the family?'

Exclude organic disease: Briefly check what investigations she has had, what were the conclusions of the various doctors she had seen and ascertain whether there were any positive findings.

Identify relevant psycho-social stressors
Identify any links regarding the onset of symptoms to any personal or social history. There may be difficulties in their relationships or at work. 'Do you think you may have been under stress when your pain began? What was the stressful situation?'

Identify psychiatric disorder
Assess current mood with an emphasis on the biological symptoms of depression, panic disorder and anxiety. Include a brief risk assessment.

For a diagnosis of somatisation disorder, there must be a history of somatic complaints for at least 2 years or more that cannot be explained by any detectable physical conditions. Preoccupation with symptoms causes persistent distress and leads the patient to seek repeated consultations (three or more). There is persistent refusal to accept reassurance.

In hypochondriac disorder, there is a preoccupation with the possibility of having one or more serious and progressive physical disorders for at least 6 months.

Rapport and communication

It is important to gain the patient's trust. A sequential approach to assessment, beginning with physical symptoms and moving to psychological topics, is advised.

Conclusion

Here you can summarise what you have assessed, any information you may need and what the next steps will be:

'Mrs Ward, thank you for coming to see me today. We talked about your symptoms and your fears. You told me that your pain in...started more than 2 years ago. You also mentioned that your pain started at around the same time you went back to work after a break. You also said that your husband had to take on more work to bring in more money because the expenses have gone up with a big family. There is a possibility that this combination of stressful factors could have presented in the form of pain. I wonder if you ever thought about the symptoms in that way.' (Gill & Bass, 1997)

FURTHER READING

Gill, D. & Bass, C. (1997) Somatoform and dissociative disorders: Assessment and treatment. *Advances in Psychiatric Treatment, 3*, 9–16.

ICD-10 (1992) *Classification of Mental and Behavioral Disorders: Clinical Descriptions and Diagnostic Guidelines*. Geneva: WHO Press.

The examiner's mark sheet

Domain/ percentage of marks	Essential points to pass	✓	Extra marks/comments (make notes here)
1. Rapport and communication 20% of marks	Introduces self appropriately		
	Uses clear communication		
	Makes appropriate use of open and closed questions		
	Demonstrates an empathic and caring approach		
2. History taking 20% of marks	Asks about the chronology of events		
	Aetiological factors		
	Explores psycho-social stressors		
3. Exploring differentials 20% of marks	Explores differentials, mood disorders, panic disorder and psychoses		
	Excludes organic condition underlying pain		

4. Ascertaining diagnosis

20% of marks

Diagnosing somatisation disorder

Advises patient on the rationale for the diagnosis

5. Addressing concerns

20% of marks

Alleviates patient's anxiety and answers her questions

% SCORE _____

OVERALL IMPRESSION

5 (CIRCLE ONE)

Good Pass

Pass

Borderline

Fail

Clear Fail

NOTES/Areas to improve

STATION 1(b): DISCUSS DIAGNOSIS AND MANAGEMENT WITH THE PATIENT

> ## INSTRUCTION TO CANDIDATE
>
> You have just seen Mrs Ward in the previous station. Please discuss your findings with the patient and formulate a management plan.

(Note: This can also be a discussion with a consultant.)

ACTOR (ROLE-PLAYER) INSTRUCTIONS

You have seen the psychiatrist and have discussed your problems with him. Now you have come for further discussion to understand what the nature of your condition is. You do not think you should really be seeing a psychiatrist, as the pain is from your body, which requires further investigations from a physician. If the psychiatrist tries to explain that this could be due to psychological stress, you get angry and ask, 'Are you saying I'm crazy?' However, if the psychiatrist alleviates your anxiety and reassures you, you listen to him or her and ask for clarifications as to how the mind can cause physical health symptoms.

SUGGESTED APPROACH

Setting the scene

Introduce yourself: 'Hello, Mrs Ward, I am Dr_____, we met previously to discuss your situation.' Start with summarising the history that you have taken so far. Be clear and non-judgemental in your approach. Clarify whether the patient continues to strongly believe that her symptoms are due to undiagnosed physical disease.

'Mrs Ward, thank you for coming to see us today. We talked about your symptoms and your fears and worries. You told me that your pain...started more than 2 years ago. You have been to see your doctors and other specialists for a diagnosis; so far, they have not been able to find an underlying disease to explain your symptoms. You also mentioned that it started at around the same time that your husband had to take on more work to bring in more money because the expenses had gone up with the growing family.'

Explain your diagnosis

Be clear that you have taken the patient's complaints seriously, neither accepting a physical cause nor conceding that it was 'all in their mind'. Focus on the symptoms and their impact on the patient, rather than on the diagnosis.

'All of us have aches and pains at different times. There are some that will get better on their own, and there are those that will need to be investigated for a cause. Sometimes even after investigations, there are no physical causes of the pain. Many people have this kind of pain that cannot be medically explained. They can still be explained psychologically, but we need to think about causes that are not just physical. This does not mean that your symptoms are imaginary or that you are making them up.'

The mind and body link

Explain the link between bodily symptoms and the mind in as simple terms as you can. You can use the computer software and hardware analogy or any other analogy that would work for the patient.

'It is not uncommon to think that our minds and bodies work separately. In fact they are linked to each other...[use an appropriate analogy]. You mentioned that your symptoms started around the same time your husband found this extra work. While it may have been the right decision because of the additional money it brought, it also meant that he was not around at home over the weekend to help you take care of the children. This could have caused psychological stress which is likely to have presented as bodily pain. I wonder whether you have thought about your complaints in that way.' (Gill & Bass, 1997)

General advice

Help the patient to understand stress and identify the sources of stress in their life. Provide advice on lifestyle changes, including a gradual increase in exercise-based activities and relaxation.

Self-help

Self-help is one way of achieving control of a patient's problems. It may enable the symptoms to become less of a problem and lead to a much improved quality of life.

Medical treatment

Comorbid depression or anxiety will need to be treated appropriately with medication, if necessary.

Psychological treatment

Both individual and group cognitive behavioural therapy are useful for the treatment of somatisation disorder of different types. The main focus is on changing the patient's cognitions and behaviour.

In some cases, brief psychodynamic psychotherapy has also been effective.

FURTHER READING

Burton, C. (2003) Beyond somatisation: A review of the understanding and treatment of medically unexplained physical symptoms MUPS. *British Journal of General Practice*, 53(488), 231–9.

Gill, D. & Bass, C. (1997) Somatoform and dissociative disorders: Assessment and treatment. *Advances in Psychiatric Treatment*, 3, 9–16.

The examiner's mark sheet

Domain/ percentage of marks	Essential points to pass	✓	Extra marks/comments (make notes here)
1. Rapport and communication 20% of marks	Introduces self appropriately		
	Uses clear communication		
	Makes appropriate use of open and closed questions		
	Demonstrates an empathic and caring approach		
2. Diagnosis 20% of marks	Explains the diagnosis of somatisation disorder		
	Explains the rationale for the diagnosis		
3. Explanation 20% of marks	Explains the link between mind and bodily symptoms in a way that the patient understands		
4. Addressing concerns 20% of marks	Alleviates patient's anxiety and answers her questions		
	Able to reassure angry patient		
5. Management 20% of marks	Able to explain various treatment options		
	Demonstrates knowledge on treatment strategies for somatisation disorder		

% SCORE _____

_____
5

OVERALL IMPRESSION
(CIRCLE ONE)

Good Pass

Pass

Borderline

Fail

Clear Fail

NOTES/Areas to improve

STATION 2(a): GENERALISED ANXIETY DISORDER

INSTRUCTION TO CANDIDATE

This is Mrs Arnold, a 53-year-old married woman, who has been seeing a counsellor in primary care as she is stressed and anxious most of the time. The patient does not feel that the sessions have been helpful and the GP phones you and describes her being persistently anxious with little let up in her symptoms. He has tried to identify triggers without success and hopes you will be able to advise further. She attends with her husband and you see them together with her consent.

Assess this woman and consider the differential diagnosis.

ACTOR (ROLE-PLAYER) INSTRUCTIONS

You are very nervous from the start.

You are nearly in tears.

You insist that your husband is present with you for the assessment.

You keep holding his hand and often seek his support.

SUGGESTED APPROACH

Setting the scene

Introduce yourself and thank the couple for coming to see you today. Direct your questioning to the patient, but keep the husband involved in the dynamics.

'I'd like to ask you what's been happening and I've been told you're comfortable to talk with your husband here. I understand that you've been feeling anxious, is that correct? Could you tell me what things make you feel anxious? What does the anxiety feel like?' Start with open questions as usual and then become more focussed in your approach.

Completing the task

Elaborate the history of anxiety

Your assessment should turn to generalised anxiety disorder from the history provided and a differential diagnosis for anxiety symptoms should be considered. You should elaborate on the onset of symptoms, exacerbating factors, relieving factors and the impairments that the symptoms cause.

'Mrs Arnold, your GP informed us that you are stressed and anxious all the time. Could you tell us more about your anxieties? What is your main concern? How did it start? Are your symptoms present all day long? What is a typical day like?'

Primary symptoms of anxiety

Primary symptoms of anxiety are present most days for at least several weeks at a time and usually several months. Symptoms usually involve:

- Apprehension – worries of future misfortune, feeling on edge and difficulty concentrating
- Motor tension – fidgeting, tension headaches, trembling and unable to relax
- Autonomic overactivity – sweating, tachycardia, tachypnoea, dizziness and dry mouth

Normal worry

People with generalised anxiety disorder (GAD) tend to have more worries. There is also little reprieve from their anxiety. Often they will report a history of long-standing worry as reported here. The worry is all-consuming and it is difficult to focus on other issues. It is ruminative and uncontrollable, with individuals unable to stop themselves worrying, despite an acknowledgement that they worry too much. In GAD, there are also the manifestations of continuous tension (psychological [e.g. irritability and nervousness] and physical [e.g. muscle tension and headache]). These features are often enough to cause significant disruption to social and employment activities.

Medical illness

Ask about features of hyperthyroidism and other chronic physical ill health. Examples include:

Cardiovascular – angina, arrhythmias and heart failure

Endocrine – hyperthyroidism, carcinoid and adrenal gland dysfunction

Neurological – encephalopathies, head injuries and intracerebral lesions

Respiratory – asthma, chronic obstructive pulmonary disease and hypoxia

Mental illness

Consider and attempt to exclude anxiety related to psychosis, depression, dysthymia and personality disorders (anxious and dependent). Try to differentiate between GAD, obsessive compulsive disorder (OCD), panic disorder, agoraphobia, social phobia, specific phobia, post-traumatic stress disorder (PTSD) and adjustment disorder.

'Mrs Arnold, you told us how your anxieties started with stress. Could I check if you were ever low in mood before your anxieties started? Have you had any strange experiences that you could not explain? Or was there something weighing on your mind all the time? Do you avoid leaving home?'

Medication

Take history of current medication use that is likely to mimic/exacerbate anxiety symptoms:

Stimulants – amphetamines and aminophylline

Anticholinergics – benztropine and procyclidine

Sympathomimetics – ephedrine (cold remedies) and epinephrine

Anti-psychotics – related to akathisia

Others – levodopa, bromocriptine and baclofen

Substance misuse

The use of amphetamines, cocaine, hallucinogens, alcohol and sedative hypnotics can lead to anxiety.

Withdrawal – benzodiazepines (BZD), alcohol, narcotics, hypnotics and barbiturates

Diet – caffeine intake, monosodium glutamate and vitamin deficiencies

Differential diagnosis

Differentiating GAD from dysthymia can be clinically challenging. Both are associated with dysphoric mood, and patients with GAD often present initially with depression as a consequence of their anxiety. Unlike PTSD and adjustment disorders, in GAD there is usually the absence of a significant life event or trauma. Unlike specific phobias, the anxiety is broad and persistent.

GAD is a common form of anxiety, particularly in primary care. It affects women more than men (2:1) and is commonly associated with other psychiatric morbidities. It is a chronic condition and up to a quarter of sufferers will develop panic disorder. In *Diagnostic and Statistical Manual of Mental Disorders*, Fourth edition (DSM IV), the distinction between GAD and normal anxiety is explained by anxiety that is excessive and difficult to control with significant impairment or distress.

Risk assessment

GAD is often associated with depression. These patients tend to be more treatment resistant, and comorbid depression increases the suicide risk.

FURTHER READING

ICD-10 (1992) *Classification of Mental and Behavioural Disorders: Clinical Descriptions and Diagnostic Guidelines.* Geneva: WHO Press.

Massion, A.O., Warshaw, M.G. & Keller, M.B. (1993) Quality of life and psychiatric morbidity in panic disorder and generalised anxiety disorder. *American Journal of Psychiatry, 150,* 600–7.

The examiner's mark sheet

Domain/ percentage of marks	Essential points to pass	✓	Extra marks/comments (make notes here)
1. Rapport and communication 20% of marks	Introduces self appropriately		
	Uses clear communication		
	Makes appropriate use of open and closed questions		
	Demonstrates an empathic and caring approach		
2. History taking 20% of marks	Asks about chronology and progression of events		
	Attempts to identify any triggers and aetiology		
3. Diagnosis 20% of marks	Able to demonstrate the diagnosis as GAD		
4. Differential diagnoses 20% of marks	Considers differentials – other psychiatric disorders and organic causes		
5. Management 20% of marks	Able to explain various treatment options for GAD to patient and reassures them		
	Demonstrates knowledge of the bio-psycho-social approach in treatment		

⇑ **% SCORE** _____

___ **OVERALL IMPRESSION**

5 (CIRCLE ONE)

Good Pass

Pass

Borderline

Fail

Clear Fail

NOTES/Areas to improve

STATION 2(b): GENERALISED ANXIETY DISORDER – AETIOLOGY

INSTRUCTION TO CANDIDATE

Mr Arnold asks if he can see you alone for a moment. His wife agrees and is happy for you both to discuss her case. He explains that he has little understanding of what it all means and wants to know what causes someone to be 'like this'. He acknowledges that she has always been a little cautious about things, but that it had become so much worse over the last few years. He had hoped she would be able to 'pull herself together', rather than having to see a psychiatrist.

Explain to Mr Arnold what causes this condition.

ACTOR (ROLE-PLAYER) INSTRUCTIONS

You are keen to support your wife.

You are anxious as to whether she will ever get better, as this is affecting your lives.

You want some help for your wife, as this has gone on for a long time.

SUGGESTED APPROACH

Setting the scene

The link here would not demand an introduction, but rather to pick up on the situation as the wife exits the scenario: 'You asked to talk about how this could have happened to your wife. Tell me what it is you would like to know and I'll do my best to answer your questions.

Was there a specific reason you didn't want Mrs Arnold to be here? Sometimes it is difficult to discuss things openly with loved ones. Was there anything that you thought might upset her?'

Completing the task

Explanation about generalised anxiety disorder
The explanation should be given in simple terms.

'As I explained to you both, I believe your wife has a condition called generalised anxiety disorder. This belongs to a family of anxiety disorders. These conditions are common and widespread, but we are still not exactly sure what causes generalised anxiety disorder or other anxiety disorders. I'll explain to you what the current thinking is on how these conditions develop and if at any time you have questions or don't understand, please interrupt me.'

Biological
Genetic: there is little evidence for a genetic influence in GAD and it is unlikely to have a specific genetic or familial basis. Studies have shown that children of GAD mothers were no more likely to be anxious than counterparts with unaffected mothers. However, other studies have shown higher rates of GAD in families, but this may reflect the influence of a shared environment.

Pathophysiological: certain chemical systems in the brain called neurotransmitters have been implicated as having a role in anxiety. There are various such compounds, such as serotonin, noradrenaline, glutamate, gamma-aminobutyric acid (GABA) and cholecysto-kinin. Currently, there is limited evidence for one neurotransmitter having a dominant role in GAD. The benzodiazepine receptor has also been implicated.

Other: so far, there are no consistent neuroimaging findings in GAD. There is a circuit in the brain which runs from our adrenal gland on top of our kidneys to certain brain regions, and these auto-regulate each other by feedback mechanisms. There are some suggestions that this hypothalamic–pituitary–adrenal axis changes in functionality, which plays a role in the stress response. Studies have suggested that the stress hormone cortisol may be increased for prolonged periods of time in people with GAD.

'Anxiety is like worry or fear that has become a problem because they are too strong, making you uncomfortable and stopping you from doing things in your life. Some of us seem to be born that way. Research seems to suggest that we can inherit anxiety from our parents. Little is known about its precise aetiology. There may be a common vulnerability shared with other anxiety and affective disorders.'

Psycho-social factors
Cognitive–behavioural theory: according to this school of thinking, people with GAD respond inappropriately to perceived dangers. They selectively attend to negative stimuli around them and doubt their own ability to cope with them. Other cognitive models include worry as a cognitive avoidance, beliefs about the benefits of worry (worrying leads to avoidance of danger) and low self-efficacy (anxiety due to the belief that one is unable to exercise control over events).

Psychodynamic: no specific model has been developed for GAD, and theorists believe that anxiety in general is a symptom of unresolved conflicts from developmental stages.

Childhood: there is some evidence that early loss or separation from a parent is seen more than would be expected in GAD cases. Individuals with GAD have described their relationships with their parents as overprotective, controlling, rejecting and dysfunctional. However, these are not specific to GAD.

Life events: despite the usual gradual onset of GAD, increased stress and life events can be precipitants.

Information on risk
As part of your assessment in the previous station, you will probably have enquired about suicidal ideation. You could follow that up here with the husband, but could also discuss the risks associated with comorbid depression, alcohol or substance misuse, if appropriate. Similarly, risks associated with BZD dependence could come up if treatment issues are raised by Mr Arnold.

Mr Arnold is looking for answers and the lack of definite causality might leave him feeling disgruntled. You should explain that whilst the research evidence does not allow us to be certain of what causes GAD, we have a good understanding of the condition itself and how we should treat people. This might lead him to ask about management.

'The earlier GAD is treated, the more effective therapy is likely to be. Unfortunately, most people tolerate the anxiety for years before they come to see us. The treatment is a combined psychological approach and medication.'

FURTHER READING

Cowley, D.S. & Roy-Byrne, P.P. (1991) The biology of generalised anxiety disorder and chronic anxiety. In Rapee, R.M. and Barlow, D.H. (eds), *Chronic Anxiety. Generalised Anxiety Disorder and Mixed Anxiety-Depression*. New York, NY: Guildford, pp. 52–75.

The examiner's mark sheet

Domain/ percentage of marks	Essential points to pass	✓	Extra marks/comments (make notes here)
1. Rapport and communication 20% of marks	Introduces self appropriately		
	Uses clear communication		
	Demonstrates an empathic and caring approach		
	Able to communicate complex theories in simple way		
2. Psycho-social model 20% of marks	Able to simplify the various psychological and social factors implied in the aetiology of GAD		
3. Biological model 20% of marks	Able to explain the brain changes associated with GAD in a simple manner		
4. Diagnosis 20% of marks	Able to describe what GAD entails in jargon-free language		
5. Addressing concerns 20% of marks	Able to address husband's concerns and answer questions		
	Demonstrates knowledge of the bio-psycho-social approach in treatment		

% SCORE _____

___
5

OVERALL IMPRESSION

(CIRCLE ONE)

Good Pass

Pass

Borderline

Fail

Clear Fail

NOTES/Areas to improve

○ SINGLE STATIONS

STATION 3: PHOBIA

INSTRUCTION TO CANDIDATE

This 28-year-old taxi driver has a painful tooth but is refusing any dental intervention. He has not been to a dentist for 15 years.

Meet him and explain how you intend to help him.

ACTOR (ROLE-PLAYER) INSTRUCTIONS

You are in serious discomfort from toothache that started last night.

You are holding one side of your face with your hand all the time.

You fear needles.

You avoid going to hospitals and GP appointments for fear of needles.

SUGGESTED APPROACH

Setting the scene

Introduce yourself and acknowledge that the patient is in discomfort or in pain.

'I'm sorry to hear that you're in some discomfort with your tooth. Can you tell me what happened? Why haven't you seen a dentist for so long? What do you think would happen if you saw a dentist?'

Completing the task

Tease out specific phobia

It is important to tease out what the anxiety relates to. In the dental situation, is it the fear of a specific dental procedure, needles, blood, pain, anaesthesia, choking, losing control or acquired infections such as HIV? Does it relate to the dentist, white coat, his equipment or chair?

According to the International Classification of Diseases, 10th Revision (ICD-10) diagnostic guidelines, a specific (isolated phobia) requires all of the following for a definite diagnosis:

- The psychological or autonomic symptoms must be a primary manifestation of anxiety, and not secondary to other symptoms, such as a delusion or obsessional thought.
- The anxiety must be restricted to the presence of the particular phobic object or situation.
- The object or situation is avoided whenever possible.

Rule out other complications

This is a management station, but establishing the diagnosis and understanding the nature of his avoidance will allow you to appropriately plan his treatment. It is important, therefore, to ask screening questions for evidence of psychosis and affective, neurotic and somatoform disorders.

Enquire about any previous or current psychiatric ill health. Ask whether he has any physical health problems (e.g. thyroid dysfunction) and about caffeine and substance misuse. Ask if he would allow you at some point in the future to speak with his partner/family/friend for more information.

Management

You quickly identify that this gentleman has a specific dental phobia related to a fear of needles. You need to explain in lay terms what you think is happening and how you suggest he is treated.

'Based on what you have told me today, I believe you have what we call a specific phobia. This means that you are not usually anxious about things in your day-to-day life, but are worried specifically about the needles dentists sometimes use. Some people are petrified of spiders, and this is the same sort of thing. Because we dislike spiders or needles, we'll do anything to avoid them. Even the thought of it can make people feel anxious and panicky and sometimes, when confronted by the object, they can have panic attacks. Specific phobias are not uncommon; some suggest that about one in ten of us are affected at some point in our lives. The good news is that we can help and the most effective form of treatment is a psychological approach.'

Psychological treatment

Behavioural approaches are generally accepted as the most effective, although cognitive therapy is also used on occasion.

Exposure-based treatment: usually involves gradual exposure *in vivo*. The patient is exposed to various aspects and parts of the feared object or situation in an organised hierarchy of increasing difficulty. Initially, the patient might be shown pictures of a dentist and syringe and then videos with situations of increasing use of the object. The next step might be to visit the dentist and once again to grade the exposure from the waiting area until the patient is able to sit in the dentist's chair. The anxiety response should eventually habituate.

Systematic desensitisation: is seldom used today and involves using the imagination to picture the feared object or scenario whilst undergoing progressive muscle relaxation. This technique uses the mechanism of reciprocal inhibition.

Modelling: is employed by many therapists alongside exposure-based treatment, in which they will demonstrate how to manage the exposure to the feared object or situation. They might, for example, hold a syringe and then ask the patient to do the same.

Medical treatment

The role of medication is limited and no drug can be confidently recommended, particularly for regular treatment. When psychology has failed or when patients have associated anxiety disorders, selective serotonin reuptake inhibitors can play a role. BZDs should be used with caution because of the high risk of dependence, but are given for time-limited relief of severe and disabling anxiety. In flying phobia, for example, they can be used with good effect for essential journeys.

Resistance from patient

The risk in this scenario relates to his oral hygiene and how a prolonged and serious neglect of his dentition could put his health at risk.

Should he decline assistance following your consultation, the concern would be that any future dental work would be more complicated. Clearly, the earlier he attends, the better. The use of motivational interviewing techniques here can be helpful in preventing resistance.

'You agree that your fear of needles is irrational, and yet you are declining any procedure on your tooth from this very fear. Suppose you do not have the procedure: what do you think is the worst that will happen to you?'

FURTHER READING

ICD-10 (1992) *Classification of Mental and Behavioural Disorders: Clinical Descriptions and Diagnostic Guidelines*. Geneva: WHO Press.

Strauss, C.C. & Last, C.G. (1993) Social and simple phobias in children. *Journal of Anxiety Disorders*, 2, 141–52.

The examiner's mark sheet

Domain/ percentage of marks	Essential points to pass	✓	Extra marks/comments (make notes here)
1. Rapport and communication 20% of marks	Introduces self appropriately Uses clear communication Demonstrates an empathic and caring approach		
2. Phobia 20% of marks	Able to identify specific phobia Demonstrates knowledge of criteria for phobia		
3. Differentials 20% of marks	Able to explore other neurotic disorders as differential diagnoses		
4. Management 20% of marks	Able to explain various psychological treatments for phobia to patient Clarifies the role of medication		
5. Addressing resistance 20% of marks	Able to make the patient reflect on the dangers of avoidance and demonstrates the risks		

% SCORE _____

___
5

OVERALL IMPRESSION

(CIRCLE ONE)

Good Pass

Pass

Borderline

Fail

Clear Fail

NOTES/Areas to improve

STATION 4: OBSESSIVE COMPULSIVE DISORDER

INSTRUCTION TO CANDIDATE

You have just finished a discharge planning meeting for a patient with OCD. There were a number of healthcare professionals present, including some students. One of the student nurses asks if you have a moment to answer some questions. Although you are busy, you agree to spend a few minutes teaching.

She asks you how you make a diagnosis of OCD and what the future holds for this patient. Speak to her and answer her queries.

ACTOR (ROLE-PLAYER) INSTRUCTIONS

You are an eager student nurse.

You profusely apologise for taking the doctor's time.

You have seen a few clients with OCD in your placement so far.

You would like to know about the diagnosis and how OCD is managed.

SUGGESTED APPROACH

Setting the scene

Keep the conversation informal and professional.

'Hello, I'm Dr_____, I didn't catch your name at the meeting. I'd be delighted to talk to you about obsessive compulsive disorder. It's great that you've shown an interest. You had some specific questions which we'll talk about. Please feel free to interrupt or ask questions as we go along. Tell me, do you know anything about OCD already?'

Completing the task

How do you make a diagnosis of OCD?

As its title suggests, OCD is characterised by obsessions and compulsions. These take the form of obsessional thoughts and compulsive acts, together with anxiety, depression and depersonalisation in varying proportions.

The individual will usually consider their obsessions to be illogical or 'ego-dystonic'. It is important diagnostically to explore whether thoughts are overvalued or delusional.

Obsessions are usually described as recurrent thoughts, impulses and/or images that are experienced as uncontrollable. They are experienced with significant distress so the individual is desperate to deal with them in some way.

Mental (covert) compulsions usually involve silent counting, use of numbers/calculations, imagining a certain situation or repeating a particular thought a certain number of times. Prevention of harm to themselves is a common explanation for mental compulsions.

If asked about demographics, in 65% of the population, onset is prior to 25 years of age; in 15%, onset occurs after 35 years of age.

According to psychodynamic theory, OCD is a regression from the oedipal to the anal phase of development.

Obsessions can present as:

• Obsessional thoughts – repetitive intrusive words, ideas or beliefs, usually unpleasant
• Obsessional ruminations – repetitive, circular internal debates, often over simple issues

- Obsessional imagery – imagined visualised scenes, often repulsive or sexual
- Obsessional doubts – about actions not having been adequately performed (e.g. closing a door or switching off a gas stove)
- Obsessional impulses – to carry out socially unacceptable acts (e.g. shouting in public areas)

Compulsions present as:

- Overt behaviours that the individual feels driven to do in response to an obsession
- Repetitive, stereotyped and seemingly purposeful actions

Compulsions are repetitive behaviours or unobservable mental acts that are performed in response to an obsession, often according to strict rules. There are attempts to resist, as they are recognised as irrational. Commonly, they involve checking, cleaning and counting. As with obsessions, compulsions are ego-dystonic, persistent and intrusive. Compulsions can be associated with a sense of relief, but this is short lived, so the act is repeated.

ICD-10 criteria
According to the diagnostic guidelines, a definitive diagnosis of OCD requires the following: obsessional symptoms or compulsive acts, or both, on most days for at least 2 weeks, which must be distressing and interfere with activities.

Obsessional symptoms should have the following characteristics:

- Must be recognised as the individual's own thoughts or impulses
- At least one thought or act that is still resisted unsuccessfully
- The thought of carrying out the act must not in itself be pleasurable
- The thoughts, images or impulses must be unpleasantly repetitive

What does the future hold for an OCD patient?
OCD tends to be a chronic illness for the majority of people. There are three generally agreed outcomes:

- A fluctuating course with lifelong remissions (complete or partial) and relapses (reports of 2%–45%)
- Constant, largely unchanging chronic course (15%–60%)
- Progressive, deteriorating course (5%–15%)

Spontaneous and lasting remissions are rare. Some studies have shown that even after a 10–20-year remission, people can still relapse. It follows that it is a condition that rarely affords complete recovery, but lies dormant. Stressful life events are likely to contribute to relapses.

Despite this, some longitudinal studies have shown improvement in the severity of OCD in approximately two-thirds of cases; 70% of 'mild' cases improve after 1–5 years; and 33% of severe (hospital-admitted) patients improve after 1–5 years.

Poor prognosis is associated with:

- Longer duration of illness
- Greater initial severity of illness
- Early age of onset
- Unmarried status
- Presence of obsessions and compulsions
- Marked magical thinking
- Delusions
- Poor social adjustment and social skills

Better prognosis is associated with:

- Short duration of illness
- Clear precipitating event
- Mild symptoms
- Absence of childhood symptoms or abnormal personality traits
- Absence of compulsions

Risks of OCD

Often, patients with OCD are secretive about their symptoms and do not seek psychiatric input for years, sometimes decades. Approximately a third of OCD patients have comorbid depression, and severe depression is associated with a higher relapse rate. There is an associated suicide risk with OCD.

Differential diagnosis

It is important to mention that in making the diagnosis of OCD, one has to exclude other psychiatric illnesses in which OCD symptoms may be a feature:

Depression

Phobias

Personality disorder (anankastic)

Schizophrenia

Tourette's syndrome

FURTHER READING

Goodman, W.K. (1999) Obsessive–compulsive disorder: Diagnosis and treatment. *Journal of Clinical Psychiatry*, *60*(Suppl. 18), 27–32.

ICD-10 (1992) *Classification of Mental and Behavioural Disorders: Clinical Descriptions and Diagnostic Guidelines*. Geneva: WHO Press.

Veale, D. (2007) Cognitive behavioural therapy for obsessive compulsive disorder. *Advances in Psychiatric Treatment*, *13*, 438–46.

The examiner's mark sheet

Domain/ percentage of marks	Essential points to pass	✓	Extra marks/comments (make notes here)
1. Rapport and communication 20% of marks	Introduces self appropriately		
	Uses clear communication		
	Demonstrates professional behaviour when dealing with a nursing student		
2. Diagnosis 20% of marks	Demonstrates knowledge of criteria for diagnosis		
	Explains the role of differential diagnoses		

⇧ 3. Symptoms
   20% of marks

Able to explain the various phenomenologies of obsessions and compulsions

4. Management
   20% of marks

Able to explain various treatment strategies, both psychological and pharmacological

5. Addressing concerns
   20% of marks

Able to address student's questions

Able to provide information in a succinct manner, yet covers all of the important points

% SCORE _____

___
5

OVERALL IMPRESSION

(CIRCLE ONE)

Good Pass

Pass

Borderline

Fail

Clear Fail

NOTES/Areas to improve

Child and adolescent psychiatry

O LINKED STATIONS

STATION 1(a): SCHOOL REFUSAL

INSTRUCTION TO CANDIDATE

Sacha Gurani is an 11-year-old girl who was referred by her GP to Child and Adolescent Mental Health Services (CAMHS). Her mother is concerned about persistent school refusal that started 3 months ago. Sacha previously refused to attend school, but her mother was able to make her go using a variety of coercive strategies that no longer work.

Take a history from Sacha's mother and establish a differential diagnosis.

ACTOR (ROLE-PLAYER) INSTRUCTIONS

You are worried about your daughter's increasing school refusal.

You've tried taking away toys, games and the television, but this no longer helps.

You are afraid of being blamed as the school is threatening legal action and you don't know what to do.

You are forthcoming as long as you do not feel blamed.

SUGGESTED APPROACH

Setting the scene

Begin by introducing yourself and explaining the purpose of the meeting: 'Hello, I'm Dr_____, a child psychiatrist. I've been asked to see you as your GP was worried about Sacha's school attendance. Could you tell me about your concerns?'

History of presenting complaint

Time of onset and course of school refusal and associated symptoms

Severity of symptoms

Associated events (bullying, accidents and other life events)

Factors exacerbating or ameliorating symptoms

School days attended in past month

Whether non-attendance is pervasive or specific to certain days/subjects/teachers

Reasons for refusal as perceived by the mother

Reasons for refusal as perceived by the young person, if known (mother's view)

Associated distress in young person and important others

Impact of symptoms on school, friendships, family relationships and leisure

Ask specifically about symptoms of separation anxiety:

- Worrying about: separation or being taken away, being alone or something unpleasant happening to attachment figures
- Refusing to: go to school, sleep alone or sleep in a strange place due to worries
- Checking if attachment figures are OK at night
- Reporting: nightmares about separation, aches, pains, feeling sick or signs of distress on separation

Establishing differential diagnosis

Screen for social phobia: avoidance or fear of social situations (meeting other people or doing things in front of other people).

Screen for agoraphobia: avoidance or fear of crowds, public places, travelling alone or being far from home.

Screen for depression: low mood, low energy and anhedonia.

Differentiating from truancy: truancy is:

- Egosyntonic: Is Sacha upset about not attending school?
- Wilful: Is Sacha free from pressure in her decision not to attend?
- Sometimes associated with other antisocial activity.
- Often hidden: Parents may have been unaware for some time.

Differentiating from a physical illness:

- Take a thorough medical history and note any symptoms of physical illness at present: is there a link with school refusal?
- Are there symptoms typical of school refusal (headaches, sore throat or stomach aches)?
- Do the symptoms arise at times of separation, when the child is at home or when the child settles at school?

Screening for associated disorders

Consider the following:

- Global or specific learning problems (persistent worries about school performance)
- Depression (poor concentration, sleep difficulty and somatic complaints)
- Autism spectrum disorder (ASD) (social awkwardness and withdrawal, social skills deficits, communication deficits, repetitive behaviours and adherence to routines)
- Attention deficit hyperactivity disorder (ADHD) (restlessness, inattention and impulsivity)
- Conduct disorder/oppositional defiant disorder

Risk assessment

Screen for risk using the questions below. If a significant level of risk is suggested, this should prompt further questioning:

- Establish the nature of the coercive measures alluded to in the referral, but be careful to do so sensitively to avoid the patient's mother becoming defensive: 'Could you tell me a bit more about the way Sacha is disciplined at home?'

- Explore any bullying at school: 'Have you ever been concerned about Sacha being bullied or picked on at school?'
- Assess the nature of family relationships: 'How does Sacha get on with other family members?'
- Assess the risk of self-harm and suicide: 'Has Sacha ever tried to hurt herself? Has she ever tried to kill herself?'
- Assess the risk of violence to others: 'Does Sacha ever get into fights?'
- Establish if there is a need for child protection (is this child at risk of significant harm?)

Rapport and communication

- Start with open questions, using closed questions to clarify specific points.
- Allow the mother to initially talk without interruption.
- Provide an opportunity to ask questions.
- Be courteous and polite.
- Use summaries, reflections and clarifications.
- Take a non-judgemental stance.
- Demonstrate cultural sensitivity.
- Seek consent to gather further information.

FURTHER READING

Kearney, C.A. (2008) School absenteeism and school refusal behaviour in youth: A contemporary review. *Clinical Psychology Review*, *28*(3), 451–71.

The examiner's mark sheet

Domain/percentage of marks	Essential points to pass	✓	Extra marks/comments (make notes here)
1. Rapport and communication 20% of marks	Clear communication		
	Open and closed questions		
	Empathy		
	Demonstrating patience		
2. History of presenting complaint 30% of marks	History of school refusal		
	Associated symptoms		
	Functional impact and distress		
	Exploration of separation anxiety		
3. Establishing differential diagnosis 20% of marks	Screening for anxiety and mood disorders		
	Differentiation from truanting		
	Screening for physical illness		
4. Screening for associated disorders 15% of marks	Screening for associated disorders, including autism spectrum disorders and conduct disorders		

⇑ 5. Risk assessment
 15% of marks

Assesses risk from others, including punishment by mother

Assesses risk to self and to others

% SCORE _____

___

5

OVERALL IMPRESSION

(CIRCLE ONE)

Good Pass

Pass

Borderline

Fail

Clear Fail

NOTES/Areas to improve

STATION 1(b): EXPLAINING A DIAGNOSIS

> ## INSTRUCTION TO CANDIDATE
>
> After completing your initial assessment of the young person, you reach a working diagnosis of separation anxiety disorder of childhood (SAD).
>
> **Briefly explain SAD to Sacha's father.**
>
> **Propose investigations and management for a preliminary diagnosis of SAD and explain the prognosis.**

ACTOR (ROLE-PLAYER) INSTRUCTIONS

You share concerns about Sacha refusing to go to school.

You worry about how scared she is to be away from her family.

You are concerned, however, about something being missed and Sacha becoming physically unwell.

You are worried about the longer term if things do not change.

SUGGESTED APPROACH

Setting the scene

'On the basis of our discussion so far, it appears that the most likely diagnosis is separation anxiety disorder of childhood. This is a preliminary diagnosis and we need to do some more investigations to make the final diagnosis. Before we continue, I'd like to ask you if you have heard of this condition before. What would you like to know about it by the time we finish talking?'

Explaining SAD

SAD is a condition in which the fear of separation from home or attachment figures causes significantly more anxiety than expected in a typical child. There is anxiety about harm coming to the child or to their attachment figures. It begins in early childhood and is different from normal separation anxiety in being unusually severe or continuing beyond the usual age period. It also causes significant problems in the child's daily activities (e.g. going to school).

Refusal to go to school often occurs at the time of change of school and after a period of legitimate absence from school (such as holidays or illness). SAD is common and affects approximately 4% of children. It is more common in girls than boys (2:1).

Proposing further investigations

In this scenario, you have not seen the young person yet, so of course the first thing to propose is an assessment of the young person.

Consider the assessment setting, chaperone (usually a parent), colleagues that might accompany you and arranging a suitable time. It may help to structure information gathering using a bio-psycho-social model.

Biological
- Arrange information gathering and physical investigations.
- Document headaches and abdominal complaints in order to establish the baseline and differentiate from side effects of medication if used in the future.
- Developmental conditions associated with SAD include dyspraxia, sensory impairment and language disorders.
- Consider the features of hyperthyroidism, migraine, asthma, seizures, lead intoxication and excessive caffeine.
- Consider non-prescription drugs with side effects that mimic anxiety, including diet pills, antihistamines and cold medicines.
- Prescription drugs with side effects that can mimic anxiety include asthma medication, sympathomimetics, steroids, selective serotonin reuptake inhibitors (SSRIs) and antipsychotics (akathisia and neuroleptic-induced SAD).

Psychological
- With parental consent, contact the mental health professionals that the young person has previously seen.
- Consider psychometric testing for global or specific learning problems.

Social
- Contact school (teachers, special educational needs coordinators, educational psychologists, mentors and learning support workers as applicable) with parental consent. Investigate learning profile (does she have an Education, Health and Care Plan?), quality of interpersonal relationships (including bullying), specific relationship problems and features of emotional or disruptive disorders in the school setting.
- Contact social services with parental consent. Look for previous contact with the family and evidence of child protection or child in need proceedings.

Outlining treatment options

Emphasise the importance of collaborative approaches – engage both child and family and comment specifically on the multidisciplinary nature of any treatment.

Establish the goals of the treatment. If the primary goal is dealing with school refusal, then returning the child to school at the earliest opportunity should be the stated target. In view of the relatively short duration of school refusal, a rapid reintroduction to school should be the aim.

The two main therapeutic approaches used to treat school refusal underpinned by SAD are cognitive therapy and operant behavioural therapy. Both draw on functional analysis of the behaviour and make use of family resources. In practice, behavioural and cognitive techniques are frequently combined. Cognitive behavioural therapy (CBT) has been shown to be superior to waiting list controls.

Treatment components are:

- Psycho-education for parents and teachers.
- Helping Sacha to return to school as quickly as possible. A graded (albeit rapidly so) rather than abrupt reintroduction is the method that is most commonly used.
- Rewarding Sacha with praise and tangible rewards for achieving the goals. The rewards used should be mutually agreed by parent and child in advance.

Pharmacological treatment
There have been small, random allocation studies of SSRIs and imipramine showing some benefit, and their use may be considered if CBT fails.

Home education
This could be considered in a tiny minority of patients with school refusal with refractory SAD.

Discussing the prognosis

The prognosis of SAD is good, with 80% of children getting better within 18 months. The long-term consequences of SAD are not well established, but it is possible that having SAD puts children at risk of developing anxiety and depressive disorders in adulthood.

Rapport and communication

Many parents of children with SAD feel disheartened, angry or guilty. These feelings need to be acknowledged and hope instilled. Some parents might insist on the physical nature of the somatic symptoms. Candidates should not argue about this, but propose a cooperative approach, trying various treatment options and assessing outcomes together. That said, excessive medical investigations should be resisted, as they are usually unhelpful and may be traumatic.

A good candidate will be sensitive to the family's culture, wishes and goals. They should also take a whole-system approach that engages a range of professionals and family members.

FURTHER READING

Ehrenreich, J.T., Santucci, L.C. & Weiner, C.L. (2008) Separation anxiety disorder in youth: Phenomenology, assessment, and treatment. *Psicologia Conductual*, 16(3), 389–412.

The examiner's mark sheet

Domain/ percentage of marks	Essential points to pass	✓	Extra marks/comments (make notes here)
1. Rapport and communication 20% of marks	Avoids jargon Allows for questions Sensitivity to family's views		
2. Explaining SAD 30% of marks	Characteristic features and prevalence of SAD		
3. Proposing further investigations 20% of marks	Excludes physical causes of anxiety Discusses gathering information from school		
4. Outlining treatment options 15% of marks	Collaborative approach Psycho-education CBT and operant behavioural therapy Limited role of medication		
5. Discussing the prognosis 15% of marks	Links to later anxiety		

% SCORE _____

___ **OVERALL IMPRESSION**

5 (CIRCLE ONE)

Good Pass

Pass

Borderline

Fail

Clear Fail

NOTES/Areas to improve

STATION 2(a): MOOD DISTURBANCE

INSTRUCTION TO CANDIDATE

You are assessing Richard Chip, a white British 17-year-old referred to a day patient unit from a local community team. He presented with a period of deterioration in school performance and increasingly uncharacteristic behaviour, with social withdrawal, loss of usual interests and irritability. He reports feelings of people laughing at him and sometimes has 'a horrible feeling' as if he were a 'puppet.'

Take a history of the presenting complaint and past psychiatric history.

Test any delusional beliefs.

ACTOR (ROLE-PLAYER) INSTRUCTIONS

You feel very low and empty inside and do not really want to talk to anyone.

You have lost interest in most things and cannot motivate yourself anymore.

You feel that the whole world is against you and closing in.

You are suspicious of the doctor, although they can put you at ease if sensitive.

You are not suicidal, but you do not worry about dying.

SUGGESTED APPROACH

Setting the scene

Begin by introducing yourself and explaining the purpose of the meeting: 'Hello, I'm Dr_____, one of the psychiatrists. I've been asked to see you today because your GP is concerned about your mood. Could you tell me if there's anything you're worried about?'

Rapport and communication

Start with open questions and use closed questions to clarify specific points, initially allowing the patient to talk without interruption. Use summaries, reflections and clarifications and reassure despite their initial suspiciousness.

The patient may feel offended or upset by you trying to clarify the nature of their symptoms. You can try to avoid this by suggesting that you are going to ask some questions that may seem strange or out of the ordinary. These questions are part of a usual psychiatric examination and you ask these of every person you see. If Richard is offended nonetheless (he may indicate this by asking 'Do you think I'm mad?'), you should not enter into arguments. A sensible way forward is to acknowledge that you asked the question in a way that offended and reframe it without backing down. 'Some young people have these experiences. Has it ever happened to you?'

History of presenting complaint

Establish the following general aspects of the history of the presenting complaint:

Onset: what, when, how and why (precipitants)

Course: fluctuations, alleviating and exacerbating factors and remedial action taken

Impact: on school/work, leisure, friendships and family

Distress: how distressed the young person is as a result of the symptoms

Take a targeted history for recent symptoms of depression:

Low mood

Loss of interest

Decreased energy

Loss of self-esteem

Excessive guilt

Suicidal thoughts/behaviour

Poor concentration

Psychomotor agitation or retardation

Sleep disturbance

Change in appetite

You should also explore the functional impairment caused by Richard's symptoms:

'How much has your [elicited symptoms; e.g. sadness/irritability/loss of interest] upset or distressed you?'

'Has your sadness/irritability/loss of interest interfered with:
- How well you get on with the rest of your family?
- Making and keeping friends?
- Learning and class work?
- Playing, hobbies, sports or other leisure activities?'

'Has your sadness/irritability/loss of interest made it harder for those around you (family, friends, teachers, etc.)?'

Background history

Past psychiatric history
- Age at which disturbance was first noted
- Previous depressive symptoms
- History of psychiatric symptoms (especially depressive, psychotic or [hypo]manic), duration and treatment

Developmental history
- Developmental delays
- School attainment
- Distress at separation from parents
- Evidence of global or specific learning problems

Medical history
- Medical differential: Hypothyroidism, mononucleosis, anaemia, malignancy, autoimmune diseases, head injury, hypoglycaemia and vitamin deficiency
- Medication mimicking depression: Stimulants, corticosteroids, clonidine, beta-blockers, diuretics and withdrawal of stimulants and benzodiazepines

Family history
- Psychiatric disorders (depression, suicidal behaviour, anxiety, psychosis and bipolar illness), criminality, substance misuse and medical illness
- Perceived family relationship: discordant or supportive?
- High expressed emotions
- History of intrafamilial abuse

Social situation
- Social adversity
- Recent loss and other life events
- Drugs and alcohol use
- Interests and hopes
- Criminality
- Reciprocal social interactions, friendships and bullying
- Romantic relationships and sexual orientation
- Protective factors such as supportive family networks

Risk
- Risk of self-harm and suicide
- Risk of non-engagement
- Risk of violence to others

Exploring comorbidities

Screening for anxiety disorders:

Are there symptoms of anxiety (biological, cognitive and behavioural)?

In what situations do they arise?

Are they distressing and impairing?

Screening for substance misuse:

Onset, nature, amount, frequency, context, features of dependence (psychological and physical), impact and distress

Differentiating symptoms from psychosis

Richard reports that other people laugh at him. Such statements might represent:

1. An idea of reference
2. An overvalued idea
3. A paranoid delusion

To be a delusion, his belief should be:

- Held beyond a shadow of doubt
- Not shared by others
- Preoccupying and of personal importance
- Held against evidence to the contrary

Richard also reports feeling 'like a puppet.' It is important to determine if this indicates the presence of:

1. Delusion of control
2. Derealisation/depersonalisation phenomena

To be depersonalisation/derealisation, the following features must be present:

- Feeling of unreality
- Unpleasant quality
- Non-delusional (see above)
- Loss of affective response

ADDITIONAL POINTS

See http://www.dawba.com for the Development and Well-Being Assessment (Goodman et al., 2000), which includes useful questions on establishing the presence of low mood.

FURTHER READING

Goodman, R., Ford, T., Richards, H. et al. (2000a) The development and well-being assessment: Description and initial validation of an integrated assessment of child and adolescent psychopathology. *Journal of Child Psychology and Psychiatry, 41*, 645–655.

The examiner's mark sheet

Domain/ percentage of marks	Essential points to pass	✓	Extra marks/comments (make notes here)
1. Rapport and communication 20% of marks	Clear communication Avoids stigmatising language Uses techniques such as reassurance to put patient at ease		
2. History of presenting complaint 30% of marks	Presenting symptoms Symptoms of depression Functional impairment		
3. Background history 30% of marks	Explores risk, especially self-harm and suicide and risk to others Social circumstances and past history		
4. Exploring comorbidities 10% of marks	Screening for anxiety disorders and substance misuse		
5. Differentiating symptoms from psychosis 10% of marks	Tests strength of beliefs and whether delusional Explores depersonalisation		

% SCORE _____

___
5

OVERALL IMPRESSION
(CIRCLE ONE)

Good Pass

Pass

Borderline

Fail

Clear Fail

NOTES/Areas to improve

STATION 2(b): EXPLAINING TREATMENT AND PROGNOSIS

INSTRUCTION TO CANDIDATE

Following your assessment, you have diagnosed a severe depressive episode. You have already discussed the diagnosis with Richard and his family.

> **Explain the treatment plan and prognosis to Richard's mother.**
>
> **Do not worry if you arrived at a different diagnosis – continue on the basis that this was depression as above.**

ACTOR (ROLE-PLAYER) INSTRUCTIONS

You are worried about Richard, but glad that he is receiving treatment.

You know that talking therapy has been suggested, but do not know how this would work.

You hope it will help and want to know more.

You want to know if anything else can be done.

You want to know whether Richard will get better.

SUGGESTED APPROACH

Setting the scene

'Thank you for agreeing to see me today. You met the team recently to discuss Richard's diagnosis and I think it's important to take a few minutes to discuss how we can treat his depression and what the future holds. Does that sound OK to you?'

It would be reasonable in an exam setting to assume that Richard has given consent to speak to his mother, although you may like to explicitly state this (particularly as you are disclosing information regarding the treatment plan and prognosis).

At the beginning of the interview, you should explore Mrs Chip's hopes and expectations and establish the overall goals and framework of the treatment. Emphasise the importance of adopting a collaborative approach with other professionals and engaging the young person and family (with the young person's consent) in all decision making.

Outlining psychological therapies for depression

The two most commonly used psychological therapies for depression are cognitive behavioural therapy (CBT) and interpersonal therapy (IPT).

Ask if she knows anything about these treatments. If not, you should briefly discuss the principles, advantages and disadvantages of both, but explain that there is no good evidence that one psychological therapy is better than another. Other therapies include family therapy and psychodynamic therapy.

'CBT is a "talking treatment" for depression. It is based on the idea that what happens to us is rarely either all good or all bad and we make it good or bad by having either good or bad thoughts about it. Let me give you an example: say if a friend does not say "hello" to us; we could think he doesn't like us, or we could think he was very busy, or we could think he just didn't see us. Having a negative thought ("he doesn't like me") might make us feel sad. When we feel sad, we may stop doing things we are good at. This could make our mood even worse and we could have even more bad thoughts about ourselves.'

'During CBT, we arrange weekly or 2-weekly 1-hour sessions with a CBT therapist for at least 3 months. We then look at the kinds of thoughts that a young person has about themselves, other people or the world in general and see if these thoughts are helpful or not and if there may be a different way to see things. We also try to see if doing positive activities could help improve a young person's mood. We ask the young person to practise the skills they have learnt and keep a diary of their progress. However, CBT does not always work. In good studies, about 50% of young people who have CBT alone get better within the first few weeks of treatment. I could also give you information about useful websites and a leaflet explaining more about CBT.'

IPT is similar to CBT and is also a "talking treatment" with several 1-hour weekly or 2-weekly sessions for at least 3 months. Unlike CBT, in IPT, the therapist and the young person look mainly at the young person's relationships with other people. This is because we know that most young people with depression could do with some help when it comes to their relationships. We also know that young people tend to get depressed at the time of relationship problems. In IPT, the young person and the therapist look at ways of improving the young person's relationships and dealing with some of the bad things that may have happened to the young person. Young people talk about their feelings and learn how to manage them. They also discover ways of communicating more effectively, solving problems and managing conflicts. During the treatment, other important people in the young person's life can participate (with their consent). It is useful for young people to practise some of the skills at home and at school and to do role-plays during the sessions. I could also give you information about useful websites and a leaflet explaining more about IPT.

Outlining pharmacological therapies for depression

'Sometimes, talking therapies may not work. If after four to six sessions of therapy Richard's depression doesn't start to respond, we may need to think about medication in addition to the therapy. There are many medicines available to treat depression, but at present, only one is recommended for treating depression in young people. It is called fluoxetine or is sometimes known by brand names such as Prozac. It works by increasing the amount of a naturally occurring chemical called serotonin in our brain. We use fluoxetine to treat depression and sometimes other conditions. About two-thirds of young people with depression tend to get better. Fluoxetine takes about 2–4 weeks to work.'

'As with any other medication, young people who take fluoxetine may experience some side effects, although most young people do not get any at all. Common side effects include headaches, upset tummies, feeling sick, feeling restless, poor appetite, fever and skin rashes. Rare side effects include getting "high" in terms of mood and very rarely having suicidal thoughts and self-harming. It should not be given to young people who are allergic to it or who are feeling "high" in terms of their mood. If Richard takes any other medication, we would need to know before starting fluoxetine. If fluoxetine does work, we would recommend that he continued treatment for at least 6 months before stopping gradually. If it does not work, other medicines could be tried. About 50% of young people will get better with a second medication. I would be happy to answer your questions about the medication treatment and could also give you a leaflet with further information.'

Outlining social interventions for depression

'Social problems make young people more likely to have depression. These include poor housing, poverty, unemployment (either of a parent or of the young person), exposure to violence and discrimination on the basis of race and sexual orientation.'

'Social interventions that can help in depression include educating family members and teachers about depression, dealing with bullying, establishing a healthy lifestyle with healthy food, sleep and exercise and helping the young person and the family improve their health and quality of life. In order for social interventions to be helpful, we will need to involve other people like family members, teachers and sometimes other health professionals and social workers.'

Even better than this general approach is to use examples of specific social problems that arose from the interview with Richard with relevant interventions.

Prognosis

In the short term, most young people will recover from depression. Between 60% and 90% of episodes of depression will get better within a year. There is, however, a high risk of depression recurring, with 50%–70% of young people who improve becoming unwell again within 5 years. Young people are also at risk of mental health disorders and psychosocial problems in adulthood, including anxiety and bipolar disorder, in addition to depression. Because of this, greater understanding of depression and engagement with the multidisciplinary team is extremely important.

Rapport and communication

The information above should not be used as a script given didactically to Richard's mother. Instead, encourage her to ask questions and constantly check her understanding. Even when explaining treatment, you should not be speaking continuously for more than a few moments at a time. Be sensitive to the family and the young person's wishes and goals and aim for a collaborative approach that involves family members and a range of professionals.

Mrs Chip may be alarmed by the reported increase in suicidality with SSRI treatment. Explain that while there is some evidence that treating young people with a drug like fluoxetine increases the risk of having suicidal thoughts and suicidal behaviour, there is no evidence of an increased risk of suicide. The risk of developing suicidal thoughts and behaviour is very low with fluoxetine and the vast majority of young people do not develop this. There is evidence that the benefits of fluoxetine treatment outweigh the side effects, and state that you will ensure that there is regular and frequent monitoring of Richard's symptoms in place during the first few weeks of treatment; for example, this might be once a week for the first 4 weeks. Mrs Chip could also call your team during office hours or contact a duty psychiatrist in the local A&E out of hours if she is concerned about any of the symptoms.

> **FURTHER READING**
>
> Thapar, A., Collishaw, S., Pine, D.S., & Thapar, A.K. (2012) Depression in adolescence. *The Lancet*, 379(9820), 1056–67.

The examiner's mark sheet

Domain/ percentage of marks	Essential points to pass	✓	Extra marks/comments (make notes here)
1. Rapport and communication 20% of marks	Asks encouraging questions and checks understanding		
	Avoids jargon		
	Confidently addresses questions		

2. Outlining psychological
   therapies for depression
   20% of marks

   Clear description of
   evidence-based
   psychological
   therapies

3. Outlining pharmacological
   therapies for depression
   20% of marks

   Clear description of
   evidence-based
   pharmacological
   therapies

4. Outlining social
   interventions for depression
   20% of marks

   Description of relevant
   interventions (e.g. at
   home and school)

5. Prognosis
   20% of marks

   Evidence-based
   discussion of likely
   outcomes

% SCORE _____

___ **OVERALL IMPRESSION**

5 (CIRCLE ONE)

Good Pass

Pass

Borderline

Fail

Clear Fail

NOTES/Areas to improve

STATION 3(a): SUICIDALITY

INSTRUCTION TO CANDIDATE

Nadia Burrell is a 16-year-old young lady who presented to A&E at 2 a.m. this morning following an overdose of 16 paracetamol tablets. She is accompanied by her mother. Nadia was at a friend's home when she took the overdose after a fight. She was admitted overnight and is now medically fit for discharge. Nadia was seen by a social worker, who expressed no immediate concerns.

Assess the risk of suicide and violence.

Conclude by making a brief risk summary and formulation to the examiner in the station – the examiner will listen but will not discuss the case with you.

YOU ARE NOT REQUIRED TO FORMULATE A MANAGEMENT PLAN

ACTOR (ROLE-PLAYER) INSTRUCTIONS

You were angry when you took the overdose, having argued with your friend.

You wanted to show her how much she had upset you, but you feel silly now and are glad you were not hurt.

You had both been drinking and you remember physically fighting.

You have been really stressed recently, but you just want to go home now.

SUGGESTED APPROACH

Setting the scene

Introduce yourself and explain why you are meeting: 'Hello, I'm Dr____, one of the psychiatrists. I was hoping we could talk a bit about what's been happening so we can think about how best to help.'

Exploring circumstances of the overdose

- Method of self-harm and description of the overdose (what, how many, where, when, staggered, etc.)
- Suicidal ideation (when, what and how severe): was it impulsive?
- Suicidal intent: include patient's belief about intent, preparation before the attempt, prevention of discovery and communication before and after the attempt
- Subjective and objective lethality
- Precipitants of the overdose (e.g. interpersonal problems)
- Precursors of the overdose: explore stressful life events (including number, types and perceived degree of control)
- Explore interpersonal conflicts, losses (e.g. death or parental separation) and physical illness
- Associated features: self-harm or use of drugs and alcohol
- Reasons for the overdose (wanting to die, trying to escape from impossible situation, making others feel sorry, punishing others or communicating distress)
- Reasons for living (future plans, responsibility to family, moral objections to suicide or fear of suicide)

Assessing factors relevant to risk of suicide and violence

Explore historical/contextual factors that elevate the risk of suicide and self-harm:

- Previous self-harm
- Previous suicidal attempts using violent methods
- Use of prescribed medication (especially SSRIs and benzodiazepines)
- Familial suicidal behaviour
- Familial psychopathology/substance misuse
- Family discord
- Exposure to suicidal behaviour
- History of antisocial behaviour
- History of physical illness
- Recent discharge from services
- Family members expressing concern about suicide
- Gay, lesbian or bisexual orientation

Explore factors that elevate the risk of violence:

- History of violent behaviour
- History of non-violent antisocial behaviour
- Early onset of violence
- Minimisation/denial of previous violence
- Disengaging from services
- Familial violence/criminality/substance misuse
- Family members expressing concern about violence
- Poor school achievement
- 'Delinquent' peer group
- Peer rejection
- Poor parenting
- Community disorganisation

Explore other factors associated with the risk of violence and suicide:

- Substance misuse
- History of emotional, physical or sexual abuse/exploitation
- Exposure to violence
- History of accidental injuries
- Recent life events
- History of self-neglect
- History of impulsive behaviour
- Social or cultural isolation
- Social adversity
- Poor daily living skills
- History of psychiatric illness

Assess protective factors:

- Good family relationships
- Problem-solving ability
- Peer support
- Pro-social behaviour
- Good social skills
- Good self-esteem
- Sense of control over life
- Positive school experiences
- Resilience to stress
- Positive attitude to treatment
- Positive attitude towards authority

Screen for substance misuse

These are suggested questions to screen for the presence of substance misuse based on Kiddie-Sads-Present and Lifetime Version (K-SADS-PL) (Kaufman et al., 1996). Please see 'Further Reading' for information.

> How old were you when you had your first drink?
>
> What is your favourite thing to drink?
>
> Do you have a group of friends you usually drink with, or do you usually drink alone?
>
> Where do you usually drink?
>
> How old were you when you started to drink regularly, say two drinks or more per week?

In the past 6 months, has there been at least 1 week in which you had at least two drinks?

Let me know if you have used any street drugs before, even if you have only tried them once. Which ones have you used?

In the past 6 months, what is the most you have used? Every day or almost every day for at least 1 week? Less? More? Was there a time when you used more?

Mental state examination

Although a mental state examination is not explicitly requested in the instructions, it forms part of the assessment of risk. These features may be particularly relevant:

- Signs of previous self-harm
- Evidence of self-neglect
- Psychomotor retardation or agitation
- Withdrawal, irritability, distractibility or apathy
- Poor eye contact, threatening body language, crying or tension
- Irritable, low or anxious mood
- Blunt or incongruous affect
- Hopelessness, self-blame, inappropriate guilt, helplessness, worthlessness or poor self-image
- Current attitude towards the overdose
- Current suicidal fantasies, thoughts or plans
- Current violent fantasies, thoughts or plans
- High level of distress
- Feeling out of control
- Low empathy/remorse
- Evidence of passivity or paranoid delusions
- Evidence of hallucinations
- Poor concentration or distractibility
- Poor insight

Risk summary and formulation

Make sure to leave 1 or 2 minutes at the end of the station for this. Rather than repeating every fact elicited, it is important to show that you have a system for thinking about risk. One way of doing this is to intersect (risk to self, risk to others and risk from exploitation) with (protective factors, risk factors), whilst adding a timeline (short-term and long-term risk).

For example, factors that increase risk of future self-harm are a history of two attempts (including this one), alcohol use, the presence of marked family discord and a family history of self-harm. Protective factors are the presence of a network of supportive friends and that all past acts of self-harm have been impulsive, of low objective lethality and self-disclosed. Use the same approach for risk to others and risk from exploitation.

A concluding statement might use the following structure: 'In summary, there is a mild/moderate/high short-term risk of self-harm/violence and mild/moderate/high long-term risk of self-harm/violence moderated by treatment engagement.'

Rapport and communication

It is important to acknowledge Nadia's feelings and empathise with any distress. She may initially be reluctant to engage with the assessment, in which case it might be easier to focus on the 'what, when and how' more than the 'why'. Avoid asking too many questions, instead using open questions to start and then guiding the conversation through the various relevant areas.

FURTHER READING

http://www.psychiatry.pitt.edu/sites/default/files/Documents/assessments/ksads-pl.pdf

Kaufman, J., Birmaher, B., Brent, D., Rao, U., Flynn, C., Moreci, P., Williamson, D. & Ryan, N. (1997) Schedule for affective disorders and Schizophrenia for school-age children – Present and Lifetime Version (KSADS-PL): Initial reliability and validity data. *Journal of the American Academy of Child and Adolescent Psychiatry*. 36, 980–988.

Ougrin, D., Tranah, T., Leigh, E., Taylor, L. & Asarnow, J.R. (2012) Practitioner review: Self-harm in adolescents. *Journal of Child Psychology and Psychiatry, 53*(4), 337–50.

The examiner's mark sheet

Domain/ percentage of marks	Essential points to pass	✓	Extra marks/comments (make notes here)
1. Rapport and communication 20% of marks	Empathy and acknowledges distress Demonstrating patience		
2. Exploring circumstances of the overdose 30% of marks	Situation leading up to overdose Method of self-harm Explores intentions		
3. Assessing factors relevant to risk of suicide and violence 30% of marks	Previous self-harm and suicidal behaviour Other related risk and protective factors Substance misuse		
4. Mental state examination 10% of marks	Evidence of depression or psychosis		
5. Risk summary and formulation 10% of marks	Clear framework for organising risk and protective factors		

% SCORE _____

___

5

OVERALL IMPRESSION

(CIRCLE ONE)

Good Pass

Pass

Borderline

Fail

Clear Fail

NOTES/Areas to improve

STATION 3(b): ENGAGING A PARENT

INSTRUCTION TO CANDIDATE

You have now interviewed Nadia and the team decision is that she is fit for discharge with urgent community follow-up. However, her mother indicates that she is in two minds about the need for community follow-up, as things now appear to be OK and the family want to move on. Nadia is also ambivalent and stated she will only attend follow-up appointments if accompanied by her mother.

Assess her mother's views and explore the importance of community follow-up with her.

Nadia has consented for you to discuss her treatment plan with her mother.

ACTOR (ROLE-PLAYER) INSTRUCTIONS

You do worry about Nadia, but think this is probably just 'a phase'.

She is not that bad and you think she just needs to learn how to deal with life.

You do not think she is 'mad' and you do not like the idea of her having to see psychiatrists.

You are willing to listen if the doctor is not patronising.

SUGGESTED APPROACH

Setting the scene

Introduce yourself and explain the purpose of the meeting. Ask about Mrs Burrell's views on her daughter and what she feels should happen. Gain a baseline understanding of her beliefs and concerns.

Explaining community follow-up

The points to cover here are:

Being 16, Nadia is presumed to have the capacity to make decisions about her treatment.

Nonetheless, it is good practice to involve family members in making decisions.

Parental support is one of the best predictors of engagement with follow-up.

British clinical guidelines require professionals to offer 7-day follow-up to all young people who have self-harmed. This is to monitor risk and to offer treatment to those who require it.

Establishing 'pros' and 'cons' of attending community follow-up

Start with the 'cons' by exploring in detail the disadvantages of attending community follow-up. Common reasons for a reluctance to attend follow-up appointments include stigma, inconvenience, desire to put the episode behind the family and having previously had negative experience of contact with health professionals.

Then move on to the 'pros'. Explore the good things about attending community follow-up. Common reasons for attending appointments include a wish to understand problematic behaviour and reduce the risk of further self-harm, a desire to improve relationships and a hope that the young person will learn new ways of dealing with problems.

Enhancing parental motivation to attend follow-up

Several techniques may be used here. The example below is based on motivational interviewing techniques (Rollnick & Miller, 2002).

'On a scale of 0–10, with 0 having no motivation to attend follow-up and 10 having no doubts about attending, where are you right now?'

Having obtained a summary score for the overall motivation you can develop this part by exploring different elements of motivation.

'How important is it that you and Nadia attend the follow-up appointments?'

Not at all important					Very important					
0	1	2	3	4	5	6	7	8	9	10

'How come your score is not 0 – tell me more about it. Why else? What would need to happen for you to move up one point?'

You could use the same principles to ask:

'How confident are you that you can attend the follow-up appointments?'

'How ready are you to attend the follow-up appointments?'

Practical techniques to maximise attendance at follow-up

The following practical arrangements increase the likelihood of attending follow-up appointments and you could therefore talk with Mrs Burrell about using them:

- Fixing the follow-up date and time at the initial assessment
- Arranging mutually convenient times when possible (taking into account the young person's and other family members' commitments, like school, college or work)
- The assessor providing the follow-up personally
- Making a telephone call or sending a letter prior to follow-up appointments
- Explaining the reasons for follow-up
- Explaining possible treatment options beyond the initial follow-up session
- Thinking through possible obstacles (transport, child care and ease of access)

Rapport and communication

You may be faced with an ambivalent mother who is reluctant to attend the follow-up appointments primarily for stigma-related reasons. Take a cooperative stance and stick to facts rather than opinions. It may be helpful to dispel some myths. You could say that you see some young people who have mental illness and some young people who do not, but who could do better with psychological or social support. You could also say that most people benefit from developing their potential in a supportive environment and that you work with other professionals who have a range of skills and expertise. Your team also works with other organisations that are not part of the mental health services (e.g. counselling services and educational advisors), whose expertise may be called upon if required. Decisions about further treatment (if recommended) will usually be made in collaboration with the family members. You could also give Mrs Burrell written information about your service and leave some time to answer questions.

Taking a cooperative stance:

- Avoid direct confrontation and arguments
- Express empathy
- Emphasise self-efficacy
- Instil hope
- Use open questions
- Affirm positives
- Provide reflections
- Use summaries

FURTHER READING

Rollnick, S. & Miller, W.R. (2002) *Motivational Interviewing*, 2nd edn. New York, NY: The Guilford Press.

The examiner's mark sheet

Domain/ percentage of marks	Essential points to pass	✓	Extra marks/comments (make notes here)
1. Rapport and communication 30% of marks	Collaborative stance Emphasises positive approach Addresses concerns around stigma		
2. Explaining community follow-up 20% of marks	Monitors risk and offers appropriate treatments		
3. Establishing 'pros' and 'cons' of attending community follow-up 20% of marks	Discusses both advantages and disadvantages of follow-up		
4. Enhancing parental motivation to attend follow-up 15% of marks	Motivational techniques to improve likelihood of engagement		
5. Practical techniques to maximise attendance at follow-up 15% of marks	Discusses practical techniques that may help attendance		

⇧ **% SCORE** _____

___ **OVERALL IMPRESSION**

5 (CIRCLE ONE)

Good Pass

Pass

Borderline

Fail

Clear Fail

NOTES/Areas to improve

STATION 4(a): SELF-HARM

INSTRUCTION TO CANDIDATE

Salim Jahani is a 15-year-old boy who presented to A&E after self-harming by cutting his arm with the blade from a pencil sharpener. He was brought in by his teacher after they noticed the cuts. His parents have now arrived at the hospital. Salim has received treatment for superficial cuts and can now be discharged from a medical point of view.

Take a focussed history of the reasons for self-harm.

Assess Salim's mental state.

Perform a brief risk assessment.

ACTOR (ROLE-PLAYER) INSTRUCTIONS

You are being bullied and it is making you miserable.

You do not know what to do and have not been able to tell anyone.

You are embarrassed about being in hospital but will gladly talk about the bullying as long as you feel safe.

SUGGESTED APPROACH

Setting the scene

Begin by introducing yourself and explaining the purpose of your meeting: 'Hello, I'm Dr_____, one of the psychiatrists. I was hoping to find out what happened.'

Exploring circumstances of self-harm

Find out about the self-harm:

What did the patient use to cut themselves with and from where did they obtain it?

Where on themselves did they cut? Was it once or several times? How deep were the cuts and what sort of medical attention, if any, did they need?

Was the self-harm impulsive or planned?

Where were they? Were they alone? How did they come to be in hospital?

What was the purpose behind the self-harm? Was it to relieve tension or to signal distress, or was there suicidal intention?

Did the patient harm themselves in any other way (including simultaneous suicidal acts such as an overdose)?

Explore possible precipitants by asking Salim about things that might have upset him and that may have led to him wanting to hurt himself. Consider possible difficulties in the following areas:

Explore life at home:

Who lives at home? What is the patient's relationship like with their parents and other family members? What about other intrafamilial relationships?

Are there fights at home? Is there any evidence of domestic (verbal, physical or sexual) abuse that they might be witnessing or experiencing?

Are there problems with the home itself (e.g. overcrowding or problems with the fabric of the home) that their family might be worried about?

Are there other stresses in the family (e.g. with money, ill health or unemployment)?

Explore life at school – this may be particularly relevant given that the patient was at school when they harmed themselves:

What is the patient's academic achievement like?

Do they get on with their teachers?

Do they have friends? How many? How close are they? Do they only see them in school or outside as well? What things do they do together and what can the patient talk to them about?

Is the patient being bullied? If so, by whom? What is the nature of the bullying? For how long has it been going on? Have they told anyone, and if so, what happened as a result?

Explore other areas of the patient's life:

Have there been any difficulties occurring in social settings outside of school and home (e.g. in after-school clubs, with friends or with extended family)?

Are they worried about relationships? Are they in a relationship, would they like to be or have they recently had a break-up? What is their sexual orientation and do they worry about this? Is there any evidence of sexual abuse or exploitation?

Have they been in trouble about anything and are they worried about this? Is there any criminal activity or involvement with gangs?

Are they using drugs or alcohol?

Background history

Past psychiatric and medical history – it is particularly important to include or exclude illnesses that might be leading to self-harm.

- Previous history of self-harm, including suicidal thoughts and acts
- History of psychiatric symptoms, including depression and anxiety
- Chronic illness causing pain or disability
- Medications

Family history
- As above, plus family history of psychiatric disorders or other problems causing stress to the patient (e.g. physical illness or substance misuse)

Developmental history
- Evidence of developmental delay or learning problems
- Evidence of difficulties with social communication or ADHD that may be contributing to stress

Assessing mental state
- Current mood and reactivity of affect
- Symptoms associated with low mood, including feelings of worthlessness, guilt, helplessness or loss of hope for the future
- Hallucinations (in different modalities), including persecutory voices leading directly or indirectly to self-harm
- Evidence of delusional thoughts, thought interference, abnormalities in thought content or formal thought disorder
- Difficulties in concentration or cognitive deficits
- Insight into the nature of these difficulties, as well as their possible causes and potential treatment

Assessing risk

It is useful to consider risk in different domains (e.g. risk of self-harm and suicide, risk of vulnerability and self-neglect, risk to other people, risk from others, etc.) and both immediate and longer-term risks.

Risk of harm to self

Was cutting a one-off or part of a pattern of self-harming behaviour? Have there been thoughts, plans or acts of a suicidal nature?

What are the patient's thoughts regarding self-harm now? Do they regret their actions, and if so, why?

What are the protective factors?

Is the patient putting themselves at risk in any other way (e.g. going out alone late at night or using drugs or alcohol)?

Risk from others

Is the patient at risk of being harmed by anyone else (including bullying, physical, emotional and sexual abuse, exploitation and neglect)?

Risk to others

Does the patient pose any risk to others (e.g. through retaliating for being harmed by them)?

Rapport and communication

Salim may be reluctant to talk, particularly if the benefits of talking are not clear to him. The key to building trust may lie in acknowledging his distress and picking up on cues about what is causing it. Explain that it is part of your role to find out about and help deal with these problems.

If Salim is being harmed by someone else, he may be reluctant to disclose this and may only want to do so on the condition that it is kept secret. Avoid promising absolute secrecy and explain the limits of confidentiality in terms of sometimes having to tell other people if someone might come to harm. Reassure Salim, however, that even if this does become necessary, it is your role to help keep him safe.

FURTHER READING

National Institute for Health and Care Excellence Clinical Guideline 16 – Self-harm in over 8s: Short-term management and prevention of recurrence: https://www.nice.org.uk/guidance/cg16

Ougrin, D., Tranah, T., Stahl, D., Moran, P. & Rosenbaum Asarnow, J. (2015) Therapeutic interventions for suicide attempts and self-harm in adolescents: Systematic review and meta-analysis. *Journal of the American Academy of Child and Adolescent Psychiatry*, 54(2), 97–107.

The examiner's mark sheet

Domain/ percentage of marks	Essential points to pass	✓	Extra marks/comments (make notes here)
1. Rapport and communication 20% of marks	Builds trust through empathic approach Maintaining confidentiality		
2. Explores circumstances of self-harm 25% of marks	Method of self-harm and intentions Stressors at home, school, etc.		
3. Background history 20% of marks	Psychiatric and medical history Relevant family history		
4. Assesses mental state 15% of marks	Assesses mood Assesses psychotic features		
5. Assesses risk 20% of marks	Assesses risk from others Assesses risk to self and to others		

% SCORE _____

_____
5

OVERALL IMPRESSION
(CIRCLE ONE)

Good Pass

Pass

Borderline

Fail

Clear Fail

NOTES/Areas to improve

STATION 4(b): ADDRESSING BULLYING

INSTRUCTION TO CANDIDATE

After meeting with Salim, it has become apparent that he is being bullied at school and this is one of the most significant triggers of his self-harm. With Salim's consent, you are now meeting with his father.

Explain your findings in relation to bullying and self-harm regarding Salim's finding.

Discuss how to address the bullying.

Respond to any concerns that Mr Jahani may have.

ACTOR (ROLE-PLAYER) INSTRUCTIONS

You were aware that Salim had not been his usual self recently, but this came as a surprise.

You are shocked and angry to hear about the bullying.

You do not understand why no one knew about it and want to know what can be done now.

You also want to know what can be done to stop Salim from self-harming.

SUGGESTED APPROACH

Setting the scene

Begin by introducing yourself and explaining your role. Salim's father did not bring him to hospital, so first find out what he knows about what has happened. It will be useful to start by checking his understanding of the situation and what might have led to Salim's presentation before explaining what you have found.

Explaining bullying and self-harm

Having identified the degree of understanding that the patient's father already has, briefly summarise the presentation. Acknowledge that a fuller assessment will be useful in due course.

Explain the circumstances of the patient's presentation and the background of other self-harming acts. Describe the triggers of self-harm, focussing particularly on bullying. Discuss also the presence or absence of symptoms that may be associated with the self-harm, such as those related to anxiety or depression.

Addressing bullying

Check with the patient's father what is already known about the bullying, whether it has already been reported and what interventions are already in place.

Explain that while the school will need to get more information about what is happening, it is important to listen to the patient and take him seriously, as he may be feeling frightened, ashamed, embarrassed or guilty. There are many reasons as to why children are bullied, and they often think it is their fault, so they should be reassured that this is not the case.

It is necessary to have a good understanding of where and how the bullying is taking place. Is it solely on school property or with peers from school, or are other people involved? Bullying can take numerous different forms, including through the use of text messages, online forums and social media, and all of these need to be addressed.

All schools are required to have an anti-bullying policy in place, and the first step will be to contact them so that they can investigate what is happening. Simply bringing attention to the bullying is enough to stop it in many cases. Talking to the young person about ways to minimise bullying can also be useful; for example, how to react if they are called names or places that they should avoid.

The patient may also need emotional support from the school nurse or counsellor. In Salim's case, the bullying has led to self-harm and he may need further help and treatment from the CAMHS.

Responding to concerns

At the outset of the interview, it will be helpful to ask if the patient's father has any questions or concerns that need addressing. Some of the concerns that may arise could include:

Why the patient harms himself:

If the patient has not given their own explanation, you might describe how some young people find that self-harm helps to relieve stress and manage difficult emotions.

Whether there are any other treatments, such as medication or psychological therapies, which may be helpful:

Treatments depend on the exact aetiology, but most importantly will include intervening with bullying and other stressors.

Counselling may be helpful, and other psychological therapies and medications may be indicated in cases of underlying diagnoses such as depression.

What to do if he continues to self-harm and how best to manage this safely:

You will be working with the patient to try to find alternatives to self-harm, although in the short term, some young people who have been self-harming for a while find it difficult to stop, and it can then be useful to try techniques that reduce the dangerousness of self-harm.

What to do if self-harm escalates into suicidal thoughts or acts:

One aspect might be to use distraction techniques in order to avoid sustained suicidal thoughts.

Acknowledge that it can be frightening and explain that if the parents are concerned, they should always get in touch or, during out-of-hours time periods, take the patient back to A&E.

Rapport and communication

If there are many questions or concerns, it may sometimes be necessary to say that time is limited and that only some of these concerns can be addressed presently. It may be useful to make a list if there are very many questions. Explain that you will be able to meet again later to discuss any outstanding concerns and suggest starting with the most significant ones first.

FURTHER READING

Vreeman, R.C. & Carroll, A.E. (2007) A systematic review of school-based interventions to prevent bullying. *Archives of Paediatrics and Adolescent Medicine, 161*(1), 78–88.

The examiner's mark sheet

Domain/ percentage of marks	Essential points to pass	✓	Extra marks/comments (make notes here)
1. Rapport and communication 25% of marks	Clear communication Empathy		
2. Explaining bullying and self-harm 25% of marks	Explains details of self-harm Explains details of bullying and other triggers and associated symptoms		
3. Addressing bullying 30% of marks	Discusses different types of bullying Anti-bullying policies and support in school and elsewhere		
4. Responding to concerns 20% of marks	Addresses concerns effectively and efficiently		

% **SCORE** _____

OVERALL IMPRESSION

4   (CIRCLE ONE)

Good Pass

Pass

Borderline

Fail

Clear Fail

NOTES/Areas to improve

○ SINGLE STATIONS

STATION 5: LEARNING DISABILITY

INSTRUCTION TO CANDIDATE

Philippa Abrahams is a 17-year-old woman who has been exposing herself to young children at a local school. A number of the school's parents have become concerned and have notified the police and the school's head teacher.

The young woman has a history of learning disability. She has shown sexually inappropriate behaviour, which has improved somewhat over the years. Her foster parents report ongoing challenging behaviour and have reported a history of self-harm.

She attends a special school where she boards for 3 days a week and you have been asked to assess her there by staff at the school. Parental consent has been obtained. You first arrange an interview with a member of staff at the young woman's residential placement.

Take a history of her behaviour.

Establish the possible aetiology and perpetuating factors.

ACTOR (ROLE-PLAYER) INSTRUCTIONS

You have known Philippa for about a year – she has always been challenging, but recently things have become much worse.

You are not sure why this is, but you are worried about the escalation with the police becoming involved.

You do not think that anyone has hurt Philippa in the placement, but if pressed, acknowledge that you cannot know for sure.

SUGGESTED APPROACH

Setting the scene

Introduce yourself to the member of staff. Establish how long the informant has known Philippa and how often they have had contact with her. Explain that you have been asked to find out a bit more about the nature of the difficult behaviours Philippa displays.

Exploring details of concerning behaviours

Identify key problem behaviours, getting specific examples of each:

What is 'sexually inappropriate behaviour'?

What is 'challenging behaviour'?

What is 'self-harming behaviour'?

Have these behaviours all become issues over the same time period? If not, what was the order in which they developed?

Establish for each problem behaviour:

Time course: onset and subsequent progress

Current frequency (e.g. monthly pattern linked to menstrual cycle)

Antecedents (e.g. change of carer, presence of a certain member of staff, certain time of day or sound)

What it looks like

Associated features (e.g. seeming to be in pain or epileptic phenomena)

Consequences

Any possible positive (i.e. brings about something pleasant) or negative (i.e. takes away something unpleasant) reinforcers?

How do others react?

What has been tried so far – any good?

Has it ever been a problem before?

With particular reference to sexual behaviours:

What are the behaviours (self-exposure, touching or masturbation)?

How do staff react now?

Access to children in foster home

How do these relate to past sexually inappropriate behaviours?

Is Philippa ever unsupervised in such a way that she might be vulnerable to maltreatment by others?

With particular reference to self-harm:

Has this required medical attention?

Does it take a particular or stereotyped form which may indicate a specific syndrome (e.g. Lesch–Nyhan syndrome)?

To what extent are these behaviours threatening the tenability of current foster and educational placements?

Why does Philippa have foster carers?

Is there a documented history of sexual or physical abuse?

Exploring aetiological and perpetuating factors

Is it known if Philippa has a mild, moderate or severe learning disability?

Is there a known cause for this (e.g. perinatal infection/neurogenetic syndrome)?

Does Philippa have functional expressive language? To what extent can Philippa understand language?

What are Philippa's abilities with regards to activities of daily living (e.g. toileting, feeding, bathing and mobility)?

Assess presence of possible mental/physical health problems:

Is Philippa physically well?

Does she take any prescribed medications?

Have there been any altered physical symptoms recently (altered bowel habits, fever, etc.)?

Is Philippa behaving as if in pain?

Is Philippa menstruating? When was her last menstrual period? Has she had a pregnancy test?

Ask about withdrawal, altered sleep/appetite, tearfulness, activity levels and uncharacteristic behaviour

Note: It is increasingly difficult to confidently establish the presence of psychopathology as learning disability (LD) worsens, especially in non-verbal populations. However, LD is clearly associated with elevated rates of mental illness.

It may help conceptually to formulate Philippa's behavioural problems. One way of doing this is to consider factors in a 3 × 3 grid of 'predisposing, precipitating and perpetuating factors' and 'biological, psychological and social aetiologies'. This can aid in distilling information in order to 'establish the possible aetiology and perpetuating factors', as instructed in the brief.

An example might be:

Predisposing: Severe LD, with chronic experience of physical and sexual abuse before entering care

Precipitating: Unidentified dental abscess, possible depressive illness and change of carer

Perpetuating: Ongoing pain from tooth, behaviour negatively reinforced by it leading to Philippa being 'calmed down' with the provision of one-to-one attention and favourite food

Risk assessment

Although not specifically requested, significant risks are evident in the candidate brief, and this should prompt the need for some exploration of risk.

Risk of self-harm:

Is this self-injurious behaviour? This tends to be stereotyped and most commonly skin picking, wrist biting, etc.

Is this better understood as purposeful, thought-out acts with the desire to end life (not incompatible with milder LD)?

Risk from others:

Has Philippa been maltreated?

Is she ever left unsupervised?

Is there any concern about those who supervise her?

Risk to others (of physical and/or sexual assault):

Frequency and severity of past behaviour

Are particular people targets of this behaviour?

To what extent can Philippa understand the impacts of her behaviour on others?

Are these behaviours planned and goal directed or, for example, is Philippa hitting people unintentionally whilst resisting restraint?

Rapport and communication

You will be asking a lot of questions, but recognise that as the staff member only sees Philippa in one setting, they may not know how she is more generally. They may, however, have been told more about Philippa and they should be well placed to comment on recent changes in behaviour.

It is very important to find out about whether Philippa may have been subjected to any harm, but this also needs to be conducted in a sensitive manner.

FURTHER READING

Oliver, C. & Richards, C. (2015) Practitioner review: Self-injurious behaviour in children with developmental delay. *Journal of Child Psychology and Psychiatry*, 56(10), 1042–54.

Xenitidis, K., Russell, A. & Murphy, D. (2001) Management of people with challenging behaviour. *Advances in Psychiatric Treatment*, 7, 109–16.

The examiner's mark sheet

Domain/ percentage of marks	Essential points to pass	✓	Extra marks/comments (make notes here)
1. Rapport and communication 20% of marks	Asks about abuse in a sensitive and non-judgemental manner		
2. Exploring details of concerning behaviours 30% of marks	Nature and onset of each behaviour Response of others to behaviours		
3. Exploring aetiological and perpetuating factors 30% of marks	Neuropsychiatric and medical history Physical symptoms		
4. Risk assessment 20% of marks	Explores possibility of abuse Risks associated with behaviours		

% SCORE _____

_____ **OVERALL IMPRESSION**

4   (CIRCLE ONE)

Good Pass

Pass

Borderline

Fail

Clear Fail

NOTES/Areas to improve

STATION 6: AUTISM SPECTRUM DISORDER

INSTRUCTION TO CANDIDATE

You are at work and have been approached by a receptionist who informs you that a local journalist is at reception. They are writing a piece on a local child with autism who has been excluded from one of the local schools. As part of the article, they would like an expert opinion on autism.

Your consultant is not available, and having spoken with the Trust's public relations department, you agree to meet the journalist briefly to make a comment about autism.

The journalist knows not to ask you any political questions.

Talk to the journalist and give an overview of the condition. The journalist wants general advice on what parents who are concerned about a child should do.

ACTOR (ROLE-PLAYER) INSTRUCTIONS

You do not know much about people with autism other than that they do not like being around others.

You want to make sure that your article is accurate, but want to get 'soundbites' that readers will find easy to understand.

You will become confused if the doctor uses too much medical jargon.

You want to get a good story, so try to exaggerate what the doctor is saying.

SUGGESTED APPROACH

Setting the scene

Begin by introducing yourself and explaining your role. Ask the journalist what in particular they would like to know about autism. Be clear that whilst you are not an expert in this field, you are happy to cover key aspects, referring them to sources such as the National Autistic Society if they need further information. Ask where the information will go and state that you would like to see how you are being quoted before the article is printed.

Clinical characteristics

ASD is characterised by problems from early childhood with social interaction and communication. These include verbal and non-verbal communication, such as eye contact and body language, as well as developing and maintaining relationships with others. Repetitive patterns of behaviour or movement, an insistence on 'sameness' and inflexible adherence to routines and highly fixated interests that are unusual in intensity or focus are also seen. Some people with autism may be very sensitive to things like particular sounds or textures.

Symptoms are typically apparent from the second year of life and interfere with social development and other areas of functioning.

Epidemiology and aetiology

Estimates of the prevalence of ASD have increased dramatically over recent years. Recent reports suggest a prevalence rate of between 1% and 2% in the United Kingdom, meaning that one or two in every 100 people has ASD. It is approximately four times more common in males than females.

Contrary to some concerns that this increase may be due to an environmental factor (e.g. the measles, mumps and rubella vaccination – now clearly disproved as a cause of ASD), the altered prevalence seems to reflect a change in how we diagnose the condition and the fact that children who would have been diagnosed with other disorders (e.g. learning disability or specific language problems) are now considered to have ASD.

The neurobiological basis of ASD is still not well understood, but there is some evidence of early brain overgrowth and developing abnormalities in parts of the brain that are used when we have to interact with others or to plan and control our behaviour.

In 10%–15% of cases, ASD is seen in the context of a medical disorder that is thought to be causal (e.g. tuberous sclerosis, phenylketonuria or Smith–Lemli–Opitz syndrome). The remaining 90% are considered 'idiopathic'. Some non-specific risk factors have been identified, however, including older parental age and lower birth weight.

Idiopathic autism has the highest heritability of all multifactorial psychiatric disorders, with heritability estimates of up to 90% or more. ASD is familial and the recurrence risk for ASD or related developmental conditions in siblings is 10%. Recent thinking regarding genetic risk is that, in some instances, many small genetic factors act synergistically to generate risk for the disorder, while in others, an abnormality within a single larger stretch of DNA imparts risk.

Approximately 70% of those with ASD also have another psychiatric disorder (e.g. anxiety, ADHD, obsessive compulsive disorder or psychosis). Approximately half have a learning disability and 20% also suffer from epilepsy.

Screening and diagnosis

Concerned carers of children should contact their GP or health visitor in the first instance. The 'National Plan for Autism' recommends that if concerns remain after this, a general developmental assessment should be completed by paediatricians, and if ASD is still suspected, then a specialist team should see the child.

Specific instruments exist to help with screening, as well as a number of specialised diagnostic tools that help establish whether or not a child has ASD. It is also important to distinguish ASD from other conditions such as deafness, generalised LD, specific developmental disorder of language, ADHD, attachment disorder, selective mutism and schizotypal disorder.

Treatment and prognosis

Although there is no 'cure' for ASD, a lot of help is available. General support is important for children and families (e.g. access to voluntary agencies, provision of good information about ASD and making sure educational placement is right).

Some treatments try to support people with ASD in learning new skills or to directly teach them strategies for communication. It seems that the earlier that these are begun, the better, but there is not yet enough data to be clear as to what is the 'active element' in these psycho-educational interventions, or for whom they work best.

There is no evidence that dietary supplements or medication can be reliably used to improve the core features of ASD, although in some instances, medicine can help with the challenging behaviours that can be seen in ASD.

ASD is lifelong. In the majority of cases, impairment persists and extra support is needed into adulthood.

Rapport and communication

Communicate in lay terms, remembering that this is for the wider public. Use examples to describe characteristics, but be clear that ASD is a heterogeneous disorder and that it is difficult to make generalisations. Each individual is unique. It is also important to be clear about what is *not* known about ASD, and to communicate this if necessary. If required, direct the journalist towards other sources of information, such as the National Autistic Society.

FURTHER READING

UK National Autism Plan: http://www.autism.org.uk/about/diagnosis/children/recently-diagnosed/national-plan-children.aspx

Volkmar, F.R., Lord, C., Bailey, A, Schultz, R.T. & Klin, A. 2004. Autism and pervasive developmental disorders. *Journal of Child Psychology and Psychiatry, 45*(1), 135–70.

The examiner's mark sheet

Domain/ percentage of marks	Essential points to pass	✓	Extra marks/comments (make notes here)
1. Rapport and communication 20% of marks	Clear communication, avoids jargon Acknowledges own limits		
2. Clinical characteristics 20% of marks	Explains characteristics using diagnostic criteria Uses illustrative examples		
3. Epidemiology and aetiology 20% of marks	Explains epidemiology with recent evidence Multifactorial aetiology Comorbid conditions		
4. Screening and diagnosis 20% of marks	Recommendations for screening Explains how diagnosis is established		
5. Treatment and prognosis 20% of marks	Explains available support and treatment Long-term prognosis		

% SCORE _____

___ **OVERALL IMPRESSION**

5 (CIRCLE ONE)

Good Pass

Pass

Borderline

Fail

Clear Fail

NOTES/Areas to improve

STATION 7: MEDICALLY UNEXPLAINED SYMPTOMS

INSTRUCTION TO CANDIDATE

Sarah Mason is a 9-year-old girl who was admitted via A&E complaining of a sudden loss of sensation and movement in both of her legs.

She has been fully investigated over the past week by the paediatricians and no clear medical cause for her symptoms could be identified. She was discussed with your liaison psychiatry consultant, who wondered if she might have a conversion disorder. A joint meeting has been arranged for 2 weeks' time, when this would be discussed with Sarah, her family and the paediatricians. Your consultant is currently on leave.

The receptionist informs you that Sarah's father is in the department. He is very angry and is saying that his child is not mad or faking it.

Take a history from the father and answer his questions.

Discuss the next steps with him.

ACTOR (ROLE-PLAYER) INSTRUCTIONS

You are worried about your daughter, but angry that her condition is not being taken seriously.

You are scared that she will get worse if not properly treated.

You do not understand why you are seeing a psychiatrist: you think that the paediatricians have given up and are now claiming that she is faking it.

You are prepared to talk if the doctor is sensitive and you feel they are listening to your concerns.

SUGGESTED APPROACH

Setting the scene

Do not interrupt the father, who may be angry at first; let him air his grievances. Thank him for coming to see you and demonstrate an understanding attitude ('I can see you are very upset...of course this must be a concern for you'). Contextualise your meeting. Explain that your consultant is away, and that whilst you have not been directly involved in Sarah's care, you are keen to help. You will try to address his questions and concerns and plan the next steps in preparation for the consultant's return.

'Many thanks for clarifying things for me. In order to best help, I will need to ask you quite a few questions. As time is limited, please forgive me if I appear to be rushing you. We can always arrange to meet again in the near future.' This is a generally helpful line in CASC scenarios in which tempers are high and there is a lot to cover.

History relevant to somatoform and conversion disorders

Gather basic information about Sarah's symptoms:

Timing of onset – sudden/gradual?

Overall course since onset – worse/stable/improving?

If fluctuating, are there any factors that seem to be associated with worsening/improvement?

Has she ever had these symptoms before? What happened then?

What does the family think has caused the symptoms?

Do they feel that they are due to a physical disorder?

If so, is there one they are particularly worried about?

Are their concerns shaped by specific prior experiences of illness (e.g. affecting another relative)?

How does Sarah explain the symptoms?

Has she been preoccupied with the possibility that she has a specific disease?

Has she ever expressed any bizarre/unusual beliefs in relation to them (e.g. nihilistic beliefs/passivity experiences)?

How distressed is she by them? Is there evidence that she has 'la belle indifférence' (a degree of distress that seems surprisingly low given the nature of the symptoms)?

Has she ever witnessed similar symptoms in other people (e.g. father)?

What is the impact of Sarah's symptoms? What can/cannot she do? Is there any secondary gain (e.g. cannot go to school where she is being bullied)?

Have the symptoms been preceded by any clear life event/stressor (e.g. family break-up, exams, victimisation, etc.)? Does Sarah have any recognised physical health problems? Does she take any prescribed medications?

Background history

Screen for:

Mood disorders

Anxiety disorders

School/home psycho-social history:

Who is in the household?

Is there a history of physical/mental health problems?

Are there tensions in the home setting?

What is Sarah's academic and social functioning at school?

Risk assessment:

Are there any factors that increase the risk of Sarah having experienced recent abuse? Is there any past history of self-harm?

It is a good idea to make sure that you ask a few screening questions about risk in any station. A good initial question might be: 'Do you have any concerns about Sarah's safety?' Sarah's symptoms could have been preceded by an adverse life experience, which may include experiences of abuse.

Addressing concerns

It is important to address the father's concerns that you might think that Sarah is 'mad' or 'faking it'. Useful things to say in response to these questions include:

- Her experiences are clearly very real for her, and understandably worrying for her family. It is highly unlikely that she is faking it.
- However, physical investigations have not found a clear cause.
- All of the physical illnesses that are usually considered to be causes of Sarah's symptoms have been ruled out.
- The important thing to recognise is that she is still impaired due to problems with walking, so we need to think of what to do next.
- It is impossible to be 100% sure that there is no physical contribution to her problems, but we know that sometimes psychological factors are very important.
- In the absence of an obvious physical cause (and treatment that any such diagnosis might suggest), an alternative approach that can often be very useful is to think of how these factors can influence the body.

  Note: You may want to use somatic features of anxiety as an example. They are common experiences and provide a concrete instance of how our emotional state can affect our physical state.

- For some people, without them knowing it, troubles and stress can influence their body in such a way that things like altered sight, altered ability to move limbs and even fits can occur.

Planning the next steps

Thank the father for coming and let him know that you will discuss your meeting with your consultant and the rest of the multidisciplinary Paediatric Liaison Mental Health team. Tell the father that detailed plans will need to be based on joint working between Sarah, her family and the clinicians on the paediatric ward (including many professionals in addition to paediatricians [e.g. physiotherapists and nursing staff]). You will need to work closely with paediatricians and ongoing assessment will be required.

Treatment addresses underlying stresses and focusses on obstacles to the patient getting better. By slowly encouraging increasing activity, the patient is able to regain confidence and independence. Both individual and family therapy may be helpful.

Rapport and communication

There is a lot to get through in a short space of time, but it is important to give Sarah's father space to vent and always to be polite, respectful and calm.

Managing anger in others can be worked into many stations, so it is a good idea to develop skills in this area. These also come in handy in the real world, of course! The essence is to be calm, measured and non-confrontational and to demonstrate that you care about what the other person is saying and have taken their concerns seriously. Additional strategies should come into play if the person becomes abusive, threatens assault or wants to lodge a complaint.

It is difficult to screen for such 'internalising' disorders in a reliable and valid manner via an informant. For exam purposes, it would be reasonable to ask, 'Have you been worried about Sarah's mood recently? Do you feel she has been particularly low? Do you think she is troubled by anxiety?'

When addressing concerns, make sure to check for understanding and ask the father if he has any further questions.

FURTHER READING

Eminson, D.M. (2007) Medically unexplained symptoms in children and adolescents. *Clinical Psychology Review*, 27(7), 855–71.

The examiner's mark sheet

Domain/ percentage of marks	Essential points to pass	✓	Extra marks/comments (make notes here)
1. Rapport and communication 30% of marks	Empathy and space to vent frustration		
	Addresses concerns		
	Collaborative approach		
2. History relevant to somatoform and conversion disorders 20% of marks	Explores nature and course of symptoms		
	Patient's and family's explanations of symptoms		
	Functional impairment		
3. Background history 20% of marks	Comorbidities		
	Psycho-social history		
	Risk assessment		
4. Addressing concerns 20% of marks	Answers concerns confidently and sensitively		
	Avoids confrontation		
	Explains link between stress and physical symptoms		
5. Planning next steps 10% of marks	Multidisciplinary working		
	Gradual increase in activity		

% SCORE _____

OVERALL IMPRESSION

5 (CIRCLE ONE)

Good Pass

Pass

Borderline

Fail

Clear Fail

NOTES/Areas to improve

STATION 8: ATTENTION DEFICIT HYPERACTIVITY DISORDER

INSTRUCTION TO CANDIDATE

GP Referral Letter

Dear Doctor,

Re: Simon Harrington, 8 years old. 17 Evershaw Road, SE19, London

I would be grateful for your opinion on this child who has become increasingly difficult for his mother to manage.

Past medical history: otitis media, gastroenteritis, right fibula fracture.

Medication: none.

His mother is asking for a psychiatric opinion. I have examined him today and he appears a physically fit and healthy child. Of note, he smelt of cigarettes, but denied smoking. I do not believe he has access to illicit substances such as cannabis. Your advice would be appreciated.

Yours sincerely,
Dr Jane Michaels

Simon refused to come for his appointment today and has locked himself in his bedroom.

Take a history from his mother.

Discuss the investigations you would like to perform.

Explain your likely diagnosis.

ACTOR (ROLE-PLAYER) INSTRUCTIONS

You do not know how much longer you can cope with Simon; he has always been a handful, but is increasingly difficult to manage.

He never sits still and constantly gets into trouble for talking in class.

You feel that everyone blames you, particularly when he broke his leg.

SUGGESTED APPROACH

Setting the scene

Thank Simon's mother for coming and check her understanding of why you are meeting. Tell her that you have received a letter from Simon's GP mentioning that she wanted to meet with Child Mental Health services about difficulties with Simon's behaviour.

Explain that you would like to ask her a few questions in order to try and understand things a bit better. What you discuss will be confidential. However, if your discussion raises concerns about safety, you may have to share these with other agencies in discussion with the family.

Acknowledge Simon's absence:

Who is looking after him now?

Any idea why is he refusing to attend?

History of presenting complaint

It is a good idea in any initial out-patient assessment such as this to begin by getting a sense of the child's family and school context. Quickly establish:

Who else lives in the house?

Is Simon in mainstream/special education?

How is school going? Is there any evidence that Simon might have generalised learning difficulties/specific learning disabilities?

What is the nature of the difficulties as experienced by the mother? General questions include:

What are the informant's main concerns and how long have they been an issue?

Do problems occur across all settings (e.g. home and school)?

Are they associated with impairment (e.g. suspended from school or limiting what the family can do)?

What has been tried in order to address the problems so far (include parental disciplinary methods, as well as formal support from within school or past CAMHS involvement)?

Has the input received to date been of any benefit? If so, how? If not, any ideas why not?

How does the family deal with Simon's behavioural difficulties? Is physical chastisement ever used? To what extent might his behaviours be reinforced by the responses of others (e.g. outbursts reinforced by Simon eventually being given what he wants)?

Move on to a more targeted ADHD history, focussing on:

Hyperkinesis:

High levels of physical activity

Fidgetiness

Inattentiveness:

How long can he stay on task?

Does he flit from one activity to another?

How easily is he distracted from a task?

If distracted, does he re-engage voluntarily or is prompting required?

Impulsivity:

Does he think before acting (e.g. running across the road if interested in something)?

Can he wait his turn (e.g. queuing)?

Does he blurt out answers or interrupt others when they are talking?

Establish that symptoms began prior to age 7

Do they occur across settings (i.e. home and school)?

Are they impairing (e.g. temporary exclusions from school)?

Other elements of history

Family history/care network:

Establish who is in the family and household.

Are there problems with 'stress', slow development, substance use or ongoing contact with mental health services in family members?

Has the family ever been known to Social Services?

Developmental history:

Antenatal (smoking, drugs and maternal health)

Perinatal (birth complications and need for special/intensive care)

Early milestones

First words other than 'mama' and 'dada'

First walking unaided

Previous school history:

Is there any evidence that Simon might have generalised learning difficulties/specific learning disabilities?

Has he ever been granted an Education, Health and Care (EHC) Plan (previously a Statement of Special Educational Needs)?

Comorbidities and differential diagnoses:

Many comorbidities of ADHD are also differential diagnoses. Consider and screen for the following (refer to diagnostic criteria for details of what to ask about):

Oppositional defiant disorder/conduct disorder

Generalised learning disability

Specific developmental disorder

Substance misuse

Depression

Risk issues:

You will by this stage already have some clues (e.g. how parents deal with difficult behaviour and whether Social Services have been involved), but ask more directly about risk:

Gently enquire about Simon's broken leg.

'I can imagine things can get very stressful trying to control Simon's behaviour. Do things ever get physical?'

'Does Simon ever get so angry he hits out? Has anyone ever needed medical attention as a result?'

Is Simon at risk of harm due to his impulsivity (e.g. does he have good road safety)?

Discussing investigations

Biological

You would want to arrange a meeting with the child so that you can carry out a physical examination yourself.

Physical investigations might follow (baseline height/weight in case stimulant medications are to be started, genetic investigations if dysmorphic, etc.).

Psychological

History and mental state examination are to be conducted with Simon himself.

If there is any suggestion that Simon may have a degree of unquantified learning disability, cognitive testing would be indicated, as the inattention, hyperactivity and impulsivity required for an ADHD diagnosis must be elevated relative to the developmental stage of the child (i.e. mental rather than chronological age).

If there is evidence that Simon has more specific learning problems (e.g. language delay), psychometric testing would be indicated.

Social

Questionnaires such as the Conners rating scale are widely used for checking teacher and parent observations of ADHD symptoms.

Mention that you might want to do direct school observations yourself at a later stage.

You could mention to Simon's mother that after further assessment has been carried out, there may be helpful ways in which social services could get involved.

Explaining your likely diagnosis

You may want to say that whilst further information needs to be gathered, it seems that Simon's difficulties may be due to a disorder called 'attention deficit hyperactivity disorder' or 'ADHD'. Ask if she has heard of this condition.

Explain that:

- ADHD is a term that is used to describe a group of children who have early-onset problems with hyperactivity, focussing their attention and doing things impulsively without thinking.
- The problems persist over time and occur across different settings.
- The term 'hyperkinetic disorder' is sometimes used, particularly in the United Kingdom, and is equivalent to the form of ADHD in which there are significant problems in all three areas.
- The condition affects boys more than girls.
- Both genetic and environmental factors play a role, and there is involvement of the frontal brain systems that use a chemical transmitter called dopamine.

- Some 40%–60% of cases may carry on into adulthood, and it can be associated with mental health and psycho-social difficulties in later life, but many young people learn to manage their difficulties with appropriate support.

Ask if there are any questions.

Rapport and communication

Thank Simon's mother for talking with you. Explain that in order to be certain of the nature of Simon's difficulties and how to best support him and his family, you will need to see him.

Time management is critical in a station with several components, so make sure that you address each of the questions asked of you. Rather than trying to ask everything, use a structured approach that will allow the examiner to see that you know the core information areas to be covered. For example, rather than spending 3 minutes asking several questions about distractibility, make sure you have two or three questions for each of inattentiveness, hyperactivity and impulsivity. Then, quickly establish age of onset and impact before moving on.

FURTHER READING

Taylor, D., Paton, C. & Kapur, S. (2015) *The Maudsley Prescribing Guidelines in Psychiatry*, 12th edn. London: Wiley Blackwell, p.384.

Taylor, E., Döpfner, M., Sergeant, J. et al. (2004) European clinical guidelines for hyperkinetic disorder – First upgrade. *European Child and Adolescent Psychiatry*, *13*(Suppl. 1), i7–i30.

The examiner's mark sheet

Domain/ percentage of marks	Essential points to pass	✓	Extra marks/comments (make notes here)
1. Rapport and communication 20% of marks	Empathic and non-judgemental approach		
	Responds to questions and concerns		
2. History of presenting complaint 20% of marks	Identifies concerns and exploring ADHD criteria		
	Response to behaviours		
3. Other elements of history 20% of marks	Excludes other disorders		
	Explores risk		
4. Discussing investigations 20% of marks	Tests to exclude physical and other neurodevelopmental disorders		
	Discusses gaining information from school		

5. Explaining your likely
diagnosis

20% of marks

Main characteristics
of ADHD

Likely prognosis

% SCORE _____

___	**OVERALL IMPRESSION**
5	(CIRCLE ONE)

Good Pass

Pass

Borderline

Fail

Clear Fail

NOTES/Areas to improve

STATION 9: FIRE-SETTING/ABUSE

INSTRUCTION TO CANDIDATE

Rachel Connors is a 14-year-old girl who has been brought to A&E after setting a fire in her bedroom. She has a history of previously setting fires and was sexually abused by her stepfather. The staff in A&E are concerned that she may have an underlying mental illness.

Assess for risk in relation to fire-setting.

Take a brief history to identify whether she has a mental illness.

ACTOR (ROLE-PLAYER) INSTRUCTIONS

You are irritated at being brought to hospital as you have set fires before and it is not a big deal.

You do not really want to talk but you will do so if it means getting things over with.

You recognise that fire can be dangerous, but you generally keep it under control and it helps you cope with how you are feeling.

You did not want to hurt anyone, but you were scared when the fire got out of control.

SUGGESTED APPROACH

Setting the scene

Begin by introducing yourself and addressing the task: 'Hello, I'm Dr_____, a psychiatrist. I was told that you lit a fire and I would like to talk about why you might have done that.'

Exploring circumstances of presentation

Allow the patient to respond to your introduction, although they may not be forthcoming at first. It can therefore sometimes be helpful to take a brief history of what happened, which also gives useful information about risk.

- Where was the fire lit, what materials and ignition source were used and was there an accelerant?
- What time was it, where were other people (and did they think about this?) and how was the alarm raised?
- Did they stay to watch the fire?
- How were they feeling at the time (i.e. their emotional state)?

From here, you might start to ask about why they lit the fire:

- Was it to destroy property or harm themselves or someone else?
- Do they have a fascination with fire or emergency services?
- Was it because they found something calming or tension relieving about the fire?
- Were they persuaded or coerced by someone else?

Background history

Consider if there are current social stressors that might have acted as a trigger for Rachel setting the fire (e.g. problems at school, with her family or with relationships). Find out about existing links with social services and other agencies. Does Rachel live with her family or is she in care? If the latter, find out more about her care history.

Explore particularly relevant elements of the history, some of which might be associated with increased risk of fire-setting:

- Past history of psychiatric disorder, neurological disorder or learning disability
- Relevant past medical history or family history
- Substance misuse
- History of being bullied
- History of neglect or physical, emotional or sexual abuse
- Offending history, including type of offences and whether there was violence against people or property
- History of other violent behaviour, including cruelty to animals

Assessing risk

It is important to understand Rachel's thoughts about what might have happened with the fire, whether it might have spread and particularly whether it might have endangered anyone. How much insight did she have into it and was she involved in calling for help? When assessing risk, you will need to ask about previous fire-setting, as well as checking other areas of forensic history. In terms of factors directly relating to fire, consider the following:

- History of setting fires or playing with fire
- Personal experience of fire and whether there is any symbolic significance

Remember to explore risk to self, particularly as the fire-setting may have been an act of self-harm, as well as risk to others.

Identifying possible mental illness

While most fires are set by people without mental illness, there are many possible differential diagnoses. By now, you may already have some ideas about potential underlying mental illness. Focus more on the most likely possibilities, but screen for others.

You have been told that the patient has been sexually abused and you will want to find out more about this and whether it relates to the fire-setting. Does fire remind her of what happened? Is it a way of coping with difficult emotions?

Has the abuse led to low mood and other symptoms of depression? Does Rachel experience anxiety symptoms, particularly those associated with post-traumatic stress disorder, such as reliving, hyperarousal, emotional numbing, avoidance and nightmares? Are there symptoms that are suggestive of an emotionally unstable personality disorder, such as impulsivity, unstable relationships, recurrent self-harm and affective instability?

Consider the following in differential diagnoses:

- Psychotic disorders: was the patient experiencing persecutory delusions or hallucinations that led to the fire-setting?
- Mania: was this part of a grandiose delusional belief?
- Depression: ask about low mood and other core symptoms of depression. Did fire-setting relate to relief of psychological distress or was this a suicidal act?
- Anxiety disorders, including post-traumatic stress disorder.
- Substance misuse: was the patient intoxicated?
- Learning disabilities.
- Organic brain disorders affecting cognition or personality.
- Social communication disorders.
- Conduct disorders.
- ADHD (particularly impulsivity).
- Evidence of traits consistent with an emerging emotionally unstable or antisocial personality disorder.

Rapport and communication

It may be difficult to gain Rachel's trust, particularly if she is concerned about what will happen to her. It is important to be non-judgemental and it may also help to point out that you are not part of the police. It might be useful to say that the reason that you are involved is both to understand what happened, but also to see if there is anything that you can do to help.

Approaching risk can be particularly difficult, as some of the questions may seem intrusive. It can help to acknowledge this if a sense of intrusion arises, explaining that these are standard questions that you need to ask.

Talking about sexual abuse with someone you have only just met may also be very difficult for the patient, so it might be easier to be less direct initially: 'I understand that some really difficult things have happened to you in the past. I wondered if it's something that's on your mind a lot.' Make sure that you are both clear regarding what you are talking about, however, as there may have been other things that have happened to Rachel in the past that are making her feel distressed. You could then go on to ask the patient whether the fire and these things are linked. It may not be necessary to go into every detail about the abuse, but it is important to identify whether it is connected to what is happening now. Conversely, Rachel may want to talk about what happened, and you should be receptive to this.

FURTHER READING

American Academy of Pediatrics; Stirling, J. Jr, Committee on Child Abuse and Neglect and Section on Adoption and Foster Care, American Academy of Child and Adolescent Psychiatry, Amaya-Jackson, L., National Center for Child Traumatic Stress (2008) Understanding the behavioral and emotional consequences of child abuse. *Pediatrics*, 122(3), 667–73.

The examiner's mark sheet

Domain/ percentage of marks	Essential points to pass	✓	Extra marks/comments (make notes here)
1. Rapport and communication 25% of marks	Non-judgemental approach Sensitively explores abuse history		
2. Exploring circumstances of presentation 20% of marks	Details of fire-setting Explores intentions		
3. Background history 20% of marks	Precipitants to fire-setting Relevant medical, psychiatric and forensic history History of abuse		
4. Assessing risk 15% of marks	Previous fire-setting Other risk to self or others		
5. Identifying possible mental illness 20% of marks	Screening for psychosis, depression and other disorders Explores abuse history		

% SCORE _____

OVERALL IMPRESSION

5 (CIRCLE ONE)

Good Pass

Pass

Borderline

Fail

Clear Fail

NOTES/Areas to improve

O LINKED STATIONS

STATION 1(a): ANOREXIA NERVOSA – HISTORY TAKING

INSTRUCTION TO CANDIDATE

Miss Anderson is a 22-year-old woman with an established diagnosis of anorexia nervosa who has been admitted to hospital with significant weight loss and hypokalaemia.

You are seeing her on the medical ward and have been asked to:

- **Find out about her current and past episodes of anorexia nervosa**
- **Ask about her physical symptoms**

ACTOR (ROLE-PLAYER) INSTRUCTIONS

You are initially withdrawn and unforthcoming, but gradually, with a gentle and persistent approach from the doctor, you warm up.

You give a clear account of your previous and current weight and eating history.

You have had a number of previous relapses since your teenage years, one of which resulted in hospitalisation.

You have a number of physical complications including constipation, cold intolerance and amenorrhoea.

You minimise the risks to your physical health.

SUGGESTED APPROACH

Setting the scene

Begin the task by addressing the patient by name, introducing yourself and explaining why you have been asked to see her.

'Hello, my name is Dr_____, I am one of the psychiatrists. The nurses have told me that you came into hospital because of your weight and blood results. Has somebody already told you about your blood results?' (If not, explain about her potassium being low.)

'I would like to spend some time finding out about your recent eating habits and any physical symptoms you've had. I'd also like to go into your past history a little bit and ask you about your eating and weight over the years. Would that be OK?'

Completing the tasks

Current episode

Here you are expected to screen for the features of anorexia nervosa according to ICD-10 and DSM-V criteria.

Enquire about her current body mass index (BMI). If she does not know this, what is her actual weight and height? What is her ideal weight?

How much weight loss has there been and in what time frame? (Rapid weight loss is more dangerous than gradual weight loss.)

Ask about methods of self-imposed weight loss. 'Have you been avoiding fattening foods? Do you make yourself vomit or use laxatives or diuretics to lose weight? Have you been exercising excessively to control your weight? Do you use appetite suppressants?' Purging and vomiting are associated with electrolyte abnormalities and medical complications such as hypokalaemia.

Ask about body image distortion and test for overvalued ideas. 'Do you constantly think about your weight and find it difficult not to do so? Do you consider yourself to be under-weight or overweight? Do you fear being or becoming fat?'

Explore recent stressors/precipitants. 'Have you been under more stress at home or work recently? What about your relationships? Have you had difficulties in that respect recently?'

Enquire about current engagement with the eating disorders team and any treatment. 'Have you been in touch with the eating disorders team? Do you have a care coordinator? How often have you been seeing them? Are you involved in any talking therapy? Do you take any medication? How do you find these? Are they helpful?'

Past episodes

Enquire about time of first presentation and diagnosis. 'Do you remember when you were first diagnosed and what the circumstances of you presenting to the doctor were? What were the main symptoms you had at this time? When were you initially referred to mental health services?'

Ask about her highest and lowest ever weights.

Ask about the methods she usually uses to control her weight, including calorie restriction, exercise, vomiting/purging and appetite suppressants.

Enquire about historical stressors precipitating relapse. 'What kinds of difficulties have led to you becoming more unwell in the past?'

Explore her history of treatment and engagement with services. 'How many relapses of your eating disorder have you had over the years? Have you ever been admitted to an eating disorders unit? How long for? What treatment did you require? Have you ever needed an enforced feeding regime? Have you previously been admitted to a medical ward like this one for problems relating to your eating and weight? What previous psychological treatment have you had?' (Ask about family therapy, cognitive behavioural therapy (CBT) and interpersonal therapy.) 'What previous medication (both psychiatric and physical) have you taken?'

Ask about comorbid psychiatric disorders and substance misuse. 'Have you ever been diagnosed with mood or personality difficulties? Do you use recreational drugs? How much alcohol do you drink?'

Physical symptoms

You should ask about associated physical symptoms. Commonly, patients describe cold intolerance, light-headedness, constipation and abdominal discomfort.

Given that this patient is hypokalaemic, she may also be feeling lethargic. Similarly, if her cardiovascular function is impaired or she has comorbid depression, her energy levels are likely to be reduced.

Ensure that you ask appropriate screening questions to cover cardiovascular, gastrointestinal, neurological, endocrine, musculoskeletal, reproductive, dermatological and dental problems.

Problem solving

The likeliest problems in this station would be a reluctance of the patient to disclose information about her eating disorder. By being empathetic and patient, the 'actor' will tell you the information you require. You are not asked about management issues here, so should not run into trouble with discussions about psychiatric admission and potential use of the Mental Health Act, but this could arise in related stations.

ADDITIONAL POINTS

Anorexia nervosa (AN) has the highest mortality rate amongst psychiatric illnesses. The mortality rate for women is 0.56% per year. There is also a high associated suicide rate. Poorer prognosis is associated with low serum albumin, poor social functioning, length of illness, purging and bingeing, substance misuse and comorbid affective disorders.

AN usually presents in adolescence. It is often a chronic illness that is characterised by relapses. The majority of sufferers actively binge or purge and many will move diagnostically from the restricting type of AN to the binge/purging type or to bulimia nervosa (BN) with the passage of time.

Fewer than 50% recover fully, 33% improve and 20% remain chronically unwell.

FURTHER READING

Birmingham, C.L. & Beumont, P.J.V. (2004) *Medical Management of Eating Disorders.* London: Cambridge University Press.

The examiner's mark sheet

Domain/ percentage of marks	Essential points to pass	✓	Extra marks/comments (make notes here)
1. Rapport and communication 25% of marks	Introduces self appropriately		
	Uses clear communication		
	Makes appropriate use of open and closed questions		
	Demonstrates an empathic and caring approach		

⇧ 2. Current episode

    25% of marks

Elicits features of AN to make diagnosis – low BMI, self-induced weight loss, body image distortion, etc.

Explores recent stressors

Asks about recent engagement and treatment

3. Previous episodes

    25% of marks

Elicits duration of illness

Asks about highest and lowest recorded weights

Explores course of illness (e.g. number and severity of relapses)

Enquires about previous treatment – admissions, psychological and pharmacological interventions, contact with eating disorders (ED) community team

4. Physical symptoms/ complications

    25% of marks

Asks about current physical symptoms (e.g. cold intolerance, light-headedness/dizziness, constipation, abdominal pain, etc.)

Uses systems review approach to screen for complications (e.g. cardiovascular (CV), gastrointestinal (GI) and endocrine)

% SCORE _____

___ **OVERALL IMPRESSION**

4 (CIRCLE ONE)

Good Pass

Pass

Borderline

Fail

Clear Fail

NOTES/Areas to improve

STATION 1(b): COMMUNICATION WITH A PROFESSIONAL COLLEAGUE

INSTRUCTION TO CANDIDATE

A Sister on the medical ward contacts you for advice as she has never managed a patient with anorexia nervosa before. She wishes to know the following:

- **What should be done about feeding her?**
- **How should staff engage with her?**
- **How will her mental health difficulties be managed?**

ACTOR (ROLE-PLAYER) INSTRUCTIONS

You are anxious because your nursing team is finding it difficult to manage the patient.

You feel stressed because a number of your nurses are complaining about their lack of support from psychiatric staff.

You are very eager to have explicit instructions on how to manage the patient's feeding and psychological needs.

You welcome suggestions for additional support such as Registered Mental Health Nurse (RMN), one-to-one observations and a visit from the psychiatrist to educate the nursing staff in eating disorders management.

You feel relieved and reassured if the doctor has given clear advice and offered you and your team support.

SUGGESTED APPROACH

Setting the scene

Begin the task by introducing yourself, clarifying the nurse's name and position and confirming the reasons you have been called.

'Hello, my name is Dr_____, I am one of the psychiatrists. Can I ask your name and confirm that you are the Sister on the medical ward looking after Miss Anderson? I have just assessed Miss Anderson, the young lady admitted with hypokalaemia and weight loss in the context of anorexia nervosa. Am I right in saying that you would like some advice on how to manage her?'

Completing the tasks

Approach to feeding

Here, you need to provide clear, step-by-step advice on how to manage the medical situation, with particular emphasis on nutritional support.

You should include the following key medical information and management advice:

- ECG in the context of hypokalaemia and possible ongoing cardiac monitoring.
- Rehydration and correction of electrolytes, especially potassium in this case.
- Dietician referral for specialist input with re-feeding.
- Nutritional rehabilitation should begin with 1000–1600 kcal/day and be increased slowly up to 3000 kcal/day so long as there is no evidence of peripheral oedema or heart failure.
- Monitor for other re-feeding complications such as hypophosphataemia (due to an increase in metabolic demands) and, more rarely, gastric dilatation with abdominal distension, pain and perforation.
- Little and often feeding (e.g. six small feeds per day) is recommended so that the patient is not over-faced with large amounts of food. A soft diet is usually appropriate, with liquid feeding via a NG tube used for severely emaciated patients.

You would like her to be transferred to an Eating Disorders Unit with a specialist multi-disciplinary team, but this can only take place once she is medically stable.

You should confirm with the Sister that the hypokalaemia has been corrected and all other relevant investigations have been done.

Approach to patient

Such patients often evoke mixed feelings amongst staff, who have limited experience of managing them. Joined-up team-working is vital and should include effective communication between nursing staff in order to avoid splitting and ensure that consistent care is provided.

You should offer to spend time with the staff, supporting and educating them about anorexia nervosa.

Specific advice might include observing the patient for attempts to purge or vomit up to 2 hours after eating and ensuring that they do not have access to diuretics, laxatives or stimulants.

Psychiatric management

You explain that she will require a full mental health and risk assessment whilst she is on the ward.

Regular mental state examination for comorbidities including depression, obsessive compulsive and anxious, dependent and perfectionistic personality traits is important.

Screening for drug and alcohol misuse should also be carried out.

Based on the initial assessment, it may be necessary to commence or reinstate anti-depressant medication.

If risk of self-harm and/or suicide is felt to be high, then the patient may require continuous one-to-one nursing observations either with a Healthcare Assistant (HCA) or registered mental health nurse (RMN).

It may also help to mention that you will be asking the ED team's clinical psychologist to assess the patient for individual therapy. This psychologist is likely to be a further source of support and guidance to the ward staff.

A discussion about what to do if the patient refuses food may be required. Patients with AN often refuse food, treatment and/or hospitalisation, and where there is significant risk of medical deterioration as a consequence of malnutrition, use of the Mental Health Act becomes necessary. If so detained, the patient can be treated without her consent, and this includes tube feeding (as feeding is 'ancillary' to the mainstay of treatment for mental disorder).

ADDITIONAL POINTS

Investigations should include full blood count (FBC), liver function tests (LFT), serum creatinine, urea and electrolytes (U&E), calcium, magnesium, phosphate, electrocardiogram (ECG) and bone density scan.

The following may necessitate a medical admission in AN:

- Cardiovascular, hepatic or renal compromise
- ECG changes – a variety of ECG changes, including sinus bradycardia, ST depression and a prolonged QT interval
- Reduced pulse (<40 bpm) or low blood pressure (<90/60) (<80/50 in children)
- Low blood glucose, potassium, sodium, phosphate and magnesium
- High sodium
- Reduced body temperature
- Dehydration, oedema, hypoproteinaemia and profound anaemia
- Rapid weight loss, exhaustion and severe lack of energy

The examiner's mark sheet

Domain/ percentage of marks	Essential points to pass	✓	Extra marks/comments (make notes here)
1. Communication with professional colleague 25% of marks	Introduces self appropriately		
	Uses clear communication		
	Demonstrates adequate professional support		
	Allays anxieties regarding management of a difficult patient		
2. Advice and support – approach to feeding 25% of marks	Gives clear and methodical advice		
	Covers rehydration and electrolyte correction		
	Suggests referral to dietician		
	Gives explanation and advice on re-feeding syndrome		
3. Advice and support – approach to patient 25% of marks	Acknowledges nursing staff frustrations and anxieties		
	Advises a unified and consistent nursing approach		
	Offers to provide support and education on AN to the nursing team		
	Suggests specific intervention such as nursing observations for purging/vomiting		
4. Psychiatric management 25% of marks	Explains screening for comorbidity		
	Covers risk assessment		
	Outlines possible interventions – medication, psychology and one-to-one observations		
	Discusses use of Mental Health Act (MHA) and planned transfer to ED unit		

% SCORE _____

___ **OVERALL IMPRESSION**

4 (CIRCLE ONE)

Good Pass

Pass

Borderline

Fail

Clear Fail

NOTES/Areas to improve

⭘ SINGLE STATIONS

STATION 2: ANOREXIA NERVOSA – DIETARY AND WEIGHT HISTORY IN A FIRST PRESENTATION

INSTRUCTION TO CANDIDATE

You are working as the on-call psychiatry senior house officer (SHO) in a general hospital.

Miss Jones is an 18-year-old dancer with a 3-year history of low weight and amenorrhoea for the last 12 months. She has been admitted to hospital overnight with gastritis and mild haematemesis. The medical team are concerned about her low BMI and have asked you to assess her.

Your task is to take a weight and dietary history in order to reach a diagnosis.

ACTOR (ROLE-PLAYER) INSTRUCTIONS

You initially say that you would prefer not to speak to 'another doctor', but can be persuaded to open up if the psychiatrist is empathic and caring towards you.

You have perfectionistic and obsessional traits, which manifest themselves in your approach towards dancing.

You downplay the concerns of the doctor regarding your recent physical symptoms.

You are very determined to get to your ideal weight.

You exercise excessively, avoid carbohydrates and fattening foods and have started to use laxatives to control your weight.

SUGGESTED APPROACH

Setting the scene

Begin the task by addressing the patient by name, introducing yourself and explaining why you have been asked to see her.

'Hello, my name is Dr_____, I am the on-call psychiatry doctor today. I understand that you came into hospital last night because of stomach discomfort. How are you feeling now? The medical doctors were concerned about your weight, which is why they've asked me to see you. Would it be OK for me to spend some time with you, finding out about your weight and eating habits?'

Completing the tasks

Weight loss history

Enquire about her current BMI. If she does not know this, what is her actual weight and height? What is her ideal weight?

How much weight loss has there been and in what time frame? (Rapid weight loss is more dangerous than gradual weight loss.)

Ask about her highest and lowest ever weights.

When did she first decide that she wanted to lose weight? Has she ever had a stable weight?

Ask about steps taken to lose weight, including:

- Avoidance of certain foods: 'Have you been avoiding fattening foods?'
- Purging: 'Do you make yourself vomit or use laxatives or diuretics to lose weight?'
- Exercise: 'Have you been exercising excessively to control your weight?'
- Compensatory behaviours such as bingeing: 'Do you ever overeat to compensate for periods of not eating at all?'

Dietary history

You should enquire about restrictive, avoidant and altered eating habits. When did these begin? What are they specifically?

You need to find out about her current dietary practices. Is she vegan or vegetarian? What does she actually eat? Ask about different food groups, amounts, restrictions and rituals (cutting, separating and mashing). Does she chew food without swallowing it?

Take a typical 24-hour diet history, starting with breakfast and including lunch, dinner and snacks. Include details such as the number of slices of toast, brown or white bread, with or without butter. In addition, ask about milk with cereals and in drinks. Is this skimmed? How much does she use?

Ask her about calorie-counting. Does she know the calorific content of each of her meals? How many calories does she aim to consume each day?

Ask about meal times. Is she missing meals? Does she eat alone or with others? Does she prepare meals for others but not eat with them?

Screening for a diagnosis

Here, you are expected to screen for the features of anorexia nervosa according to ICD-10 and DSM-V criteria. By now, you should know her BMI and have a sense of her weight and dietary history, but you still need to ask about body image distortion and test for overvalued ideas with questions such as:

- Do you constantly think about your weight and find it difficult not to do so?
- Do you perceive yourself as fat or thin? Do you fear being or becoming fat?
- When you look in the mirror, what do you see? Do you dislike your body? If so, in what way?
- What would happen if you could not control your weight?
- Does losing weight make you feel good?
- Have others ever commented on your weight? If so, who and what have they said?

ADDITIONAL POINTS

Cognitive distortions

You may elicit cognitive distortions during the course of the interview, either in this or other ED stations. Where relevant, discussions about CBT may follow. Examples of classic cognitive distortions in anorexia nervosa include:

- 'If I put on a pound, none of my clothes will fit me' (magnification).
- 'If I put on even a pound in weight, I will lose my friends as they'll think I'm ugly' (catastrophizing).

Risk

Although not specifically asked, consider the risk component in all stations where possible. Does she have insight into the effect her eating restriction is having on her physical health? What does she believe will happen if she continues to lose weight?

How does she explain the reasons for her admission to a medical ward?

If she appears low in mood, a few screening questions for low mood and suicidality would be prudent.

Substance misuse

Some patients will use psychostimulants such as cocaine to help them lose weight. It is important to ask about substance misuse in this station, including alcohol. Dependence or intoxication may account for any behavioural change.

The examiner's mark sheet

Domain/ percentage of marks	Essential points to pass	✓	Extra marks/comments (make notes here)
1. Rapport and communication 25% of marks	Introduces self appropriately		
	Uses clear communication		
	Makes appropriate use of open and closed questions		
	Demonstrates an empathic and caring approach		
2. Weight loss history 20% of marks	Elicits current BMI		
	Asks about extent and rate of weight loss		
	Asks about highest and lowest recorded weights		
	Enquires about different methods of weight loss		
3. Dietary history 20% of marks	Asks about specific dietary restrictions		
	Takes a 24-hour diet history		
	Asks about calorie-counting		
	Enquires about meal times/rituals		
4. Screening for a diagnosis 20% of marks	Elicits features of AN to make diagnosis – low BMI, self-induced weight loss, body image distortion, etc.		
5. Additional points 15% of marks	Elicits cognitive distortions		
	Screens for risk of self-harm/ suicide and elicits level of insight		
	Enquires about substance misuse		

STATION 3: BULIMIA NERVOSA – COMMUNICATION AND EXPLANATION TO A RELATIVE

INSTRUCTION TO CANDIDATE

You are a junior doctor working for the Community Eating Disorders team.

Mrs Tomkins, a 34-year-old woman, has been referred to you by her GP. She has been concerned about her weight for many years and believes that she is overweight. As a teenager, her school teacher told her parents that he was concerned she may have anorexia nervosa, but she was never formally diagnosed and did not receive any specialist treatment. She is now a successful barrister working in a high-pressure job, and it appears that this may have led to an abnormal eating pattern.

Her husband has asked to see you first, alone. He wishes to know the following:

- **Does his wife have bulimia, and if so, what caused it?**
- **What can be done to help her?**

You should assume that the patient has given her consent for you to discuss things with her husband.

ACTOR (ROLE-PLAYER) INSTRUCTIONS

You are very concerned about your wife, who you say has been preoccupied with her work for the last 6 months, and you think she is depressed.

You desperately want to know if your wife has an eating disorder and what has caused this.

You have noticed a change in your wife's eating behaviours, including that she refuses to eat certain foods and no longer wishes to go out for meals with friends.

You suspect that your wife may have been making herself vomit, as you have occasionally heard her in the bathroom.

You want to know what the best available treatment for your wife is and how likely this is to be effective.

SUGGESTED APPROACH

Setting the scene

Begin the task by introducing yourself, confirming the identity of Mr Tomkins (as the husband of the patient) and clarifying why he wishes to see you.

'Hello, my name is Dr_____, I am one of the psychiatrists working in the eating disorders service. Thank you for coming to see me today. I understand that you would like to speak to me about your wife, Mrs Tomkins, and have some specific questions that you would like answering, is that correct?'

Completing the tasks

Does she have bulimia nervosa?

It is very important that you avoid using medical jargon and speak in lay terms as much as possible. Although it is unlikely that the patient's husband will know all of the answers to your questions, a useful approach would be to take him through the ICD-10 diagnostic criteria for bulimia, asking him if he recognises the features in his wife whilst explaining what they mean:

1. Persistent preoccupation with eating and craving for food; overeating large amounts of food in short periods of time.
2. An attempt to counteract the fattening effects of food by one or more of: vomiting, purging, starvation and drugs (e.g. appetite suppressants, diuretics or thyroid analogues)
3. Specific psychopathology and/or history, including a morbid dread of fatness, low threshold for self-induced weight loss and previous history of anorexia nervosa. Other features of BN can include normal weight (atypical bulimia) and irregular menstrual periods.

Next, you should provide an explanation of bulimia; for example:

'Bulimia refers to episodes of uncontrolled excessive eating or "binges" with the consumption of a large amount of food in a short period of time and a loss of self-control. After a binge, actions are taken to counteract any weight gain, such as the person making themselves sick or using other methods, such as water tablets, to lose weight. Often, individuals with bulimia are slim or even underweight for their height.'

First, ask him if he recognises anything in his wife from what you have described above, and then ask him whether he has noticed any of the following characteristics or behaviours associated with BN:

- Calorie-counting
- Weighing herself frequently
- Feelings of anxiety, loneliness, boredom and depression
- Binges exacerbating feelings of self-loathing, disgust and poor self-esteem
- Difficulty eating in front of others

What caused the bulimia? (Aetiology)

You now explain that you would want to see his wife before you can be certain about the diagnosis and that you would also like to carry out some tests (e.g. blood) to exclude a physical cause of her presentation.

If she does indeed have BN, there are a number of factors that are thought to increase the risk of developing such a disorder. You should take Mr Tomkins through the following factors in turn:

- Social factors: a cultural emphasis on slimness, media pressures, associations with particular professions and dieting fashions.

- Family factors: genetic influences are important, such that first-degree relatives of individuals with BN have an increased risk of developing an eating disorder. Family environment is also important, particularly where other members of the family have had issues with food or have been critical of eating, weight or body shape.
- Personality factors: the presence of certain personality traits or characteristics, including perfectionism, impulsivity, mood lability, thrill-seeking and dysphoria associated with rejection, have been linked to developing an eating disorder.
- Life events: significant life events, such as relationship break-ups, can trigger the onset of bulimia in up to 70% of cases. Childhood sexual abuse as well as parental neglect, loss, indifference or separation have all been suggested as risk factors in BN.
- Depressive symptoms: people often turn to food as a comfort when they feel depressed or low in self-esteem. It is possible that bulimia starts off this way when people feel unhappy with their lives and themselves. The guilt associated with bingeing then often leads to vomiting or purging.

What can be done to help her? (Treatment)

You might start by explaining that the treatment of eating disorders such as bulimia consists of three main elements: psycho-education, psychological therapy and pharmacological management (medication).

You can now take Mr Tomkins through each of the main strands of treatment, giving him the opportunity to ask questions along the way.

Psycho-education

This involves being given information on a number of important issues, such as the physical consequences of repeated bingeing and vomiting and the inappropriate use of prescribed and over-the-counter medicines, as well as the long-term effects of being underweight. It might also include advice on how to limit binges and the use of self-help materials (e.g. books such as *Getting Better Bit(e) by Bit(e)*). NICE guidelines suggest an evidence-based self-help programme as the first step in the treatment of BN. Healthcare professionals have a role to play in providing direct encouragement and support to patients undertaking this self-help programme, as this may improve outcomes. This may be sufficient treatment for a limited subset of patients.

Psychological therapy

A number of psychological approaches have been used in the management of bulimia, including:

- Cognitive behavioural therapy: This is the most studied modality and is claimed to be the treatment of choice for BN. You might want to explain the basic principles of this therapy and the focus of challenging associated cognitive ('thinking') distortions in an attempt to modify behaviour. An experienced therapist or one specialising in eating disorders is needed in such cases.
- Interpersonal therapy: This is a short-term, focussed psychotherapy where the main goal is to help patients identify and modify current interpersonal difficulties. It was adapted from the treatment of depression by Fairburn (1997).
- Family therapy: This is often less effective in bulimia than anorexia. It probably has a greater role in patients of younger age, for whom family factors may be more relevant.

Therapy might also be useful in addressing feelings of loneliness and boredom, anxiety and depression and low self-esteem.

Pharmacological treatment

NICE guidelines (2004) state that adults with bulimia may be offered a trial of the selective serotonin reuptake inhibitor antidepressant, fluoxetine, as an alternative or additional first-line management strategy. Such medication can help to reduce the frequency of binge eating and purging episodes, and these benefits are usually rapidly apparent. Medication is not recommended in the treatment of adolescents with BN.

ADDITIONAL POINTS

Comorbidities

- The incidence of borderline personality traits is higher in bulimia than anorexia nervosa.
- Half of patients with anorexia meet the criteria for bulimia.
- A third of patients with bulimia have a history of anorexia and another third have a history of obesity.
- In 25% of bulimia cases, there is benign enlargement of the parotid gland.

Risk

- Where there is a risk of self-harm or if community treatment has been unsuccessful, a psychiatric admission can be arranged. This is not without risk in itself, as patients can sometimes worsen. Therefore, admissions are usually kept short.
- It is also important to exclude comorbid substance misuse, particularly when considering a treatment plan.
- Oesophageal rupture (Boerhaave's syndrome) is a complication that is associated with vomiting after eating.

REFERENCE

Fairburn, C.G. (1997) Interpersonal psychotherapy for bulimia nervosa. In D.M. Garner and P. E. Garfinkel (Eds.), *Handbook of Treatment for Eating Disorders*. (pp. 278–294). New York, NY: Guilford Press.

FURTHER READING

Laird, B. C. & Treasure, J. (2010) *Medical Management of Eating Disorders*, 2nd edn, Cambridge: Cambridge University Press.

NICE guidelines for eating disorders, January 2004. www.nice.org.uk/guidance/cg9

Schmidt, U. & Treasure, J. (1993) *Getting Better Bit(e) by Bit(e)*. London: Lawrence Erlbaum Associates.

Semple, D. & Smyth, R. (2013) *Oxford Handbook of Psychiatry*, 3rd edn, Oxford: Oxford University Press.

The examiner's mark sheet

Domain/ percentage of marks	Essential points to pass	✓	Extra marks/comments (make notes here)
1. Rapport and communication 25% of marks	Introduces self appropriately		
	Uses clear communication		
	Allows patient's relative the opportunity to ask questions		

2. Explanation and diagnosis of bulimia 20% of marks	Gives a clear explanation of the problem and avoids using too much medical jargon
	Elicits features of bulimia from husband's account
3. Aetiology of bulimia 20% of marks	Covers relevant risk factors, including psycho-social, family and personality factors and adverse life events
4. Treatment of bulimia 20% of marks	Approaches management using the bio-psycho-social model
	Covers self-help, psychological therapies and medication options
	Offers a simple explanation of CBT (best evidence for bulimia)
5. Additional points 15% of marks	Discusses comorbidities and risks

% SCORE _____

___ **OVERALL IMPRESSION**

5 (CIRCLE ONE)

Good Pass

Pass

Borderline

Fail

Clear Fail

NOTES/Areas to improve

Chapter 5
Addiction disorders

Mark Parry

O LINKED STATIONS

STATION 1(a): OPIOID DEPENDENCE

INSTRUCTION TO CANDIDATE

Mr Smith, a 22-year-old gentleman, has been referred to you by his probation officer (PO) for help with his illicit drug use. You are assessing him in an out-patient clinic.

Evaluate Mr Smith for illicit drug use. Please make notes if you wish as in the next station you will be discussing Mr Smith's problems and treatment with his probation officer.

ACTOR (ROLE-PLAYER) INSTRUCTIONS

You use many illicit substances, including heroin, cannabis and alcohol.

You tend to underplay your drug-seeking behaviour.

You are reluctant to divulge information about your petty crimes.

You seem very guarded in answering the doctor as you think he works for the police.

You slowly begin to tell the doctor the details if he or she is reassuring and empathic.

SUGGESTED APPROACH

Setting the scene

Introduce yourself and start the station by thanking the patient for coming to see you. Enquire about reasons for seeking help, whether on his own accord or subject to a Drug Treatment and Testing Order (DTTO) or a Drug Rehabilitation Requirement (DRR). Explain that you will need to ask him details of his legal and illicit drug use and associated problems if any.

Completing the tasks

After the introductions, ask what substances he has been using recently, including legal and illicit drug use, type, method of administration, quantity and frequency.

C: I understand that you have been using drugs for some time, please can you tell what you have been using recently? (Drug use in the last 6 weeks is the most pertinent.)

Pt: I have been using heroin.

C: Are you using anything else; for example, alcohol or cannabis?

Pt: I drink alcohol occasionally, couple of pints once or twice a week, I smoke skunk once in a while.

One should be familiar with the street names of illicit drugs (please refer to the table below); however, street names for illicit drugs often change quite rapidly, so if in doubt, ask the patient what drug the street name refers to.

Common street names/types of some illicit drugs	
Amphetamines	Speed, uppers
Benzodiazepine	Temazzies and jellies (temazepam), vallies (diazepam)
Cannabis	Dope, weed, skunk, hash, grass
Cocaine	C, Charlie, coke, snow, crack and bones (crack cocaine)
Heroin	H, horse, smack, brown
LSD	Acid
MDMA (ecstasy)	E, XTC, hug drug, Adam

C: We can discuss use of the alcohol and cannabis later on, shall we first look into your heroin use? Please tell me how much heroin you use and how you use it.

Enquire into the details of the amount of heroin used, the frequency of use and the route of administration (whether smoking, snorting or injecting). Some users may not be able to quantify the amount; enquire into the amount of money spent; the street price and the quality of heroin varies and is usually approximately £40 per gram. Many users may smoke (chase) as well as injecting the drug. Ask about first use, pattern of use and any periods of abstinence/treatment.

Some patients are vague when giving details. It is important to obtain the basic information of their drug use. Ask what is the least amount they can get by on over a 24-hour period. It is important to establish that they experience withdrawal symptoms, as it is these that establish whether they are physically dependent; for example, by asking 'How do you feel when you stop taking drugs, even briefly?' It is not uncommon for patients either to understate or overstate their use for whatever reason.

State that it will be necessary to obtain a sample of urine (or alternatively a sample of saliva) for drug testing. This is extremely important to note that while a sample that is positive for opioids does not prove opioid dependence, a negative sample disproves a diagnosis of opioid dependence. Drug testing must *never* be omitted.

Explore the following:

- Criteria for dependence: These are the same as for alcohol. The withdrawal symptoms associated with heroin and other opioids are:
  - Aches and pains, anxiety, stomach cramps, nausea, hot/cold flushes, runny nose, yawning, gooseflesh, sweating, tremors, dilated pupils, restlessness, tachycardia, diarrhoea, vomiting, muscle twitches
- Use of other illicit drugs and alcohol.
- Medical complications: any accidental overdoses, abscesses/infections, blood-borne viral diseases (hepatitis B and C, HIV).
- Psychiatric complications/comorbidities: anxiety, depression, post-traumatic stress disorder (PTSD), etc. When psychiatric symptoms are present, try to establish whether they predate and/or persist during periods of abstinence. Do not go into details of psychiatric history; remember the task of the station.
- Psycho-social complications: relationships and social and occupational functioning. Briefly explore what are the predisposing, precipitating and maintaining factors.
- Forensic history: the fact that he has been referred by the probation officer indicates involvement with the Criminal Justice System (CJS). Ask how he was funding his drug habit. Often, drug users resort to crimes in order to fund their drug use. Briefly ask about previous offending and criminal records.

Problem solving

Individuals referred by the CJS may have been coerced into treatment; they may view the health professionals as part of the CJS. It will be important to emphasise that you are not part of the CJS, but will have to work closely with the CJS. If the individual is not motivated, one may have to use the motivation enhancement techniques to improve motivation. Use of a non-confrontational approach is essential when dealing with these individuals, who are often complex and difficult to engage.

The examiner's mark sheet

Domain/ percentage of marks	Essential points to pass	✓	Extra marks/comments (make notes here)
1. Communication and empathy 20% of marks	Introduces self appropriately		
	Uses clear communication		
	Makes appropriate use of open and closed questions		
	Demonstrates an empathic and caring approach		
2. Details of illicit drug use 20% of marks	Elicits the names of illicit drugs		
	Asks about the amount and timings of drug usage		
	Asks about symptoms of dependence		
3. Exploring high-risk behaviours 20% of marks	Asks about needle sharing and safety precautions during drug usage		
	Asks about forensic and criminal history		
	Asks about mixing various drugs from the street		
4. Physical health complications 20% of marks	Elicits symptoms of infections		
	Asks about accidental overdoses		
	Elicits any deterioration in carrying out activities of daily living		
5. Psychiatric comorbidity 20% of marks	Elicits depressive symptoms		
	Screens for risk of self-harm and suicide		
	Elicits level of insight		

% SCORE _____

___ **OVERALL IMPRESSION**

5 (CIRCLE ONE)

Good Pass

Pass

Borderline

Fail

Clear Fail

NOTES/Areas to improve

STATION 1(b): DISCUSSION WITH PROBATION OFFICER

INSTRUCTION TO CANDIDATE

You have seen Mr Smith in the previous station. You are now required to meet his probation officer to discuss his treatment options. You have obtained consent from Mr Smith regarding this discussion.

ACTOR (ROLE-PLAYER) INSTRUCTIONS

You want to know about the treatment options for Mr Smith's condition.

You ask how long these treatments will take and what are the expected outcomes.

You wish to know if this will work and keep Mr Smith out of trouble.

You ask what might happen if he starts using illicit street drugs again and how to find out about this.

SUGGESTED APPROACH

Setting the scene

Introduce yourself and state that you have the client's consent for sharing information. Enquire whether the probation officer has any particular questions or information they wish to obtain before you get into the details. The discussion would be shaped by your earlier assessment and the information you gathered.

Completing the tasks

Outline the principles of opioid dependence treatment, which would include pharmacological and structured psycho-social interventions in a multidisciplinary setting.

Pharmacological treatment

Regarding opioid detoxification or maintenance, explain the important factors, such as patient choice, motivation and engagement, length and pattern of use and previous treatments. Remember to avoid medical terms and explain in layman's language. 'Detoxification is done over 2–4 weeks gradually by replacing with prescription medicines such as methadone or buprenorphine. This is then followed by a medication called naltrexone, which in turn will block the effects of opioid drugs. Other medications such as lofexidine and non-steroidal pain relief can be used to give relief from withdrawal symptoms such as muscular pain.'

If maintenance (substitute prescribing) is chosen, then patients are stabilised either on methadone or buprenorphine and supervised prescription/administration is sometimes continued for many years. Regular monitoring with drug testing through urine/salivary analysis is mandatory in order to prevent misuse of the prescription and to detect on-top use of illicit drugs. The idea behind substitute prescribing is stabilisation (the relief and prevention of withdrawal symptoms, allowing the patient not to have to rely on street heroin), prevention of the harm associated with injecting, reduction of criminal activity and engagement in treatment.

Psycho-social intervention

Substitute prescribing or detoxification on their own do not have much value; these should be part of a treatment plan which will include structured psycho-social interventions such as individual/group therapy, provision of suitable accommodation, support from family, friends and self-help organisations such as Narcotics Anonymous.

PO: What can we do to help?

C: We need to work closely alongside statutory and non-statutory agencies, including health, social services, the Criminal Justice System and voluntary sector, in order to cater to the needs of these often complex patients. Despite best efforts, a significant number of patients relapse. Needle exchange, education about safe sex and injecting behaviour, screening for blood-borne viruses, vaccination against hepatitis B and nutritional advice are some of the harm minimisation strategies for those who continue to use illicit drugs. An important concept is relapse prevention; a toolkit is made up of a combination of various pharmacological and psycho-social interventions.

FURTHER READING

Department of Health (England) and the Devolved Administrations (2007). *Drug Misuse and Dependence: UK Guidelines on Clinical Management*. London: Department of Health (England), the Scottish Government, Welsh Assembly Government and Northern Ireland Executive.

Ghodse, H. (2010) *Ghodse's Drugs and Addictive Behaviour: A Guide to Treatment*, 4th edn. Cambridge: Cambridge University Press.

WEBSITES

http://www.talktofrank.com/

http://www.nta.nhs.uk/uploads/nta_care_planning_practice_guide_2006_cpg1.pdf

The examiner's mark sheet

Domain/ percentage of marks	Essential points to pass	✓	Extra marks/comments (make notes here)
1. Communication and empathy 20% of marks	Introduces self appropriately Uses clear communication Makes appropriate use of open and closed questions Demonstrates an empathic and caring approach		
2. Details of pharmacological treatment 20% of marks	Explains the rationale for various prescribed treatments Explains the role of substitute prescribing Explains the time period and long-term options of treatment		
3. Explaining psycho-social interventions 20% of marks	Talks about individual and group-based therapies Talks about multidisciplinary working Explains the role of voluntary organisations and community-based social programmes		
4. Addressing the queries of the probation officer 20% of marks	Being mindful of dealing with someone of a different profession Allows the officer to ask questions Clarifies if there are any doubts or further questions		

5. Harm minimisation strategies

20% of marks

Explains role of education

Mentions needle exchange programmes

% SCORE _____

___ **OVERALL IMPRESSION**

5 (CIRCLE ONE)

Good Pass

Pass

Borderline

Fail

Clear Fail

NOTES/Areas to improve

STATION 2(a): PHYSICAL EXAMINATION OF DRUG INTOXICATION/WITHDRAWAL STATE

INSTRUCTION TO CANDIDATE

Mr Johnson, a 25-year-old gentleman, has been brought to the Section 136 Suite at a Psychiatric Unit. The police who detained him report that he appeared confused and was found wandering on the streets. He is unable to provide any sensible information, but is settled enough to allow a physical examination. There are no informants for obtaining a collateral history. Do not elicit a history from the patient.

Carry out a physical examination for signs and symptoms of drug intoxication/withdrawal state.

Make notes if you wish as in the next station you will be discussing Mr Johnson's differential diagnosis and immediate management plan with the Consultant Psychiatrist over the phone.

ACTOR (ROLE-PLAYER) INSTRUCTIONS

You are very confused and agitated.

You appear very distracted and you can see some small insects crawling on the chair.

You cannot pay sustained attention to the doctor.

You cannot walk in a straight line and you seem as if you are going to fall a couple of times.

Though you are confused, you should cooperate with the doctor when he examines you.

SUGGESTED APPROACH

Setting the scene

Introduce yourself and explain to the patient that you need to carry out a physical examination on him. If the patient appears confused/does not understand your explanation, try again; do not rush into the examination if he resists your examination.

C: I am a doctor and I need to examine you. Is that OK? I would like to check your pulse, blood pressure and temperature first. I'll explain what I'm doing as I go along. You shouldn't experience any discomfort at any time, but let me know if you are uncomfortable at any point. Do you understand me?

Completing the tasks

After explaining the task, proceed to carry out relevant mental state examination (MSE) and systematic physical examinations, including general and systems examinations. If the instructions are that you should provide a commentary of what you are doing, do so (it may be beneficial to do so even if there are no such instructions), demonstrating to the examiner what you are doing.

'I am going to observe you for a minute or so, to understand what is going on...'

General examination: observe the general appearance, behaviour (any agitation or increased or decreased physical activity), conscious level (alert, drowsy or confused), self-care (dress and grooming), movements (voluntary and involuntary) and comprehension.

'I am now going to examine your heart and then your lungs and stomach; for this, I will have to come a bit closer to you, I hope that this is OK...I will then proceed to test your nerves.'

Systems examination includes:

- Cardiovascular: pulse, blood pressure and auscultation of precordium
- Respiratory: respiratory rate, pattern of respiration (regularity and depth) and auscultation of chest (lungs)
- Abdomen: jaundice, scars, distended veins, tenderness, palpation for mass, liver and spleen.
- Nervous system: higher mental functions (consciousness, orientation, memory, speech, etc.), cranial nerves (mainly pupils and nystagmus), motor and sensory deficits, coordination and gait.
- MSE: reactions, evidence of perceptual abnormalities, behaviour suggestive of delusions and mood state.

Be familiar with the features of various drug intoxication and withdrawal states; some of these are summarised below.

Alcohol

Intoxication: tachycardia, hypertension, mydriasis (dilated pupils), skin flushing, slurred speech, impaired coordination, nystagmus and gait disturbance.

Withdrawal: tremors, sweating, increased temperature, tachycardia, dilated pupils and diaphoresis. Seizure and delirium tremens are not uncommon.

Look for consequences of long-term excessive alcohol use – virtually any organ in the body could be affected:

- Gastrointestinal system: poor nutritional state, anaemia, hepatomegaly and liver failure signs such as jaundice, oedema and spider naevi
- Nervous system: peripheral neuropathy, Wernicke's encephalopathy (WE; ataxia, nystagmus and confusion) and Korsakoff syndrome (memory impairment)
- Cardiovascular system: high blood pressure and alcoholic cardiomyopathy
- Musculoskeletal system: proximal myopathy (proximal muscle weakness, shoulder and hip).

Opioids

Intoxication: varying degrees of clouded consciousness, pinpoint pupils and respiratory depression.

Withdrawal: sweating, nausea, vomiting, diarrhoea, abdominal cramps, myalgia, bone pains, dilated pupils, rhinorrhoea and insomnia.

Stimulants (cocaine and amphetamines)
Intoxication: euphoria, agitation, increased pulse and blood pressure, sweating, tremors, confusion, dilated pupils, hyperactivity, seizures, stroke, cardiac arrhythmias (irregular heartbeat) and sudden death can occur.

Withdrawal: dysphoria (crash), anxiety, hypersomnolence, paranoid ideation and hallucinations.

Benzodiazepines
Intoxication: drowsiness, ataxia, dysarthria, nystagmus and hypothermia.

Withdrawal: irritability, anxiety, insomnia, hypersensitivity to stimuli, tremor, hypotonia and hyporeflexia and seizures.

Cannabis
Intoxication: dry mouth, red eyes, impaired perception and motor skills, decreased short-term memory, paranoia, mood swings and, rarely, hallucinations.

LSD
Intoxication: dilated pupils, high body temperature, increased heart rate and blood pressure, sweating, loss of appetite, sleeplessness, dry mouth, tremors, flashbacks and perceptual abnormalities.

Look for factors associated with illicit drug use, such as needle track marks, thrombosed veins and a perforated nasal septum.

Problem solving

This will be a challenging station. You will need to be selective in your assessment and focus on the task. (If the patient is uncooperative, try to carry out as much of the examination as possible; try the Kirby's examination of an uncooperative patient.)

Form your opinion from the general reaction, attitude, posture, hygiene, dressing and behaviour towards staff. Look out for symptoms and signs of resistance, evasiveness and irritability/apathy. Look for any abnormal movements (retardation/overactivity), facial expressions and conscious levels (alert, attentive, placid, vacant, aversive, perplexed and distressed), emotional state and indication of mood fluctuations (tears/smiles). See if the eyes are open or closed; if open, do they follow the examiner's movements or are they fixed in terms of eye contact, and if closed, does the patient resist attempts to open the eyes? Observe the pattern and content of speech (mute, slow/retarded, over-talkative, relevance and coherence) and reactions to what is said or done. Examine the muscular reactions (rigidity and resistance).

The examiner's mark sheet

Domain/ percentage of marks	Essential points to pass	✓	Extra marks/comments (make notes here)
1. Communication and empathy 25% of marks	Introduces self appropriately		
	Uses clear communication		
	Considers the use of chaperone		
	Demonstrates an empathic and caring approach		

2. Demonstrates to examiner the salient features of physical examination

   25% of marks

   Either by talking through with the patient what the examination involves or stating what signs are being looked for

3. Systematic and relevant physical examination

   25% of marks

   Demonstrates methodical examination of systems

   Considers Wernicke's encephalopathy and examines for the signs

4. Mental state examination and brief cognitive examination

   25% of marks

   Systematic approach to MSE

   Demonstrates examination of cognitions/orientation

% SCORE _____

_____ **OVERALL IMPRESSION**

4 (CIRCLE ONE)

Good Pass

Pass

Borderline

Fail

Clear Fail

NOTES/Areas to improve

STATION 2(b): DISCUSSION WITH CONSULTANT

INSTRUCTION TO CANDIDATE

You have examined a confused patient during your period on call. You have noted that the patient has gait abnormalities; he is agitated, disorientated and experiencing visual hallucinations. You are about to speak to the on-call consultant psychiatrist over the phone.

Please discuss your findings with the consultant.

You will be asked about the differential diagnosis and immediate management.

ACTOR (ROLE-PLAYER) INSTRUCTIONS

You ask the candidate to present his or her findings.

You then ask for the differential diagnosis and why.

You are interested in knowing how the candidate is going to manage the patient.

You then ask about the long-term management plan.

You have to ask if the patient requires treatment under Mental Health Act (MHA) and why.

SUGGESTED APPROACH

Setting the scene

Introduce yourself: 'I am the doctor on-call, I wonder if I can discuss a patient who I have assessed?' The discussion will be shaped by your findings from the previously carried out assessment.

Completing the tasks

Try to present the findings in a systematic way. 'I have seen a 25-year-old man who has been brought under Section 136, as he has been confused and wandering on the streets. I notice he appears perplexed, sweating and disorientated.' Then go on to describe the positive findings of your examination. 'The patient appears distracted with poor attention span and seems to be responding to visual hallucinations. I notice profuse sweating and some mild tremors in the upper limbs. Cardiovascular examination reveals tachycardia and raised blood pressure. On examination of gait, he appears to be ataxic. Cranial nerves examination reveals...' and so on.

When prompted, discuss the differential diagnosis with points for and against. In this scenario, the differential diagnoses could be delirium tremens due to alcohol withdrawal, acute alcohol intoxication, delirium due to other systemic causes (e.g. hepatic encephalopathy due to alcohol-induced liver cirrhosis) and due to the presence of ophthalmoplegia and ataxia, one should consider Wernicke's encephalopathy. Explain that, if possible, you will try to obtain collateral information from staff/professionals and family/friends if and when they are identified and patient himself if he is to become communicative. Explain relevant tests such as urine and other body fluid drug screening and routine bloods that you will consider (be prepared to justify any of the investigations). Be familiar with the management of illicit drug and alcohol intoxication and withdrawal states, including the management of overdoses and complications such as delirium and seizures.

Consider the management in the short, medium and longer term. The short-term management will include whether the patient requires immediate hospital admission and what drug treatment and further investigation (blood tests for infection screening, electrolyte abnormalities, deranged kidney or liver functions and brain imaging and urine for infection screening and drug screening) he will require. You may be asked about what observations are required on the ward, including neurological observations if indicated.

A discussion of risk is likely to ensue and whether the patient is likely to need further assessment and/or treatment under the Mental Health Act. Be familiar with the Mental Capacity Act and the relevant safeguards under the Act. You may also be asked whether the patient needs any immediate management in the acute hospital setting before transferring him to a psychiatric hospital, and if so, why. This will again be guided by the differential diagnoses, and if you consider any acute physical health complications, then this may need treatment on a medical ward, at least in the short term.

FURTHER READING

Department of Health (England) and the Devolved Administrations (2007). *Drug Misuse and Dependence: UK Guidelines on Clinical Management.* London: Department of Health (England), the Scottish Government, Welsh Assembly Government and Northern Ireland Executive.

NICE. CR184. When patients should be seen by a psychiatrist. Delirium: Prevention, diagnosis and management. www.nice.org.uk/guidance/cg103

Royal College of Psychiatrists (2014) College Report 184. www.nice.org.uk/guidance/cg100/ifp/chapter/acute-withdrawal-from-alcohol

The examiner's mark sheet

Domain/ percentage of marks	Essential points to pass	✓	Extra marks/comments (make notes here)
1. Rapport and communication 20% of marks	Introduces self appropriately Uses clear communication Able to discuss findings in cohesive manner Demonstrates understanding of dealing with a senior colleague		
2. Positive findings 20% of marks	Elicits features of delirium Elicits positive findings in the systemic examination Complete and systematic approach in examination		
3. Differential diagnosis 20% of marks	Able to think broadly about causes of acute confusional state Able to formulate a possible diagnosis of alcohol withdrawal Able to rationalise the reasons for various differentials		
4. Management plan 20% of marks	Systematic approach in management plan Discusses relevant investigations Able to describe immediate, short-term and long-term management plans		
5. MHA and Mental Capacity Act (MCA) 20% of marks	Demonstrates understanding of the principles of the Mental Health Act and Mental Capacity Act		

% SCORE _____

_____ **OVERALL IMPRESSION**

5 (CIRCLE ONE)

Good Pass

Pass

Borderline

Fail

Clear Fail

NOTES/Areas to improve

STATION 3(a): CANNABIS AND SCHIZOPHRENIA – DISCUSSION WITH FAMILY

INSTRUCTION TO CANDIDATE

You are the junior doctor working in an in-patient unit where Mr Mark Roberts, a 19-year-old man, was recently admitted and diagnosed with schizophrenia.

You are exploring factors that were relevant to the onset of the illness and suspect that illicit drug use may have contributed to it. Mr Roberts is reluctant to talk about his illicit drug use. His mother is visiting the unit and wants to speak to you. Mr Roberts has consented for you to meet his mother and share information about him.

Gather information on Mr Roberts's illicit drug use history from his mother.

Address her concerns if she has any.

Make notes as required as you will be meeting Mr Roberts in the next station.

ACTOR (ROLE-PLAYER) INSTRUCTIONS

You have been told by ward nurses that your son has schizophrenia, but you do not know anything else and you are very worried.

You know your son has been experimenting with cannabis, but you think most kids do that nowadays.

You are sceptical about the diagnosis, not sure how cannabis can cause this and ask the doctor about this.

You appear somewhat reluctant to discuss your son's drug-taking behaviour as your family is embarrassed.

SUGGESTED APPROACH

Setting the scene

Introduce yourself and start the station by thanking the mother for coming to the ward and speaking to you. Inform her that her son has consented to the meeting occurring. Enquire about her views on his current state, treatment and the effects of the illness on herself and other carers (family/friends).

Completing the tasks

After setting the scene you might say:

C: This must be a difficult time for you. Have you been told about your son's diagnosis?

At this point, she may raise some queries about the diagnosis itself – be prepared to address those. If she has no knowledge of diagnosis, be prepared to explain this to her. Today I want to find out more about the things that may have had a role in Mark becoming unwell. There are a number of risk factors for the development of schizophrenia, and one such risk factor is use of illicit drugs. Mark has been reluctant to talk about it, I wonder whether you know anything about his drug use?

M: Well, doctor, as far as I know, Mark does not use drugs, except for cannabis.

C: Actually, cannabis is an illicit drug and can contribute to the development of mental health problems. Please can you tell me about Mark's use of cannabis?

M: I caught him smoking cannabis soon after his 14th birthday; I was not happy about it, but didn't say much as many kids nowadays smoke the stuff.

C: We know that quite a few people use cannabis, but that does not make it any less harmful. There is increasing evidence that it causes mental health problems. Do you know when Mark started using cannabis and how often he used it?

Obtain illicit drug and alcohol consumption details as outlined in the Opioid Dependence and Alcohol Dependence stations.

M: I didn't know that cannabis caused so many problems, if I only knew these things before, I could have done something about it.

C: Please don't be hard on yourself, as you said you did not know these things and probably even Mark himself didn't know about it. The important thing is how we can help Mark now to get better and remain well. It will be important for him to stay clear of all illicit drugs. Now that I know that he regularly smoked cannabis from a young age, I can talk to him about it.

M: I thought cannabis was just for fun and relaxing, can it damage one's health?

C: Although cannabis can produce relaxation, if higher amounts are consumed, it can have the opposite effect by increasing anxiety. Some cannabis users may have unpleasant experiences, including confusion, hallucinations, anxiety and paranoia, depending on their mood and circumstances. Some users may experience psychotic symptoms with hallucinations and delusions lasting a few hours, which can be very unpleasant. Even though these unpleasant effects do not last long, since the drug can stay in the system for some weeks, the effect can be more long-lasting than users realise. Long-term use can have a depressant effect and reduce motivation. Some researchers also suggest that long-term use can lead to irreversible, but minor cognitive deficits.

Problem solving

The carers may feel guilty about their role in the causation of the condition, be it the genetics, family environment, lack of supervision, and so forth. It is important to acknowledge these feelings and educate and empower them so that they contribute constructively in the care and treatment of the affected individual.

ADDITIONAL POINTS

There can be similar scenarios involving the role of genetics (family history of similar illness), compliance with medication and illicit drugs in relapse of schizophrenia, and so forth. The key skills would relate to obtaining a collateral history from carers and being sensitive to their needs.

FURTHER READING

http://www.rcpsych.ac.uk/healthadvice/problemsdisorders/cannabis.aspx

---

The examiner's mark sheet

Domain/ percentage of marks	Essential points to pass	✓	Extra marks/comments (make notes here)
1. Rapport and communication 25% of marks	Introduces self appropriately		
	Uses clear communication		
	Able to empathise with the carer in distress and guilt		
	Able to reassure carer and elicit history despite carer being reluctant		

2. History taking
   25% of marks

Elicits features of drug use/
dependence

Asks questions pertaining to amount,
type and time of various drug usages

3. Addressing
   concerns
   25% of marks

Able to show good listening skills

Able to address carer's concerns
and alleviate anxiety

Able to explain the role of
cannabis in mental health

4. Reassurance to
   mother
   25% of marks

Able to explain the role of mental
health services in further
treatment planning

Able to alleviate mother's anxiety
and provide reassurance that her
son can be helped

% SCORE _____

___ **OVERALL IMPRESSION**

4 (CIRCLE ONE)

Good Pass

Pass

Borderline

Fail

Clear Fail

NOTES/Areas to improve

STATION 3(b): CANNABIS AND SCHIZOPHRENIA

INSTRUCTION TO CANDIDATE

You meet Mark Roberts, a 19-year-old man on the ward. You are familiar with
him and know that he has been diagnosed with schizophrenia. He is no longer
displaying any active symptoms of schizophrenia and you are working towards
a discharge plan. He had been reluctant to speak about his illicit drug use,
despite his urine drug screen being positive for cannabis. You have met his
mother and discussed his cannabis use.

Educate him about the effects of cannabis on schizophrenia.

Explain how he can be helped further by mental health services.

ACTOR (ROLE-PLAYER) INSTRUCTIONS

You are Mark; you have been using cannabis regularly for a few years now. You do
not think it is a big issue, as many of your friends are doing the same.

You first dismiss the doctor's ideas that cannabis can be linked to mental health,
but when probed gently and reassuringly, you then begin to wonder if he or she
might be correct.

You wish to know what further help you can get.

SUGGESTED APPROACH

Setting the scene

Introduce yourself: 'Hello, Mr Roberts, I am Dr_____, the psychiatrist, we have met a few times in the last few days. It is good to see you doing well, I think you will soon be ready for discharge. There are a few important things that we need to talk about today. We need to discuss your cannabis use and be sure that you understand its effects.'

If the patient denies use of cannabis, you may well have to mention the positive urine drug screen and collateral history from the mother. However, it is important not to be confrontational, and you may use the motivational interviewing (MI) techniques as outlined in the Motivational Interviewing station.

Completing the tasks

Pt: Cannabis helps me to relax, most of my friends use it.

C: Cannabis helps some people to relax, but it also causes a number of problems, particularly related to one's mental health. Are you aware of this?

Pt: I am not sure.

C: Cannabis users are known to experience higher rates of anxiety, depression, paranoia and psychosis. The heavier and longer the use, the higher the chance of someone developing mental health problems. There is growing evidence that people with serious mental illness, including depression and psychosis, are more likely to use cannabis or to have used it for long periods of time in the past. Regular use of the drug has appeared to double the risk of developing a psychotic episode or long-term schizophrenia.

Use an interactive approach to explain and educate about the role of cannabis in the causation of schizophrenia and the higher risk of relapse with continued use.

C: There are alternative ways to cope with difficulties and to relax.

Pt: Sounds like it can affect my health, so is there any help for me to come off cannabis?

C: The Home Office has published a guide on how to cut down and stop cannabis use. It suggests a range of things you can do to successfully stop using, including:

• Drawing up a list of reasons for wanting to change
• Planning how you will change
• Thinking about coping with withdrawal symptoms
• Having a back-up plan

If you decide to give up cannabis yourself, you could work through the leaflet on the Talk to Frank website. Many people will be able to stop on their own. However, if you need support, join a support group; for instance, the online Marijuana Anonymous UK. You can talk to your GP or practice nurse. They can also refer you to more specialist services, such as a counsellor, support group or NHS substance misuse service.

Pt: Where can I get more help and information?

C: Talk to Frank is a website with a lot of useful information. You can order free information leaflets for different age groups, read real-life stories of other people's experiences with drugs and get reliable, factual information. The helpline is 0300 123 6600. They also have a chat line.

Decisional balance matrix

The idea is to get the patient to reflect on their use of a drug. This involves asking the patient to consider what the advantages and disadvantages are of continuing to use the drug and the advantages and disadvantages of stopping the drug. Patients are often ambivalent about their drug use – there are factors that cause them to continue (e.g. relief of stress and enjoyment of effects) and other factors that oppose the use of drugs (e.g. negative effects, cost, etc.). Patients will often become defensive about their drug use if advised to stop, even when feeling unhappy about their drug use. The aim is to get the patient to reflect and come to their own decision: whether to continue using or to stop. If the latter is decided upon, then the patient has moved along 'the cycle of change' (Prochaska and DiClemente, 2005) from pre-contemplation to contemplation.

Problem solving

Many individuals may have a history of poly-substance misuse; be familiar with the role of stimulants in the causation of schizophrenia/psychosis.

FURTHER READING

Cannabis and mental health leaflet (with references) published by the Royal College of Psychiatrists: www.rcpsych.ac.uk

Castle, D., Murray, R.M. & D'Souza, D.C. (eds) (2011) *Marijuana and Madness*. Cambridge: Cambridge University Press.

DiClemente, C.C. (2006) *Addiction and Change: How Addictions Develop and Addicted People Recover*. New York, NY: Guildford Press.

Moore, T.H.M., Zammit, S., Lingford-Hughes, A. et al. (2007) Cannabis use and the risk of psychotic or affective mental health outcomes: A systematic review. *Lancet, 370*(9584), 319–28.

Prochaska, J.O. & DiClemente, C.C. (2005) The transtheoretical approach. In: Norcross, JC; Goldfried, MR. (eds.) *Handbook of Psychotherapy Integration*. 2nd ed. New York, NY: Oxford University Press, pp. 147–171.

WEBSITE

http://stepupprogram.org/docs/handouts/STEPUP_Stages_of_Change.pdf

The examiner's mark sheet

Domain/ percentage of marks	Essential points to pass	✓	Extra marks/comments (make notes here)
1. Rapport and communication 25% of marks	Introduces self appropriately		
	Uses clear communication		
	Able to build rapport with patient		
	Able to empathise with patient who uses cannabis and being non-judgemental		
2. Explanation 25% of marks	Explains the role of cannabis in mental health		
	Draws upon evidence-based conclusions on the relationship between drugs and mental health		

3. Educating on drugs
and mental health

25% of marks

Able to alleviate the anxiety of the patient

Able to use Socratic-style questioning to explore patient's ideas to change

Able to demonstrate knowledge of drug and alcohol services, self-help groups, etc.

4. Addressing patient's concerns

25% of marks

Able to explain the role of health services in further treatment planning

Able to address patient's concerns about drug-seeking behaviour

Addresses patient's concerns on the effects of cannabis on health

% SCORE _____

___

4

OVERALL IMPRESSION

(CIRCLE ONE)

Good Pass

Pass

Borderline

Fail

Clear Fail

NOTES/Areas to improve

O SINGLE STATIONS

STATION 4: ALCOHOL DEPENDENCE – HISTORY TAKING

INSTRUCTION TO CANDIDATE

You have been asked to assess Mr Jones, a 35-year-old gentleman who was admitted to an Acute Medical Assessment Unit for severe stomach pain 2 days ago. His stomach pain has subsided and he is feeling better. The physical examination and routine investigations are essentially normal except for slightly raised mean corpuscular volume and gamma-glutamyl transferase. The medical team suspect alcoholic liver disease secondary to excessive alcohol consumption and are suggesting that he undergoes further tests. He is agitated, anxious, reluctant to have any more tests and is keen to leave the unit. The medical staff are concerned and want you to assess him. He has agreed to speak to you.

Evaluate Mr Jones for alcohol dependence.

Take an alcohol history.

You will then have to provide feedback to him.

ACTOR (ROLE-PLAYER) INSTRUCTIONS

You work as a sales executive. You usually drink socially, but for the past 6 months, you have been stressed at work and have been drinking more regularly, almost every day. You sometimes need a drink in the morning and have been told off by your boss. You were caught drink driving 2 weeks ago. Your wife is also annoyed about this as she thinks you do not want to spend time with your family. You are also worried that you are financially worse off as you have been spending more on alcohol. You think it is all due to work-related stress and you need alcohol as a way of coping. You drink mostly strong beer but sometimes whisky and vodka during the week. You now want to go home as you want a drink.

SUGGESTED APPROACH

Setting the scene

Introduce yourself, thank the patient for agreeing to speak to you and acknowledge his anxiety and any distress. Ask if it would be OK to talk about what has been happening (open question to start).

Completing the tasks

After the introductions, you might say:

C: I heard that your physical examination was OK but some of your blood tests were abnormal, what do you think might be the reason for this?

Pt: I don't know.

C: The commonest reason for these tests to be increased is excessive alcohol consumption.

Pt: I do not drink excessively.

C: Shall we look at what it is you drink? Please can you tell me what you drink each day?... Thank you for that, what about at the weekend?

Ask the patient what he drinks each day, including the brand and quantity of the alcoholic beverage. As individuals often minimise their alcohol consumption, ask them: 'Are there times and days when you might drink more than the usual amount?' It would look impressive (although not necessary), once the patient has given the details of his consumption, to calculate the units by multiplying the volume in millilitres by the alcohol by volume and dividing the result by 1000; one 500 mL can of 5% lager would be 2.5 units. Most often people consume a mixture of alcoholic beverages, in which case you should calculate units for each beverage and add them up to arrive at the total. The following is a table of commonly used quantities of beverages and approximate units of alcohol:

Beverage	Quantity	Units
Ordinary beer (3%–4%)	1 pint (568 mL)	2
Strong beer (8%–9%)	1 pint (568 mL)	4.5
Wine (12%)	1 glass (175 mL)	2
Spirits (40%)	1 pub measure (25 mL)	1

Do not get bogged down with numbers and percentages; you should get an idea of the quantity of alcohol being consumed and demonstrate that to the examiner. 'So you are telling me that in a week you consume about 2 litres of vodka and 10 pints of lager. That's approximately 100 units per week, which is far in excess of the recommended maximum of 21 units per week for men.'

Elicit the alcohol consumption details, including the age of first drink, lifetime pattern of drinking and any previous periods of abstinence/treatment, then focus on the following:

- Criteria for dependence: check for cravings, loss of control, tolerance, withdrawal symptoms, salience and excessive use despite knowledge of harmful physical or mental health consequences (refer to 'Features of Alcohol Dependence Syndrome' for specifics).
- Medical complications: seizures, delirium tremens, head injury, liver damage, etc.
- Psychiatric complications/comorbidities: anxiety, depression, PTSD, etc. When psychiatric symptoms are present, try to establish whether the psychiatric conditions are primary by enquiring whether these symptoms predated and/or persisted during periods of abstinence. Do not go into details of psychiatric history; remember the task of the station.
- Psycho-social complications: relationships, social and occupational functioning and forensic history.
- Time allowing, you could provide feedback of your assessment to the patient. You might say: 'You have told me that on average you have been drinking 100 units of alcohol per week for the last 2 years, you crave alcohol and experience shakes and sweats in the morning. Without alcohol, you feel anxious to face people. You have been warned at your workplace for being drunk on duty and your wife is threatening to leave you if you don't stop drinking. It appears you are dependent on alcohol and it has caused you a number of problems. Perhaps you need to do something about it.'

Pt: What can I do about it?

C: Ideally, you should stop drinking, and there is help available for you to achieve this. You are possibly suffering from withdrawal symptoms, which is why you are uncomfortable and may be your reason for wanting to leave the hospital. You can be prescribed medication to avoid these withdrawal symptoms. You might also need help with some of the problems associated with alcohol dependence. I will give you information on how you can access our service and also give you some leaflets. You can look through these and I'll be happy to discuss any issues with you another time. In the meantime, it's important that you undergo the further tests and assessments that have been recommended to you.

Problem solving

Individuals who consume alcohol excessively can be defensive and minimise their alcohol consumption. A gentle and non-confrontational approach often succeeds in building rapport and eliciting details of alcohol consumption and the problems associated with it. Be prepared to have a more detailed conversation about treatment options, including in-patient detoxification.

Features of alcohol dependence syndrome (more information below)

1	Stereotyped pattern of alcohol consumption
2	Salience of drinking behaviour
3	Compulsion to drink
4	Increased tolerance to alcohol
5	Repeated withdrawal symptoms on reduction of alcohol intake
6	Relief/avoidance of withdrawal symptoms with alcohol intake
7	Reinstatement after abstinence

ADDITIONAL POINTS

Focus on harm minimisation if the patient is not willing to stop drinking.

Identify predisposing, precipitating and maintaining factors for alcohol dependence.

Features of alcohol dependence syndrome: More information

1. Non-dependent drinkers drink in accordance with a variety of cues, whereas the dependent drinker drinks to avoid symptoms of withdrawal. The drinking repertoire is therefore narrowed.

2. The dependent drinker will continue to drink even though there are several negative consequences such as financial, familial and physical.

3. The individual knows that taking a drink is irrational and the action is resisted but, as in the case of compulsions in obsessive compulsive disorder, further drink is taken.

4. There are physiological and neurochemical changes (more alcohol is required to achieve the same effect). In the later stages, tolerance develops, often with loss of control over alcohol intake.

5. Shaking, trembling, anxiety, physiological craving, vomiting and seizures may occur.

6. The individual may drink throughout the night and on waking in severe cases.

7. For severe dependents, following a period of abstinence, the previous high levels of alcohol intake and tolerance can be achieved within a number of days.

FURTHER READING

Edwards, G. & Gross, M. (1976) Alcohol dependence: Provisional description of a clinical syndrome. *Br Med J, 1*(6017): 1058–61.

Raistrick, D., Heather, N. & Godfrey, C. (2006) Review of the effectiveness of treatment for alcohol problems. National Treatment Agency. Available at: http://www.nta.nhs.uk/uploads/nta_review_of_the_effectiveness_of_treatment_for_alcohol_problems_fullreport_2006_alcohol2.pdf (A very useful résumé of basic techniques used in alcohol treatment.)

The examiner's mark sheet

Domain/ percentage of marks	Essential points to pass	Extra marks/comments ✓ (make notes here)
1. Rapport and communication 20% of marks	Introduces self appropriately	
	Uses clear communication	
	Able to build rapport with patient	
	Able to elicit alcohol history in a non-judgemental manner	
2. History taking 20% of marks	Elicits information regarding alcohol intake	
	Gathers information about changes to lifestyle	
	Demonstrates knowledge of International Classification of Diseases (ICD)/Diagnostic and Statistical Manual of mental disorders (DSM) criteria for alcohol dependence	

⬆ 3. Overall
assessment

20% of marks

Elicits information on comorbid
psychiatric symptoms

Elicits any risk-taking behaviours –
driving, risk to self or others

Assesses level of insight into alcohol
consumption-related problems

4. Giving feedback

20% of marks

Provides information to patient in a
sensitive manner

Uses Socratic questioning to make
patient reflect upon alcohol use

5. Providing
information on
management

20% of marks

Discusses immediate management in
hospital and longer-term options of
treatment

Alleviates patient's anxiety and provides
reassurance

Demonstrates knowledge of strategies
for reducing alcohol consumption and
harm minimisation

% SCORE _____

___ **OVERALL IMPRESSION**

5   (CIRCLE ONE)

Good Pass

Pass

Borderline

Fail

Clear Fail

NOTES/Areas to improve

STATION 5: ALCOHOL DEPENDENCE – MANAGEMENT

INSTRUCTION TO CANDIDATE

A 45-year-old engineer has come to see you as he was found drunk on duty
and his employer wants feedback on this individual. You have obtained the
history, which reveals that he has been drinking over a bottle of spirits every
day for the last year, has been drinking during his lunch break for 6 months
and more recently started drinking in the mornings. He experiences withdrawal
symptoms if he does not drink, craves alcohol and has gradually increased his
alcohol consumption in the last 1–2 years. He blames difficult work conditions
and his relationship with his partner for his drinking. His employer has warned
him that unless he stops drinking, he will be dismissed from his job. He wants
to stop drinking and wants to know his treatment options. He does not have
obvious mental health or physical health problems.

**Discuss the treatment of alcohol dependence and any other issues raised by
the patient.**

ACTOR (ROLE-PLAYER) INSTRUCTIONS

You are aware of your heavy drinking behaviour, but you blame this on work-related stress. You are ambivalent about what your options are, but you are worried that you may lose the job if you do not stop drinking. You must ask questions as to how you can remain abstinent from alcohol and what to do if you relapse. You are also worried that if your employer knows you are seeing a doctor, this may adversely affect your chances of promotion in the future.

SUGGESTED APPROACH

Setting the scene

Introduce yourself and say, 'I am glad that you have come to see me today about your drinking and that you want to address it. I think we should discuss the options for treatment. How does this sound?'

Completing the tasks

Enquire about the aims and goals of treatment (i.e. abstinence or reduced and controlled drinking). Discuss the treatment options, including medical and psycho-social interventions, both in the short term and long term (bio-psycho-social approach). 'I wonder what prompted you to seek help for your alcohol-related problems. Are you thinking of reducing the amount of alcohol consumed or stopping completely? What do you think you will gain from this?'

Short term

Explain the rationale and principles of medically assisted withdrawal from alcohol (detoxification programme): 'We can offer a medication regime that will help you during the time when you are trying to stop drinking; let me explain this to you.'

- Management of withdrawal symptoms, most commonly with benzodiazepines (BZDs): Chlordiazepoxide is the most widely used medication; the dose can vary considerably depending on the severity of dependence, physical health, etc. The usual starting dose is 20–40 mg four times a day (QDS) and is tapered down and stopped over 7–10 days. 'Front-loading' and symptom-triggered therapy are alternatives, but are not commonly used. The aim is to minimise the discomfort of withdrawal symptoms and prevent serious complications such as withdrawal seizures and/or delirium tremens. Lorazepam or oxazepam are used in those with hepatic failure. Chlormethiazole and carbamazepine are other options, but are not commonly used in the United Kingdom.
- Vitamin supplements: 'Alcohol can affect the vitamin levels in your body and, over a period of time, causes damage to nerves. We will offer you some important vitamin preparations to protect your nervous system.' This approach consists mainly of thiamine and other vitamin B preparations, often by a parenteral route. Pabrinex, a preparation with thiamine, riboflavin, pyridoxin, ascorbic acid and nicotinamide, is administered by intramuscular route for 3–5 days; an intravenous preparation can be used in suspected cases of Wernicke's encephalopathy (WE). Vitamin supplements are administered in order to replenish the body's stores and to prevent WE and Korsakoff syndrome.
- Management of comorbid medical and psychiatric conditions.
- Psychological support prior to and during the detox.
- Setting: 'Planned treatment always works better. We can discuss where you would like to be treated, either in hospital or in your own home.' A community setting is for those with less severe dependence, no significant physical or psychiatric comorbidities and good social support; an in-patient setting is recommended for complex patients or those who failed community detox.

Long term

'We should aim to maintain abstinence; in order to achieve this, psycho-social interventions, including relapse prevention, motivational enhancement and cognitive behavioural therapy in individual or group setting, are the mainstays of treatment.'

'Pharmacological treatments can supplement psycho-social interventions and these may include drugs such as acamprosate, naltrexone and disulfiram. They act as deterrents when one tends to consume alcohol. Self-help organisations such as Alcoholics Anonymous can benefit you. If necessary, we offer advice on suitable accommodation, debt counselling, employment, etc. We will also consider family work, which is often necessary to rehabilitate and integrate the individual with the family and society.'

C: You seem to have been dependent on alcohol for about a year, but you do not have any physical or mental health problems and have a supportive family, so I think you can receive detoxification at home. I will explain and provide some leaflets about the treatment process. Detox is only a small part in giving up alcohol; it will be important for you to look into the reasons for your drinking and how to avoid drinking again, and this can be achieved through psychological help.

C: What we have discussed is confidential; your employer may ask us for a report or an opinion about your suitability to return to work, and we can only provide information to your employer with your consent. If you were to object to information being shared with your employer, we will not do so; however, that may adversely affect your employment.

Problem solving

As with other substances of addiction, relapse rates for alcohol dependence are high. Many individuals are able to achieve abstinence only after several treatment episodes. Consider residential rehabilitation for those who find it difficult to stop drinking. Consider harm minimisation strategies, such as reduced drinking, improved nutrition, vitamin supplements and social support, for those who do not want to stop drinking.

(Although management of delirium tremens or Wernicke's encephalopathy might be an unlikely CASC scenario, it would still be advisable to familiarise yourself with these topics.)

FURTHER READING

Lingford-Hughes, A.R., Welch. S. & Nutt, D.J. (2004) Evidence-based guidelines for the pharmacological management of substance misuse, addiction and comorbidity: Recommendations from the British Association for Psychopharmacology. *Journal of Psychopharmacology, 18*(3), 293–335.

Scottish Intercollegiate Guideline Network (2003) *The Management of Harmful Drinking and Alcohol Dependence in Primary Care. Clinical Guideline No 74.*

The examiner's mark sheet

Domain/ percentage of marks	Essential points to pass	✓	Extra marks/comments (make notes here)
1. Rapport and communication 20% of marks	Introduces self appropriately		
	Uses clear communication		
	Able to build rapport with patient		
	Able to discuss alcohol consumption in a non-judgemental manner		

2. Detoxification programmes 20% of marks	Explains what detox involves Discusses various settings for detox Explains the role of medications without jargon
3. Psycho-social interventions 20% of marks	Explains role of cognitive behavioural therapy and family therapy Explains social support Explains role of self-help groups
4. Long-term supportive measures 20% of marks	Provides information on long-term medical treatment Discusses long-term goals and motivation for abstinence
5. Confidentiality and reassurance 20% of marks	Alleviates patient's anxiety about confidentiality and information sharing Reassures patient that help is available and provides hope for future

% SCORE _____

___ **OVERALL IMPRESSION**

5 (CIRCLE ONE)

Good Pass

Pass

Borderline

Fail

Clear Fail

NOTES/Areas to improve

STATION 6: BENZODIAZEPINE MISUSE

INSTRUCTION TO CANDIDATE

A 35-year-old woman suffering from panic attacks and agoraphobia for several years has been referred by her GP for advice regarding her prescription of diazepam and temazepam. You are meeting her in the out-patient clinic.

Elicit a history regarding the usage of benzodiazepines. Please discuss with her the management of benzodiazepine use.

Do not take a psychiatric history.

ACTOR (ROLE-PLAYER) INSTRUCTIONS

You are meeting the doctor as suggested by your GP.

You have been using benzodiazepines prescribed by your GP for about a year for panic attacks.

When your panic attacks began you were also drinking more than usual to calm your nerves down.

You have read in the papers that these can be harmful but you cannot imagine life without the medications.

Recently you have been buying extra tablets via Internet as you are using more than prescribed.

You would like to hear more form the doctor as to how to reduce this excessive consumption of benzodiazepines.

SUGGESTED APPROACH

Setting the scene

Introduce yourself and say, 'Your GP has requested we discuss your medication, particularly diazepam and temazepam. Would that be OK? Before I can make any suggestions, I need to ask you about details of your use of these medications, please can you tell me about this.'

Completing the tasks

Enquire about the dose and duration of the BZD use and whether all of the medication is prescribed by the GP or she gets some/all of it from elsewhere. Enquire about the use of other illicit drugs and alcohol (it is particularly important to diagnose alcohol dependence if it is present). You may need to enquire briefly about the anxiety symptoms, whether the BZD use predated the panic attacks and agoraphobia and, if there were any periods in which she was free of the anxiety symptoms, what was the pattern of her BZD use? Similarly, what were the anxiety symptoms during the BZD-free period, if any?

It can often be useful to summarise, particularly towards the end of the station.

C: So you are telling me that you started having panic attacks about 3 years ago and started drinking excessively, and you soon realised the dangers of drinking after you were caught drink driving. About a year ago, your GP prescribed you some diazepam as you found it difficult to go out of the house, but you soon started taking more than what was prescribed, and you sometimes bought diazepam and temazepam from the Internet. In the last few months, you have been taking 30–40 mg of diazepam and 10–20 mg of temazepam per day and you experience panic attacks if you can't take the BZD. What would you like to do about it?

Pt: I don't want to take the diazepam or the temazepam, but I get horrible panic attacks [be sure to check that these are actually panic attacks], I can't go out of the house and I can't sleep without them, I feel so anxious without them, the very thought of not taking them makes me anxious.

C: BZDs are very good at providing short-term relief, but you soon develop tolerance and need more and more of them. Soon, you can end up becoming dependent on them. I understand you experience significant anxiety and panic, but in the long run, BZDs are not the answer to these.

Pt: What do you suggest?

C: The panic attacks and agoraphobia are best managed with another medication which is not addictive and there is good evidence that cognitive behavioural therapy is more effective than medication alone in the long run. A combination of these two is quite effective, and that leaves us with what to do about your BZD prescription.

Pt: How can I stop taking the BZDs?

C: That has to be done in a methodical way: I would suggest that the BZDs are replaced with other preparations that tend to remain in body for lengthy periods of time. This will then be gradually reduced in small increments over a period of weeks or months until you tolerate the smaller doses, eventually discontinuing all BZDs completely.

Outline the principles of medically assisted BZD withdrawal.

- Transfer all BZD and Z drug (non-benzodiazepine hypnotics) prescriptions to a long-acting preparation such as diazepam (refer to the table below for equivalent doses). It is very rarely necessary to prescribe more than 30–40 mg of diazepam as an equivalent, whatever the stated use. This is because the benzodiazepine receptors will be fully occupied at this level of prescribing. Prescribing above this level does not convey any benefits and may substantially increase risk. Additionally, it is not uncommon for patients to grossly exaggerate their use of benzodiazepines in the hope of getting a larger prescription. Prescribing excessive amounts does not alleviate the problem, it merely exacerbates it by providing extra supplies, which may be misused or diverted by selling or giving to others.

Approximate equivalent doses to diazepam 5 mg	
Chlordiazepoxide	15 mg
Lorazepam	0.5 mg
Clonazepam	0.25 mg
Nitrazepam	5 mg
Oxazepam	15 mg
Temazepam	10 mg
Zopiclone	7.5 mg
Zolpidem	10 mg

Note: This table is only a rough guide to equivalences.

- If on large doses of BZD or concomitant use with methadone/alcohol dependence, consider BZD withdrawal in an in-patient setting.
- Taper down the dose of diazepam gradually. An individual approach is needed, as patient sensitiveness can differ; in an out-patient setting, the GP can consider decreasing by 10%–25% per fortnight.
- Be cautious and seek expert advice if there are more complex psychiatric and/or physical comorbidities such as epilepsy.
- Supportive counselling/groups along with treatment of underlying conditions such as panic attacks and agoraphobia as in this patient are required.
- Urine drug screens are needed in order to monitor for misuse of other drugs and to prevent diversion of the prescribed medication; if urine screens test negative for benzodiazepines, the medication is not being taken as prescribed and may be being misused (e.g. being sold/given to others or being consumed in a binge) and prescribing should be stopped.
- A binge pattern of consumption, whereby a large amount of benzodiazepines is taken in one go, is not uncommon. In contrast to regular benzodiazepine consumption on a daily basis, there may not be a positive urine test for benzodiazepines on testing. With the binge pattern of use, physical dependence does not develop and prescribing is not advisable, as this will not alleviate the problem, but merely provide another source of benzodiazepines and exacerbate the problem.

Problem solving

At times, it may be better to prescribe/stabilise some individuals on a small dose of diazepam if they cannot be successfully withdrawn from BZD. The aim here would be to stabilise the individual's life and prevent their dealing in the illicit drug market.

FURTHER READING

Department of Health (England) and the Devolved Administrations (2007). *Drug Misuse and Dependence: UK Guidelines on Clinical Management*. London: Department of Health (England), the Scottish Government, Welsh Assembly Government and Northern Ireland Executive.

Lingford-Hughes, A.R., Welch. S. & Nutt, D.J. (2004) Evidence-based guidelines for the pharmacological management of substance misuse, addiction and comorbidity: Recommendations from the British Association for Psychopharmacology. *Journal of Psychopharmacology, 18*(3), 293–335.

The examiner's mark sheet

Domain/ percentage of marks	Essential points to pass	✓	Extra marks/comments (make notes here)
1. Rapport and communication 20% of marks	Introduces self appropriately		
	Uses clear communication		
	Able to build rapport with anxious patient		
2. History taking 20% of marks	Elicits information regarding anxiety symptoms and panic attacks		
	Elicits history of BZD usage		
	Demonstrates knowledge of criteria for dependence syndrome		
3. Overall assessment 20% of marks	Demonstrates link between anxiety disorder and BZD usage		
	Establishes dependence on BZD		
4. Discussion 20% of marks	Provides information to patient in a sensitive manner		
	Uses Socratic questioning to make patient reflect upon alcohol use		
5. Providing information on management 20% of marks	Discusses short-term and long-term management plan		
	Alleviates patient's anxiety and provides reassurance		
	Demonstrates knowledge of strategies for BZD discontinuation		

% SCORE _____

___ **OVERALL IMPRESSION**

5 (CIRCLE ONE)

Good Pass

Pass

Borderline

Fail

Clear Fail

NOTES/Areas to improve

STATION 7: MOTIVATIONAL INTERVIEWING

INSTRUCTION TO CANDIDATE

A 30-year-old woman was admitted to the acute medical ward following an overdose of prescribed antidepressant medication. At the time of admission, she was under the influence of alcohol, but 12 hours later, she has become sober and has been referred for a psychiatric assessment. You have completed your assessment and found that this patient suffers from depression and has been drinking excessively in order to cope with stress. You have found out that being under the influence of alcohol was an important factor in the overdose.

Using motivational interviewing techniques, try to motivate this patient to abstain from alcohol. You are not required to discuss the management of depression.

ACTOR (ROLE-PLAYER) INSTRUCTIONS

You are seeing the psychiatric doctor after you have taken an overdose whilst under the influence of alcohol. You have been depressed lately due to relationship difficulties and have been drinking excessively to cope. You did not plan to take the overdose, but feel that, after drinking alcohol, you lost control. You realise that your drinking is causing problems to your health and work life, but you are not sure if you want to stop drinking, as this is the only coping mechanism for you at present.

SUGGESTED APPROACH

Setting the scene

Introduce yourself and say, 'We have talked about what happened and how you got to be here, and part of that seems to be due to alcohol. I guess what I'd like to know is, what are the things you like about alcohol? What's really good about drinking for you?'

Completing the tasks

After setting the scene, you might try to assess the patient's views on excessive alcohol consumption, whether she recognises it to be a problem and, if so, whether she wants to address it. 'What do you think about your drinking pattern? Have you ever considered that it is in excess?' If she wants to address her drinking, what does she want to do? The discussion would depend upon her current stage of motivation. Described below are the stages of motivation for change and the suggested tasks relevant to the stage.

Stage of motivation for change	Suggested task
1. Pre-contemplation: does not consider the possibility for change	Raise doubt. 'Do you think you may be drinking in excess? Has it occurred to you that your alcohol consumption may be related to some of your problems?' Increase patient's perception of risks and problems with current behaviour. (Excessive alcohol consumption worsening the depression.)

2. Contemplation: ambivalence, patient considers change and rejects it	Tip the balance, evoke reasons to change, present risks of not changing and strengthen self-efficacy. 'Have you ever considered cutting down on alcohol, say if that means it could be advantageous to you? What do you think the benefits are if you decide to cut down alcohol consumption?' (Increased risk of self-harm while intoxicated.)
3. Preparation: determination, considers various strategies for change	Help patient determine best course of action. 'How do you see yourself going about reducing alcohol consumption? Have you thought what difficulties you may encounter? If so, how will you manage them?' (Discuss options of reduced drinking versus abstinence.)
4. Action: engages in particular actions designed to bring about change	Help patient to take steps toward change. 'I am pleased to see you taking such steps already towards your goal. Let us talk about how you can engage with services further to achieve your goals.' (Engage with treating team for depression and alcohol consumption.)
5. Maintenance: strives to sustain changes made in action phase	Help patient identify and use strategies to prevent relapse. 'Let us discuss what might hinder your sustained abstinence from alcohol. We can then come up with some solutions and ways of coping.' (Effective treatment of depression and coping with stress.)
6. Relapse: may have minor slips or major relapses.	Help patient renew process of contemplation, determination and action without becoming stuck or demoralised due to relapse. 'I can see you have tried hard to remain abstinent from alcohol, but for one reason or another, you have started drinking again. This happens to many people and there is no reason to despair. With the right help and motivation, you can soon be on the road to recovery.' (Re-engagement with treatment.)

In the current scenario, the patient is likely to be in one of the first three stages.

C: Do you think the overdose might have happened even if you hadn't been drinking, or do you think that it really had to do with the alcohol?

Pt: I think I just lost control for a minute, I wouldn't have lost that control if I was sober.

The principles of motivational interviewing are outlined below.

Express empathy
Expression of empathy is critical to the MI approach. When patients feel that they are understood, they are more able to open up to their own experiences and share those experiences with others. Importantly, when patients perceive empathy, they become more open to gentle challenges by the interviewer about lifestyle issues and beliefs regarding substance use.

Support self-efficacy
A patient's belief that change is possible is an important motivator to succeeding in making a change. Patients are responsible for choosing and carrying out actions for change in the MI approach, and the interviewer focusses his/her efforts on helping the patient stay motivated; supporting their sense of self-efficacy is a great way to do that.

Roll with resistance
In MI, the interviewer does not fight a client's resistance, but 'rolls with it'. Statements demonstrating resistance are not challenged. Instead, the interviewer uses the patient's resistance to further explore their views. MI encourages individuals to develop their own

solutions to the problems that they themselves have defined; the interviewer should not impose his/her ideas.

Develop discrepancy

Motivation for change occurs when people perceive a discrepancy between where they are and where they want to be. When individuals perceive that their current behaviours are not leading toward some important future goal, they become more motivated to make important life changes.

C: We have talked about your alcohol consumption and how it adversely affects your mood and makes you impulsive, but you feel it helps you cope with stress.

Pt: I know I shouldn't be drinking, especially when I am on an antidepressant. My key worker and my family have been telling me not to drink, but I was ignoring them. I guess this overdose changes that. I will have to stop drinking and look for other ways of handling the stress in my life.

C: What do you think you can do?

Pt: I will discuss with my key worker about a group programme she was talking about. She was telling me that it helps people stop drinking, I think I will attend that group, I will also attend the sessions about handling stress so that I am less likely to drink.

C: These seem to be good ideas. You have been managing your home, looking after kids and supporting your mother. You have been under a lot of stress and turned to drink. I think you are a capable person and you will be able to stop drinking, which might help improve your depression.

A useful concept is the 'cycle of change', first described by Prochaska and DiClemente (1992). Motivational interviewing is applicable when a patient is in the contemplative stage. When a patient is in the pre-contemplation stage, then it is not useful.

Problem solving

If the patient was to deny problems and did not wish to change anything, do not become despondent; try to provide information and educate them about the link between worsening depression and alcohol consumption. Use open-ended questions and MI principles.

FURTHER READING

Miller, R.W. & Rollnick, S. (2012) *Motivational Interviewing: Helping People Change (Applications of Motivational Interviewing)*. New York, NY: Guildford Press.

Sciacca, K. (1997) Removing barriers: Dual diagnosis and motivational interviewing. *Professional Counselor, 12*(1), 41–6.

http://stepupprogram.org/docs/handouts/STEPUP_Stages_of_Change.pdf

The examiner's mark sheet

Domain/ percentage of marks	Essential points to pass	✓	Extra marks/comments (make notes here)
1. Rapport and communication 20% of marks	Introduces self appropriately Uses clear communication Able to build rapport with patient		

2. History taking 20% of marks	Elicits information regarding patient's thoughts and views on their own alcohol consumption	
	Able to ascertain the patient's goals and what they would like to achieve	
3. Overall assessment 20% of marks	Able to ascertain what stage of motivation the patient is in	
	Demonstrates knowledge of the stages on motivation	
4. Discussion 20% of marks	Provides information to patient in a sensitive manner	
	Demonstrates knowledge of and conducts motivational interviewing	
5. Education on strategies to manage alcohol dependence 20% of marks	Discusses short-term and long-term management plan	
	Discusses various psycho-social treatment plans and treatment for depression with a view to reducing or abstaining from alcohol	

% SCORE _____

_____

5

OVERALL IMPRESSION

(CIRCLE ONE)

Good Pass

Pass

Borderline

Fail

Clear Fail

NOTES/Areas to improve

STATION 8: SUBSTANCE MISUSE – MANAGEMENT IN PREGNANCY

INSTRUCTION TO CANDIDATE

A 25-year-old woman with a 10-week pregnancy has been referred by the antenatal services for assessment and management of her substance misuse.

Assess her substance misuse history.

Give her advice about substance use in pregnancy.

Discuss relevant treatment options with her.

ACTOR (ROLE-PLAYER) INSTRUCTIONS

You have come to see the psychiatrist as advised by your midwife. You consume alcohol and heroin regularly, often bought from the streets. You are quite anxious as to what this is about and are worried as to whether your baby may be taken away by the social services (if the doctor mentions social services, appear shocked). You also are worried about the effects that the drugs may have on the unborn baby.

SUGGESTED APPROACH

Setting the scene

Introduce yourself and thank the patient for coming to see you. Enquire about her understanding of the referral. 'Hello, Ms_____, I am Dr_____, a psychiatrist. I gather you are expecting a baby. The antenatal clinic has advised a psychiatric review. I gather from their referral that you are using drugs, and I wonder if we can discuss this further.' If the patient looks uncomfortable or reluctant, you may add, 'I understand this is a sensitive topic to talk about, but this will be a confidential consultation. It is important because we want the best outcome for you and your baby.'

Completing the tasks

Obtain the history as outlined in the Alcohol History and Opioid Dependence stations. Specifically ask about the quantity and duration of substances she has been using during the pregnancy. Tactfully ask whether it was a planned pregnancy and who the father is. A difficult issue is asking about a history of prostitution, and this would best be done by normalising; for example, 'Sometimes I see people who have had to fund their habit by sleeping with men for money. Has anything like this happened to you?' Do not spend too much time on the history, as the scenario has other tasks as well.

An example scenario might be as follows:

C: You have been telling me that you have used heroin and alcohol daily in the last 6 months and at times taken diazepam as well, what do you want to do about it?

Pt: I am not sure, the pregnancy was unexpected, and I am not sure whether the baby is affected. What might have been the effects on the baby?

Briefly explain the effects of the substances on the foetus; the higher the doses and durations of substance intake, the greater is the risk to the foetus.

Substance	Main effects on unborn baby
Smoking (tobacco)	Miscarriage, low birth weight, sudden infant death syndrome (SIDS) and congenital defects
Alcohol	Miscarriage, foetal alcohol syndrome – low birth weight, cognitive deficits, facial abnormalities and failure to thrive
Opioids	Low birth weight, pre-term delivery and SIDS
Benzodiazepines	Cleft palate and reduced growth and brain development
Cocaine	Miscarriage, placental abruption, stillbirth, neonatal death and SIDS

C: Alcohol and drugs can affect the baby throughout the pregnancy; the sooner you stop, the less will be the effect on the baby. Continuing use of alcohol or drugs increases the risks of complications to you as well.

Treatment principles

These are broadly similar to non-pregnant drug users. Some of the additional and specific requirements are:

• Substance misuse treatment is to be fast tracked.
• Close coordination of treatment between various agencies including antenatal, substance misuse, paediatric, social services and the family.

- Support to stop smoking (tobacco), alcohol and all illicit drugs.
- Psycho-social interventions (PSIs) for tobacco smoking cessation and nicotine replacement therapy in those who do not succeed with PSIs.
- There is no safe limit for alcohol consumption in pregnancy. If detoxification is required, an in-patient setting is preferred with the least effective doses of BZD. The benefits of detoxification with BZD outweigh the risk of continued alcohol use.
- Stabilise opioid users on methadone; dose may need to be increased in third trimester due to increased metabolism. The risks to the mother and the unborn baby are least on methadone. If detoxification is planned, carry out the same with caution in the second trimester, usually 2–3 mg every 3–5 days.
- If BZD dependent, prescribe least effective dose of diazepam.
- Illicit drugs such as cocaine, amphetamines and cannabis can be safely stopped; no pharmacological intervention needed. Monitor drug use through regular screening.
- Immunise against hepatitis B and counsel about risk of blood-borne viral infections to the baby during pregnancy, childbirth and breast feeding.
- Effective pain relief during childbirth and management of neonatal withdrawal symptoms if any.
- Psycho-social interventions are of paramount importance. Often, pregnant users have substance-misusing partners, so consider family/couples therapy.

Pt: What about the effect of methadone on the baby, will it be affected?

C: Methadone treatment is safer than heroin use; compared to heroin, it seems to provide more positive outcomes for the baby's growth and reduces the risk of premature birth. We need to work closely with the obstetric team during childbirth and manage any issues then if the baby shows any signs of withdrawal from methadone after birth. There are no long-term consequences to the baby due to opiate withdrawal.

Problem solving

Some women worry that their baby may be 'taken into care' because they use drugs. Substance misuse in itself is not a reason to involve the Social Services or to assume that these individuals cannot care for their baby. However, if there is concern about the safety or welfare of the child, their involvement will be necessary. This is true for everyone, whether they use substances or not.

Many women are very ashamed of their substance misuse. It is important to convey an empathic and non-judgemental approach or you may well find the patient difficult to engage.

FURTHER READING

Department of Health (England) and the Devolved Administrations (2007). *Drug Misuse and Dependence: UK Guidelines on Clinical Management*. London: Department of Health (England), the Scottish Government, Welsh Assembly Government and Northern Ireland Executive.

http://www.rcgp.org.uk/learning/~/media/Files/SMAH/RCGP-Guidance-for-the-use-of substitute-prescribing-in-the-treatment-of-opioid-dependence-in-primary-care-2011.ashx

Lingford-Hughes, A.R., Welch. S. & Nutt, D.J. (2004) Evidence-based guidelines for the pharmacological management of substance misuse, addiction and comorbidity: Recommendations from the British Association for Psychopharmacology. *Journal of Psychopharmacology, 18*(3), 293–335.

The examiner's mark sheet

Domain/ percentage of marks	Essential points to pass	✓	Extra marks/comments (make notes here)
1. Rapport and communication 20% of marks	Introduces self appropriately		
	Uses clear communication and alleviates anxiety		
	Able to build rapport with patient and discuss sensitive topics		
2. History taking 20% of marks	Elicits information regarding patient's heroin and alcohol use		
	Able to ascertain any withdrawal symptoms and risk-taking behaviours		
3. Effect of drugs in pregnancy 20% of marks	Able to educate patient about the effects of illicit substances on pregnancy and unborn baby		
	Demonstrates empathy and gives information in a sensitive manner without alarming the patient		
4. Treatment of drug abuse in pregnancy 20% of marks	Provides information to patient about various pharmacological and psycho-social treatment options		
	Demonstrates knowledge of methadone replacement therapy		
5. Addressing concerns 20% of marks	Able to reassure the mother about the wellbeing of the baby		
	Able to address her concerns and alleviate her anxieties		

% SCORE _____

___ **OVERALL IMPRESSION**

5 (CIRCLE ONE)

Good Pass

Pass

Borderline

Fail

Clear Fail

NOTES/Areas to improve

STATION 9: SUBSTANCE MISUSE HISTORY AND MANAGING WITHDRAWAL

INSTRUCTION TO CANDIDATE

A 20-year-old man is admitted to hospital at 10 p.m. on Saturday evening. He states he is depressed and suicidal. He also says he is prescribed 50 mL of methadone as a maintenance dose daily and is experiencing opioid withdrawal symptoms. He asks that his methadone be prescribed.

> **Take a history of illicit drug use from the patient and details of the treatment he is receiving. Explain to him your plan of management. You need not discuss the symptoms of depression or suicidality.**

ACTOR (ROLE-PLAYER) INSTRUCTIONS

You are on a methadone detoxification programme, but you have also been using some heroin in addition. You do not wish to disclose this information to the doctor. You have run out of money to get more drugs and have used all of your week's supply of methadone. You have been experiencing withdrawal symptoms such as yawning, body pain, tiredness and feel anxious and low in mood. You are demanding that you ought to be prescribed more methadone or else you are going to end your life. You want to know what is going to happen next.

SUGGESTED APPROACH

Setting the scene

Introduce yourself and thank the patient for coming to see you. Enquire about his current difficulties. 'Hello, Mr_____, I am Dr_____, a psychiatrist. I gather you are not feeling very well. Can you tell me what is going on?' The patient may immediately start talking about having methadone prescribed; listen to his concerns and probe more into the drug-seeking behaviour.

Completing the tasks

You will need to take a drug misuse history, enquiring about the types of drugs used and their routes of administration, including alcohol. You will be most interested in the history covering the last 6–8 weeks. You will need to find out who from and where (Substance Misuse Service or GP) the patient is receiving methadone prescriptions. Does the patient need to visit the pharmacy to pick up their prescription and consume it under supervision? It is not uncommon for patients to continue to use illicit drugs even though they are on a prescription.

The patient may be reluctant to divulge information about their drug-seeking behaviour. In such situations, generalisation may make them feel less stigmatised. 'I understand you have been on a methadone programme; often, I come across people using other substances along with methadone. Has that happened to you?'

Enquire about the symptoms of opioid withdrawal. Begin with open-ended questions such as, 'What happened when you go without these drugs for a period of time? Do you experience anything different when there is a delay in taking drugs? What do you do then?'

You may expect to find some objective signs of opioid withdrawal (sweating, nausea, anxiety, agitation, runny nose, tremor, yawning and gooseflesh).

Other opioid withdrawal symptoms:

- Abdominal cramps
- Anxiety, irritability and dysphoria
- Back aches
- Cramps
- Diarrhoea
- Disturbed sleep
- Elevated blood pressure

- Increased sweating
- Joint pain
- Lacrimation
- Muscle spasm leading to headaches
- Nausea and vomiting
- Rhinorrhoea
- Twitching
- Urinary frequency

You will have to attempt to do a brief physical examination in order to check for tremors, pulse rate and blood pressure (if equipment is available). You may want to demonstrate to the examiner that you are observing such symptoms, 'You seem very shaky today. I can see you are sweating a lot; this sometimes happens when someone experiences withdrawal effects. Is it possible you are going through that?'

It is very important to tell the patient about drug testing of either urine or saliva. You would expect to find a positive test for methadone. If the test is negative for methadone, then this is incompatible with a history of being on methadone; this is an important point, as it would be dangerous to prescribe methadone in these circumstances as overdose and death could ensue.

If the test is positive for methadone, it does not confirm either that the patient is being prescribed methadone or that they are receiving the dose they say they are. During normal working hours, it is possible to confirm a prescription with the prescribing service or pharmacy; you may say to the patient, 'I would like to get in touch with your GP/methadone clinic to check the right amount of prescription for you.'

The safest management plan in this circumstance is to use when necessary (PRN) dihydrocodeine in order to relieve symptoms of opioid withdrawal: 30–60 mg every 6 hours PRN will help relieve symptoms of withdrawal without running the risk of causing opioid overdose. Stress to the patient that this is not a life-threatening situation, but can be uncomfortable. Explain that you will be looking at supportive measures to alleviate his discomfort. Nursing staff should observe for objective symptoms of opioid withdrawal using a chart such as the Clinical Opiate Withdrawal Scale (COWS). When possible, contact the service that the patient attends in order to confirm the information the patient has given.

Problem solving

This station may test the candidate's ability to elicit a drug history from a reluctant historian. The patient may be insisting upon getting more methadone, and the candidate has to make sure that the patient is reassured that the uncomfortable symptoms of the opioids will be addressed. It is important to demonstrate to the examiner that withdrawal symptoms of opioid are considered and adequate checks such as urine/saliva drug screening and communication with GP/pharmacy about the accuracy of prescriptions will be done as part of the management.

FURTHER READING

American Psychiatric Association (2006) *Practice Guideline for the Treatment of Patients with Substance Use Disorders*, 2nd edn. http://www.psychiatryonline.org

Drug Misuse in Over 16s: Opioid Detoxification. *NICE Guidelines [CG52]*. (2007).

The examiner's mark sheet

Domain/ percentage of marks	Essential points to pass	✓	Extra marks/comments (make notes here)
1. Rapport and communication 20% of marks	Introduces self appropriately Uses clear communication to engage with reluctant patient Able to build rapport with patient and discuss sensitive topics around drugs		
2. History taking 20% of marks	Elicits information regarding patient's drug use		
3. Withdrawal symptoms 20% of marks	Able to ascertain any withdrawal symptoms from history and physical observations		
4. Management plan 20% of marks	Able to explain to patient about the effects of withdrawal from opioids and supportive measures Demonstrates judgement and caution in prescribing further methadone		
5. Addressing concerns 20% of marks	Provides information to the patient about pharmacological measures of symptom control Demonstrates knowledge of opioid withdrawal management		

% SCORE _____

___ **OVERALL IMPRESSION**

5 (CIRCLE ONE)

Good Pass

Pass

Borderline

Fail

Clear Fail

NOTES/Areas to improve

Chapter 6

Forensic psychiatry
Marc Lyall

O LINKED STATIONS

STATION 1(a): SELF-HARM IN CUSTODY

INSTRUCTION TO CANDIDATE

As a psychiatry trainee, you have been called to assess a young woman who is in police custody charged with shoplifting. She has a history of deliberate self-harm. While in the police station, she has made superficial cuts to her forearm with a disposable razor that she had hidden.

Take a history of her self-harming behaviour and assess the risk of suicide and of further self-harm in the short term.

ACTOR (ROLE-PLAYER) INSTRUCTIONS

You are agitated and upset.

Initially, you distrust the doctor, believing that what you say will be reported to the police, but are reassured if the candidate is professional in their manner.

You have cut yourself countless times over many years, acting impulsively, often when drunk.

Today, you became despondent when arrested and cut yourself, which made you feel better.

You have a partner who is supportive.

You do not wish to kill yourself and never have.

SUGGESTED APPROACH

Display appropriate empathy

Set the scene – start with general open questions, perhaps about the patient's experience in police custody. The woman is likely to be angry, anxious and distressed – establishing trust and empathy will be necessary before an accurate assessment can be undertaken.

Explain professional role and the boundaries of confidentiality

Introduce yourself: 'Hello. I'm Dr_____, I work at the hospital as a doctor. I'm not a police officer. I've been asked to see you today because of worries that you've hurt yourself.'

Explain that the consultation between you is confidential unless something is said that you believe suggests a significant risk to someone else or the woman herself. Reassure the woman that you will not divulge what is said to the police unless you have her agreement, although there might well be pressure from the police to report what the woman said.

Explore past episodes of self-harm

Past episodes of self-harming should be explored: what were the circumstances, what was the method of self-harm (lacerating self, burning or 'head banging'), what was the intent of the self-harm, was there any planning, what was the patient's attitude afterwards?

Explore this episode of self-harm: precipitants, method of self-harm, desired outcome of self-harm and assess current ideas and intent of suicide and self-harm

A history should be taken of the current episode; in particular, what was the aim and how does the woman feel now?

The woman's access to the means to self-harm while in custody should be explored, bearing in mind that she will have been searched on reception into the custody suite, but nonetheless has managed to secrete a razor blade.

Discuss future risk of self-harm, including factors that would increase and decrease this risk

Factors affecting the future risk of self-harm should be elicited.

Predictors of repetition of self-harm include: number of previous episodes; features of personality disorder; a history of violence; alcoholism; unmarried; and being of lowest social class.

Predictors of suicide after deliberate self-harm include: evidence of serious intent; continuing wish to die; previous acts of self-harm; depressive disorder; substance misuse; dissocial personality disorder; social isolation; unemployment; older age group; and male sex.

Detailed psychiatric or substance misuse histories are not required, but these areas should be concisely explored, and some attempt should be made to assess her current level of substance misuse.

A detailed forensic history or an account of the current criminal allegation is not needed.

ADDITIONAL POINTS

Good candidates might suggest to the woman that they will gather background information from her GP and any mental health professionals who have been involved in her care to date.

Approximately a third of deaths in police custody are due to self-harm or suicide. The most common form of self-harm/suicide in custody is through the tying of ligatures.

FURTHER READING

Bouch, J. & Marshall, J.J. (2005) Suicide risk: Structured professional judgement. *Advances in Psychiatric Treatment*, 11(2), 84–91.

The examiner's mark sheet

Domain/percentage of marks	Essential points to pass	✓	Extra marks/Comments (make notes here)
1. Rapport and communication 15% of marks	Clear communication Open and closed questions Empathy Acknowledges woman's distress		
2. Explains professional role and the boundaries of confidentiality 10% of marks	Explains that you are a doctor Explains limits to 'duty of confidentiality'		
3. Explores past episodes of self-harm 25% of marks	Explores number of episodes Elicits methods used Discusses lethality of methods Explores planning Explores mental state at time of episodes		
4. Explores this episode of self-harm 25% of marks	Elicits precipitants Describes method of self-harm Explores desired outcome of self-harm Assesses current ideas and intent of suicide and self-harm		
5. Discusses future risk of self-harm, including factors that would increase and decrease this risk 25% of marks	Explores history of violence Discusses substance use-historical and current Elicits sources of support Explores symptoms of depression Assess impulsivity Describes protective factors		

% SCORE _____

___ **OVERALL IMPRESSION**

5 (CIRCLE ONE)

Good Pass

Pass

Borderline

Fail

Clear Fail

NOTES/Areas to improve

STATION 1(b): DISCUSSION WITH POLICE OFFICER

INSTRUCTION TO CANDIDATE

The woman has given her consent for you to explain her situation to the custody sergeant. Explain to the police officer your risk assessment and advise him on how to manage the situation.

ACTOR (ROLE-PLAYER) INSTRUCTIONS

You are anxious about the woman prisoner.

You want to know from the doctor if she is mentally ill.

Your main worry is that the woman might commit suicide – ask the doctor about this.

Ask the doctor what you practically can do to help.

If the doctor is not being helpful, become demanding and raise your voice.

SUGGESTED APPROACH

Communicate with a non-medically trained professional appropriately

The difficulty in this station is to communicate the woman's future risk of self-harm and suicide in a way that is understandable to the police officer and avoids discussing unnecessary details of the woman's history. The police officer's understanding of mental health issues is likely to be limited. However, they will be concerned with avoiding the woman self-harming again or attempting suicide.

Introduce yourself: 'Hello. I'm Dr_____, I'm the on-call psychiatrist and I've just been to see Ms_____. Can I speak to you somewhere privately where we won't be disturbed? Is this a good place?'

Do not use medical jargon and check the understanding of the police officer.

Explain professional role and issues around confidentiality

Giving the right amount of information, neither too little (so that the risk of self-harm/suicide cannot be managed), nor too much (so that the woman's confidentiality is unnecessarily breached), can be made easier if the rules by which the candidate is working are discussed explicitly with the police officer at the start of the discussion. The candidate might want to make clear that they can only disclose information for managing the risk that the woman poses to herself. If they are asked to comment on issues not relating to this, their response needs to be clear but polite.

Explain that the purpose of your assessment was to assess the woman's risk of suicide and self-harm in order to ensure that she receives proper medical care and explain doctor–patient confidentiality.

Ask if the patient's injuries have been assessed by the police doctor (Forensic Medical Examiner [FME]). If not, you should request that this happens.

Taking a brief account of the events surrounding her arrest and self-harm from the police officer would be useful, not least to see if this concurs with the patient's description.

Explain findings in relation to the future risk of self-harm

A formulation of risk will form the basis of your discussion with the police officer. It will be based on the history and mental state, but also factors that are likely to increase the risk of self-harm or dangerous behaviour. The following questions will need to have been considered:

- How serious is the risk?
- Is the risk specific or general?
- How immediate is the risk?
- How volatile is the risk?
- What specific treatment and which management plan can best reduce the risk?

Offer practical suggestions to manage the risk of self-harm

Giving practical advice, such as organising a search of the woman's cell, ensuring an adequate level of observation and providing advice on what factors might increase the risk of self-harm in the short term are important.

Suggest avenues through which the police officer can access further help

The police are likely to want to know whether the woman has a mental illness. If in your opinion she does, detention under mental health legislation will need to be considered.

FURTHER READING

Kent, J. & Gunasekaran, S. (2010) Mental disordered detainees in the police station: The role of the psychiatrist. *Advances in Psychiatric Treatment*, 16(2), 115–23.

The examiner's mark sheet

Domain/ percentage of marks	Essential points to pass	✓	Extra marks/Comments (make notes here)
1. Communicates with a non-medically trained professional appropriately 20% of marks	Communicates the woman's future risk of self-harm and suicide in a way that is understandable to the police officer Uses non-technical language Invites police officer to ask questions		
2. Explains professional role and issues around confidentiality 20% of marks	Explains doctor–patient confidentiality Avoids discussing unnecessary details of the woman's history		
3. Explains findings in relation to the future risk of self-harm 20% of marks	Describes risk of self-harm Describes how immediate the risk is		

⇧ 4. Offers practical suggestions to manage the risk of self-harm

20% of marks

Suggests search of the woman's cell

Discusses adequate level of observation

Gives advice on factors that might increase the risk of self-harm in the short term

5. Suggests avenues through which the police officer can access further help

20% of marks

Discusses role of FME

Explains role of local mental health team

Comments on use of mental health legislation

% SCORE _____

___ **OVERALL IMPRESSION**

5 (CIRCLE ONE)

Good Pass

Pass

Borderline

Fail

Clear Fail

NOTES/Areas to improve

STATION 2(a): DUTY TO WARN

INSTRUCTION TO CANDIDATE

This woman became depressed after her husband left her. She was extremely distressed and presented herself to accident and emergency (A&E), where she was seen by the liaison nurse.

She agreed to an informal psychiatric admission to the ward and settled extremely quickly. It was recommended that she start lofepramine (an antidepressant) at night and she has cooperated with this.

She would now like to leave hospital and return home. There are no grounds currently to detain her under the Mental Health Act.

During her admission, she disclosed detailed plans to another patient about how she intends to kill her husband.

She has a history of violence towards her husband.

Take a relevant history and mental state, assessing the risk she poses to her husband.

ACTOR (ROLE-PLAYER) INSTRUCTIONS

You are intensely angry with your husband and want to kill him.

You have detailed plans to do so.

You have thought about killing your husband in the past but have not tried to do this.

You believe that 'God' is controlling your body and commanding you to kill your husband.

You do not want to tell the doctor what your plans are, but if the doctor is tactful and empathetic, you reveal what you are thinking.

SUGGESTED APPROACH

Communicate appropriately, displaying empathy

'Hello, I'm Dr_____, I work here on the ward. I wanted to speak to you about your plans for when you leave hospital.'

The course of the interview will be largely determined by the patient's attitude to being questioned. The discussion could initially be framed as a way of planning the care package for her discharge, before later moving on to the specifics of the risk that she poses to others.

The patient might well be guarded about her plans with regard to her husband. An open and empathetic style of interviewing will be important. If the patient refuses to talk about her threats, she will need to be informed – tactfully and in a way that does not put others at risk – that she has been overheard describing what she might do to her husband. She will need to be challenged directly about these ideas.

Take a detailed account of threats

Will she disclose any plans to harm her husband? If so, what are the details of these plans? Has she considered how to harm him, when to act against him, how to avoid detection and how to defend herself against (presumably) a stronger 'opponent'? Does the patient know where her husband is living? Does she have access to weapons (e.g. guns or knives)? Is there evidence of jealousy (delusional jealousy)? Does she identify any others that could potentially be victims? Is her husband aware of the way she feels or the plans she has?

Always ask about children.

Assess past forensic history

The history needs to focus on factors that are related to the risk that the woman poses to her husband.

Has there been previous violence towards others, including her husband? Is there any forensic history?

Assess substance misuse

What is her use of alcohol and illicit drugs, especially stimulants such as cocaine and amphetamines? Has past intoxication been associated with violence?

Perform a focussed mental state examination

Look for evidence of any threat/control override symptoms: firmly held beliefs of persecution by others (persecutory delusions) or of the mind or body being controlled or interfered with by external forces (delusions of passivity).

Assess the patient for the presence of emotions that are known to be related to violence (e.g. irritability, anger, hostility and suspiciousness).

What is her level of insight? Will she comply with treatment in the community, including with medication?

Assess the risk of violence

Is there evidence of rootlessness or 'social restlessness' (e.g. few relationships or frequent changes of address or employment)? What are the protective factors against violence?

You have a duty to warn the woman's husband. Has the patient got the capacity to consent to you speaking to her husband about risk issues? If yes, would the patient consent to disclosure of the threats that she has made?

FURTHER READING

Adshead, G. (1999) Duties of psychiatrists: Treat the patient or protect the public? *Advances in Psychiatric Treatment*, 5(5), 321–28.

The examiner's mark sheet

Domain/ percentage of marks	Essential points to pass	✓	Extra marks/Comments (make notes here)
1. Communicates appropriately displaying empathy 10% of marks	Accommodates the patient's unwillingness to engage Uses tact Open and empathetic Challenges ideas expressed		
2. Takes a detailed account of threats 30% of marks	Takes a detailed history of wife's plans Considers method of proposed violence Examines degree of planning Elicits access to weapons Asks about children		
3. Assesses past forensic history 15% of marks	Ascertains if previous violence towards others, including her husband Elicits any forensic history		
4. Assesses substance misuse 15% of marks	Assesses use of alcohol and illicit drugs Elicits whether past intoxication been associated with violence		
5. Performs a focussed mental state examination 15% of marks	Examines for threat/control override symptoms Assesses the patient for irritability, anger, hostility and suspiciousness. Examines insight		

6. Assesses the risk of violence

15% of marks

Elicits protective factors against violence

Examines capacity to consent to discuss violent ideas

% SCORE _____

OVERALL IMPRESSION

6 (CIRCLE ONE)

Good Pass

Pass

Borderline

Fail

Clear Fail

NOTES/Areas to improve

STATION 2(b): DISCUSSION WITH RELATIVE

> **INSTRUCTION TO CANDIDATE**
>
> Following your interview in the previous station, you have arranged to meet with her husband, who has been asking to see you.
>
> **Discuss how you intend to manage his wife. He wants to know if he is at risk.**

ACTOR (ROLE-PLAYER) INSTRUCTIONS

You are very worried about your wife.

You have heard her talk of wanting to hurt you, which you cannot understand as you have always had a good relationship.

You understand that she is mentally unwell.

You want the best for your wife but are worried about your own safety.

You seek reassurances from the doctor that support will be available to you.

SUGGESTED APPROACH

Introduce self appropriately and display empathetic style

Introduce yourself: 'Hello, I'm Dr_____. I'm your wife's doctor.'

The man is anxious and will be looking to you for support and assistance. He is likely to be shocked and upset by his wife's threats.

Explain issue of confidentiality

Explaining to the husband the legal limitations on your ability to share information will be helpful. What he is likely to want is practical advice. However, the resources available to mental health services for aiding him are limited, as the focus of care is on his wife. This needs to be explained.

Describe risk to husband

The management of your patient depends on the level of risk, guided by the assessment carried out in the previous station.

If the patient does not want you to share the details of her clinical state with her husband, how much information needs to be shared with the husband in order to manage the risk that is posed? Only the minimum necessary to manage the risk (e.g. the circumstances in which violence is likely and how this risk could be managed) should be disclosed.

Give advice on managing the risk

Explain to her husband that you will try to persuade his wife to remain in hospital, treat any underlying mental illness, arrange temporary accommodation away from him and offer close support and monitoring through the home treatment team. Inform him that there will be ongoing, careful assessment for detention under mental health legislation.

Other options could include advising her husband to seek a non-molestation order, which could be made by a court if it was believed that the husband was at significant risk and the couple have had a child together; otherwise, legal action could be taken under the Protection from Harassment Act.

Answer questions appropriately

If the husband asks for further help, offer out-of-hours 'crisis' numbers for mental health services and advise him to inform the police urgently if he feels under threat.

ADDITIONAL POINTS

If the patient has capacity but refuses to consent to disclosure, the grounds for breaking confidentiality are a matter of judgement and involve weighing the risk of disclosing information against the risk of non-disclosure. If the matter is of overriding public interest (e.g. if there is a risk of violence), then there is a right to disclose (as described in the Royal College of Psychiatrists guidance, *Good Psychiatric Practice: Confidentiality and Information Sharing*); arguably, if the risk is considered significant and is focussed on a particular individual, there is a duty to disclose information which safeguards that individual. In essence, the question is: what would be supported by a Bolam/Bolitho test (i.e. by a reasonable body of medical practitioners based on logical evidence)?

If in doubt, the clinician should discuss with a senior colleague, their medical defence organisation or their Trust's solicitors. Whatever decision is taken will need to be justified in writing in the clinical notes.

FURTHER READING

Royal College of Psychiatrists (2012) *Good Psychiatric Practice: Confidentiality and Information Sharing*. 2nd edn. http://www.rcpsych.ac.uk/usefulresources/publications/collegereports/cr/cr160.aspx

The examiner's mark sheet

Domain/ percentage of marks	Essential points to pass	✓	Extra marks/Comments (make notes here)
1. Introduces self appropriately and displays empathetic style 20% of marks	Acknowledges the man's anxiety Offers appropriate support and assistance Uses non-technical language		
2. Explains issue of confidentiality 20% of marks	Explains legal limitations on your ability to share information		
3. Describes risk 30% of marks	Shares appropriate amount of information Discusses circumstances in which violence is likely Explains link with mental illness		
4. Gives advice on managing the risk 20% of marks	Discusses treatment in hospital and community for wife Discusses use of mental health legislation Explores arranging temporary accommodation for wife		
5. Answers questions appropriately 10% of marks	Offers out of hours 'crisis' numbers for mental health services Gives advice on informing police if husband feels under threat		

% SCORE _____

___ **OVERALL IMPRESSION**

5 (CIRCLE ONE)

Good Pass

Pass

Borderline

Fail

Clear Fail

NOTES/Areas to improve

STATION 3(a): PRISON ASSESSMENT

INSTRUCTION TO CANDIDATE

You have been asked by the prison doctor to assess a 45-year-old man in prison. He is charged with attempted murder. He has assaulted other inmates while in prison. The man has spoken to a number of prison officers about hearing the 'voice of God' commanding him to attack others.

Assess the risk of the man acting violently to others in prison.

ACTOR (ROLE-PLAYER) INSTRUCTIONS

You are annoyed at seeing the doctor and suspicious of his/her intentions.

If the doctor shows empathy, engage with him/her.

You are in prison because you attempted to kill a man you thought was poisoning you.

You have been in prison before for violence, but on each occasion you have been transferred to hospital for psychiatric treatment.

During this period in prison, you have been frightened by the voices that you hear, which make you worried for your own safety.

SUGGESTED APPROACH

Communicate appropriately and with empathy

'Hello. I'm Dr_____. I work at the hospital. I'm not a prison officer. I've been asked to see you today to see how you are. Could you tell me a little bit about what it's been like in prison? I understand that there have been some fights with other inmates – can you tell me about them?'

It is important to be empathetic and non-judgemental.

Explain professional role and boundaries of confidentiality

Confidentiality is an issue in this station. Candidates need to explain their role and be clear about their purpose in carrying out an assessment (i.e. to facilitate appropriate healthcare, not to provide information to the criminal justice system for use in any trial).

The patient is likely to be hostile and suspicious of seeing a doctor. Given his history of violence, the candidate needs to be aware of their own safety.

Explore past episodes of violence

Was the attempted murder the first incident of violence? If not, who were the victims of previous violence, what were the circumstances and what was the man's mental state at the time?

Regarding the alleged attempted murder: who was the victim, what was the man's intention, did he have symptoms of mental illness at the time (e.g. delusional beliefs/command hallucinations concerning the alleged victim), what was the degree of planning and how does he view what happened in hindsight? (Note: the man has not been convicted. He might not wish to discuss the allegation. If he does describe what happened, the candidate should give an assurance that the details of what he describes will be kept in confidence and not relayed to the police or the courts.)

In terms of the prison assaults: who were the victims and what was their link to the prisoner, was a weapon used, what was the man's motivation (e.g. does he want to be transferred to hospital) and how did the assaults end?

Elicit current ideas of violence and intent

Assess ideas, intent and plans to act violently. Look to take a focussed history and conduct a mental state examination targeted towards relevant areas.

Has the man any ideas, intent or plans for future violence? If so, who are the likely victims, when might the assaults take place, are there any protective factors that, if present, might reduce the chances of assault and are there any factors that might trigger an assault?

Perform a focussed mental state examination

A mental state examination should be conducted focussing on his level of irritability, hostility, the presence of delusional beliefs of control and persecution, beliefs about particular individuals, hallucinations (especially command-type auditory hallucinations), level of insight and, in particular, the man's attitude towards anti-psychotic medication.

Several large-scale epidemiological studies (e.g. the MacArthur risk assessment study) have found an increased rate of violence in patients with psychosis. Specific symptoms such as ideas of 'threat and control override' increase the risk of violence, as do the presence of anger and distress associated with delusional beliefs.

FURTHER READING

Buchanan, A. (1999) Risk and dangerousness. *Psychological Medicine*, *29*, 465–73.

Maden, A. (2007) *Treating Violence*. Oxford: Oxford University Press.

Mullen, P. (1997) Assessing the risk of interpersonal violence in the mentally ill. *Advances in Psychiatric Treatment*, *3*, 166–73.

The examiner's mark sheet

Domain/ percentage of marks	Essential points to pass	✓	Extra marks/Comments (make notes here)
1. Communicates appropriately and with empathy 15% of marks	Demonstrates empathy Is non-judgemental Checks patient's understanding of questions		
2. Explains professional role and boundaries of confidentiality 15% of marks	Explains limits to confidentiality Deals appropriately with patient's hostility and suspicion Is mindful of own safety		
3. Explores past episodes of violence 30% of marks	Explores victims of previous violence Elicits circumstances of previous violence Explores alleged attempted murder in details Attempts to describe mental state at the time of the alleged attempted murder Takes a detailed history of assaults in prison		
4. Elicits current ideas of violence and intent 20% of marks	Assesses ideas, intent and plan to act violently Attempts to elicit beliefs about particular individuals		

⇧

	Assesses presence of any protective factors which might reduce the chances of assault
	Attempts to elicit factors that might trigger an assault
5. Performs focussed mental state examination 20% of marks	Assesses level of irritability and hostility
	Examines for the presence of delusional beliefs of control and persecution
	Examines for command type auditory hallucinations

% SCORE _____

_____   **OVERALL IMPRESSION**

5   (CIRCLE ONE)

Good Pass

Pass

Borderline

Fail

Clear Fail

NOTES/Areas to improve

STATION 3(b): DISCUSSION WITH CONSULTANT

> **INSTRUCTION TO CANDIDATE**
>
> You have made your assessment of the man in the previous station.
>
> **Summarise your findings to your supervising consultant and discuss your proposed management plan.**
>
> The examiner in this station will take part in the role-play.

ACTOR (ROLE-PLAYER) INSTRUCTIONS

You are interested to hear about the assessment.

You want to know details of the attempted murder and the man's recent behaviour in prison.

You expect the junior doctor to be clear in their account.

If they do not use appropriate language, this makes you irritable and you become more demanding.

SUGGESTED APPROACH

Communicate appropriately

Use language that is appropriate when discussing with a professional colleague. Avoid jargon. Be precise and accurate. Respond to questions that are asked appropriately and fully.

Explain to the consultant the circumstances of you visiting the prison and that you have assessed the patient only briefly but that you are worried about the risk that he might pose to other inmates.

Accurately summarise the history and mental state examination

The consultant will need to know relevant background information about the prisoner. This will include brief details of the alleged attempted murder and information about the assaults in prison. The man's mental state should be described. Any ideas, intent or plan to be violent again also need to be conveyed.

Offer practical suggestions to manage the risk

Advice on immediate management should include a suggestion that the prisoner be placed on an enhanced observation level and that their access to potential weapons (e.g. razor blades) should be limited. If he has made threats to specific inmates, particular measures to protect them should be discussed.

An assessment of his mental health will inform future medical management. An admission to the prison healthcare wing is likely to be appropriate. He should be reviewed regularly by the prison psychiatric in-reach team. Anti-psychotic medication should be offered, although treatment cannot be enforced.

Describe longer-term risk management plan

Obtaining further history from past medical records is likely to be helpful. His solicitor might be able to provide further details of the current charge. If the man's mental state means that the court case is not going to be able to proceed, then informing his solicitor, with the prisoner's consent, would be useful.

In the longer term, he might need treatment in hospital, especially if he is refusing to accept medication. If this is needed, given the seriousness of the offence and his assaults in prison treatment, management in a secure unit will be necessary.

ADDITIONAL POINTS

The prison environment is an unusual one and, for candidates who have not visited a prison, such an environment might be hard to imagine. However, the basics of risk assessment are transferable to any environment. The management of the risk of violence, whether in prison or in hospital, has common features, notably enhanced observation and limitation of access to weapons and potential victims.

The examiner's mark sheet

Domain/ percentage of marks	Essential points to pass	✓	Extra marks/Comments (make notes here)
1. Communication 25% of marks	Uses appropriate language		
	Avoids jargon		
	Uses language that is precise and accurate		

2. Accurately summarises history and mental state examination

   40% of marks

   - Gives relevant background information including brief details of the alleged attempted murder
   - Describes assaults in prison
   - Describes current mental state

3. Offers practical suggestions to manage the risk

   20% of marks

   - Describes need for enhanced observation level
   - Discusses limiting access to potential weapons
   - Highlights need to possibly protect specific inmates
   - Discusses need for regular psychiatric review
   - Suggests that anti-psychotic medication should be offered

4. Describes longer-term risk management plan

   20% of marks

   - Discusses obtaining further history from medical records and legal papers
   - Discusses possible treatment in hospital
   - Highlights potential need for management in a secure unit

% SCORE _____

___ **OVERALL IMPRESSION**

4 (CIRCLE ONE)

Good Pass

Pass

Borderline

Fail

Clear Fail

NOTES/Areas to improve

STATION 4(a): SCHIZOPHRENIA AND VIOLENCE

INSTRUCTION TO CANDIDATE

Mr Dillon is a 23-year-old man who has recently been admitted to an in-patient psychiatric ward. He has presented with symptoms of psychosis. This morning, without any warning, he approached a nurse on the ward, Mr Griffiths, from behind and punched him repeatedly to the floor.

Assess Mr Dillon and his short-term risk of violence.

ACTOR (ROLE-PLAYER) INSTRUCTIONS

You have just assaulted a nurse on the ward where you are a patient.

You punched the man because of the way he was looking at you. You thought he was sneering and laughing at you. You are not sure why he was doing this.

Before being admitted to hospital yesterday, you were taking cocaine regularly.

You have not previously been violent.

You are puzzled by your own actions, which you regret. You are agitated and worry you will be violent again. You are happy to take medication, but worry that this will cause tiredness and you will be unable to defend yourself.

SUGGESTED APPROACH

Rapport and communication

You need to gain Mr Dillon's confidence, being non-judgemental and calm. Give him the space to talk, but also control the interview so that you can elicit the necessary details of Mr Dillon's history and mental state.

Elicit details of assault

You need to know details of what has happened on the ward. Ask Mr Dillon what happened. What was his intention? Consider how impulsive his actions were. How long has he been thinking of assaulting Mr Griffiths? Why did he act now? What did he want to achieve? What stopped him carrying on with the attack? How does he feel now? Did he want other patients to join in the assault?

Assess history of violence

Has Mr Dillon been violent like this before? If so, what were the circumstances? Who were the victims? How serious were the injuries sustained? Try and build a picture of Mr Dillon's mental state when he carried out these assaults. Was the use of substances important?

Perform a focussed mental state examination

There are many different reasons why people act violently. Some symptoms of psychosis (e.g. delusions of control and of persecution) increase the risk of violence. However, even in violence which seems directly linked to psychotic symptoms, other factors might be important (e.g. 'negative' [rule-breaking] attitudes and impulsivity) – the good candidate will try and elicit these. The clinical items (C-items) of the HCR-20 (Historical, Clinical and Risk Management Scales) are a useful aide-memoire.

As well as psychosis, look for symptoms of withdrawal from illicit drugs, intoxication and other possible physical causes of agitation.

Establish future risk

You need to establish how safe the situation now is. Is Mr Dillon likely to attack Mr Griffiths again, or another member of staff or another patient? Can he guarantee his own safety? If not, what would help him?

FURTHER READING

Baird, J. & Stocks, R. (2013) Risk assessment and management: Forensic methods, human results. *Advances in Psychiatric Treatment*, 19(5), 358–65.

The examiner's mark sheet

Domain/ percentage of marks	Essential points to pass	✓	Extra marks/Comments (make notes here)
1. Rapport and communication 15% of marks	Manages patient's agitation		
	Acts in a non-judgemental and calm manner		
	Controls interview appropriately		
2. Elicits details of assault 25% of marks	Elicits Mr Dillon's intention		
	Assesses how impulsive his actions were		
	Notes triggering factors		
	Elicits factors that stopped the attack carrying on the attack		
3. Assesses history of violence 25% of marks	Establishes past history of violence		
	Notes details of past violence		
	Assesses mental state at the time of past violence		
	Elicits the importance of use of substances		
4. Performs focussed mental state examination 20% of marks	Assesses symptoms of psychosis		
	Elicits delusions of control and of persecution		
	Assesses impulsivity		
	Assesses for symptoms of withdrawal from illicit drugs and intoxication		
5. Establishes future risk 15% of marks	Establishes how safe the situation		
	Assesses how likely another assault is		
	Establishes what factors would help reduce the risk of a further assault		

% SCORE _____

____

5

OVERALL IMPRESSION

(CIRCLE ONE)

Good Pass

Pass

Borderline

Fail

Clear Fail

NOTES/Areas to improve

STATION 4(b): DISCUSSION WITH COLLEAGUE

INSTRUCTION TO CANDIDATE

Having assessed the patient, now speak to the nurse who is coordinating the shift about your short-term management plan and your suggestions for managing the risk in the medium to long term.

ACTOR (ROLE-PLAYER) INSTRUCTION

You are an experienced mental health nurse. Today, you are in charge of the ward where one of your colleagues was assaulted.

Ask the doctor about his proposed management plan.

You are concerned about the safety of the ward, especially the ongoing risk that the patient poses to other staff members and other patients.

You should expect to have an open discussion about the situation.

The doctor should listen and respond appropriately to your concerns.

You believe that extra medication needs to be prescribed.

SUGGESTED APPROACH

Rapport and communication

You are discussing the situation with an experienced colleague. There is a need to use appropriate professional language and to show the ability to listen attentively, take on board the nurse's concerns and negotiate and agree on a management plan.

Use of medication

Your management plan should consider the use of additional medication. You need to be clear why medication is being prescribed; for example, is it for extra sedation? There should be a discussion with the nurse about the type of medication, how long it will be prescribed for and what route it should be administered by. You should consider what approach to take if the patient refuses to take medication. Consider potential side effects and physical health monitoring.

Nursing interventions, including ward placement

There should be a discussion about the level of nursing observations and whether this is the right ward for the patient presently. One possibility is for the patient to be transferred to a psychiatric intensive care unit.

Do additional safeguards, such as the suspension of leave, need to be put in place?

A 'debrief' of the patients and staff who witnessed or who were involved in the patient's violence should be organised – the other patients might well feel unsafe because of what has happened, and some might blame staff for this; other patients might feel angry towards Mr Dillon. The staff involved might need support.

Criminal justice system involvement

There might be merit in reporting the assault to the police. The advantages and disadvantages of this should be discussed.

Future risk management

The patient's risk assessment will need to be updated. An attempt will need to be made to formulate the factors that lie behind the assault so that the patient's future risk can be better understood.

FURTHER READING

Davison, S.E. (2005) The management of violence in general psychiatry. *Advances in Psychiatric Treatment*, 11(5), 362–70.

The examiner's mark sheet

Domain/ percentage of marks	Essential points to pass	✓	Extra marks/Comments (make notes here)
1. Rapport and communication	Uses appropriate professional language		
20% of marks	Shows the ability to listen attentively		
	Successfully negotiates and agree to a management plan		
2. Use of medication	Considers the use of additional medication		
30% of marks	Describes clearly why medication is being prescribed		
	Discusses type of medication, how long it will be prescribed for and what route it should be administered		
	Considers potential side effects and physical health monitoring		
3. Nursing interventions, including ward placement	Discusses level of nursing observations		
	Discusses ward placement		
	Considers suspension of leave		
30% of marks	Considers 'debrief' of the patients and staff		
4. Criminal justice system involvement	Elicits advantages and disadvantages of reporting assault to police		
10% of marks			
5. Future risk management	Indicates that the patient's risk assessment will need to be updated		
10% of marks	Attempts to formulate the factors that lay behind the assault		

⇧ % SCORE _____

STATION 5(a): EROTOMANIA

INSTRUCTION TO CANDIDATE

You have been asked to see Mr Cowan, a 45-year-old in-patient on a general psychiatric ward. Mr Cowan is thought to suffer from paranoid schizophrenia. He has unescorted leave from the ward once a day. A nurse on a neighbouring ward, Ms Williams, has told you that she has noticed Mr Cowan outside of her house when he is on leave. He has not approached her, but she has seen him several times in the last week and is concerned about her own safety. A number of 'love letters' have been left for her in the dining area of the ward. These are crudely written and unsigned, but Ms Williams suspects that Mr Cowan might be the author.

Examine relevant aspects of Mr Cowan's history and mental state and conduct a focussed risk assessment.

ACTOR (ROLE-PLAYER) INSTRUCTIONS

You believe with total certainty that Ms Williams, a young nurse on an adjacent ward, is in love with you.

You know this because of the way she looks at you and the way she speaks – you believe she looks at you in a 'special way' and you think she wants to live with you when you leave hospital.

You become upset when the doctor challenges you about your belief.

You have no intention of being violent towards Ms Williams, but would be upset if she does not love you.

You learnt where she lives by following her one day when you were on leave. You have been back to her house a few times hoping to speak to her.

SUGGESTED APPROACH

Rapport and communication

The patient is likely to resent the suggestion that his belief is mistaken. He might become agitated and aroused, challenging the doctor about the basis of their comments. You need to remain calm and focussed, acknowledging what the patient believes, but also gently seeking to challenge.

Establish delusional belief

The essence of erotomania is a delusional belief held by an individual that another person, often a stranger of higher social status, is deeply in love with them. It is essential to establish the core characteristics of a delusional belief (i.e. is it a false belief based on false evidence that is held with certainty and which is culturally inappropriate?).

To do this, you will need to elicit details of the belief from the patient and test the certainty with which it is held. 'Can you tell me why you believe that Ms Williams is in love with you? What evidence do you have for this? Are you absolutely sure that you're right? It seems unlikely to me that what you're saying is true–what's your view?'

Risk assessment

This has several parts: current intention, wider history and current mental state.

Patients who hold delusional beliefs often do not act directly on them; however, some do. You should conduct a risk assessment to try and determine if and how the patient's behaviour has been influenced by their belief and what their plans are for the future. Risk factors, such as general antisocial behaviour and having multiple delusional objects, and protective factors, such as a lack of substance misuse, should be elicited. 'Have you tried to contact her? What was her response? How do you make sense of her response?' Or: 'Why haven't you made contact with Ms Williams?'

'What is your intention now given your belief about Ms Williams?'

Test out whether the patient has any thoughts of violence towards Ms Williams. 'If Ms Williams doesn't want to see you, what will you do? Have you any thoughts of being violent towards her? What thoughts have you had?'

Explore the patient's wider history, including their social circumstances – patients without social support who are actively misusing substances, with a forensic history and who are impulsive are likely to be at particularly high risk of acting on their delusional beliefs.

Past behaviour is the best guide to future conduct. Hence, you should take a brief relationship history from the patient. How long have relationships lasted? Why have they ended? How has the patient met partners in the past? Has there been any violence or police involvement? How have relationships ended? Has the patient cohabited with a partner?

Erotomanic beliefs can arise as a part of a delusional disorder, mania or paranoid schizophrenia. There should be an attempt to explore the patient's mental state, in particular trying to establish symptoms of mania, other delusional beliefs and abnormal perceptions. Feelings of anger and rejection that are so strong that they can lead to suicidal ideas can be present and need to be elicited if present.

FURTHER READING

Mullen, P.E., Pathé, M. & Purcell, R. (2001) The management of stalkers. *Advances in Psychiatric Treatment*, 7(5), 335–42.

The examiner's mark sheet

Domain/ percentage of marks	Essential points to pass	✓	Extra marks/Comments (make notes here)
1. Rapport and communication 20% of marks	Manages patient's agitation with empathy		
	Remains calm and focussed		
	Gently seeks to challenge patient's beliefs		
2. Assessment of delusional ideas 40% of marks	Establishes the core characteristics of a delusional belief: a false belief based on false evidence that is held with certainty which is culturally inappropriate		
3. Risk assessment 40% of marks	Establishes current intention		
	Assesses current mental state		
	Explores the patient's wider history, including their social circumstances		
	Assesses past history of relationships and violence		

% SCORE _____

___ OVERALL IMPRESSION

3 (CIRCLE ONE)

Good Pass

Pass

Borderline

Fail

Clear Fail

NOTES/Areas to improve

STATION 5(b): DISCUSSION WITH COLLEAGUE

INSTRUCTION TO CANDIDATE

Having assessed Mr Cowan, you meet with Ms Williams (the nurse in question). You need to judge what to say, bearing in mind that Ms Williams is not directly involved in Mr Cowan's clinical care and your duty of confidentiality to Mr Cowan.

Inform the nurse of the situation. Provide advice in relation to support and risk management.

ACTOR (ROLE-PLAYER) INSTRUCTIONS

You are a 25-year-old nurse on a psychiatric ward.

Having seen Mr Cowan outside of your house, you are frightened about your safety.

You want to know how he found out where you live and what he wants from you.

You ask the doctor about Mr Cowan's history, including his previous relationships. If the doctor does not tell you what you believe you need to know, you become upset and try to persuade the doctor to say more.

SUGGESTED APPROACH

Rapport and communication

Ms Williams is likely to be nervous and worried about her safety. You need to be reassuring, professional and honest, while explaining the limits of what you can say about your interview with Mr Cowan. You need to tell Ms Williams enough for her to be able to keep safe, but not details that are not directly related to any threat she might face.

Explore support

Explore with Ms Williams what support she has. Does she have a partner or friends she can talk to about this stressful situation? Can her manager at work help?

Discuss risk management

You should help Ms Williams think practically about her own safety. How can she minimise her contact with Mr Cowan at work? She should involve her managers at work and potentially consider a period in an alternative unit/work environment. What should she do if she sees Mr Cowan again outside of her house? Should the police be involved? How can colleagues help her?

> **FURTHER READING**
>
> Pathé, M., Mullen, P.E., & Purcell, R. et al. (2001) Management of victims of stalking. *Advances in Psychiatric Treatment*, 7(6), 399–406.

The examiner's mark sheet

Domain/ percentage of marks	Essential points to pass	✓	Extra marks/Comments (make notes here)
1. Rapport and communication	Acts in a reassuring, professional and honest way		
50% of marks	Explains the limits of what you can say about your interview with Mr Cowan		
	Describes appropriate level of detail of information obtained		
2. Explores support	Explores with Ms Williams what personal support she has		
25% of marks	Discusses sources of support at work		

⇧ 3. Discusses risk
    management

    25% of marks

Helps Ms Williams think practically about her own safety

Considers how she can minimise her contact with Mr Cowan at work

Considers risk management plan should she have contact with Mr Cowan outside of work

% SCORE _____

                                                 ___ **OVERALL IMPRESSION**

3 (CIRCLE ONE)

      Good Pass

      Pass

      Borderline

      Fail

      Clear Fail

      NOTES/Areas to improve

O SINGLE STATIONS

STATION 6: ARSON

INSTRUCTION TO CANDIDATE

You have been called to the Emergency Department of a local hospital to see a young man who is under arrest for an alleged offence of arson. He has suffered burns but is now physically well.

Take a forensic history with particular reference to fire-setting.

ACTOR (ROLE-PLAYER) INSTRUCTIONS

You are reluctant to speak to the doctor as you are worried about being under arrest.

If the doctor is empathetic, you engage with the assessment but are anxious throughout.

You describe setting the fire because you enjoy watching flames. This gives you a sense of relief.

You have set fires for many years.

It has never been your intention to harm anyone.

SUGGESTED APPROACH

Communicate appropriately and with empathy

An important aspect of the task is to be empathetic and non-judgemental. The patient will need to be informed about the general confidentiality of the interview and reassured that information will not be disclosed to the police unless there appears to be a significant risk to a named individual.

Time might run short in this station, as the candidate needs to take a comprehensive history and the patient is likely to be a somewhat reluctant interviewee. Having a good structure in approaching the task is important: concentrate first on the present incident, and then consider past episodes.

Take a history of this episode of fire-setting, including precipitants and desired outcome

Take a history of the current incident. What happened? Was there any forethought? What degree of planning was there? Was an accelerant (e.g. petrol) used? What was the intention in setting the fire (e.g. to receive help, financial or to harm others)? Was any consideration given as to how the fire would spread? Was there any attempt at concealment? Conversely, was the fire set with the aim that it be easily discovered? Did the patient call the emergency services? Did they wait and watch the fire? Were they alone?

Explore motivations for setting fire

Assess the man's mental state at the time of setting the fire: use of substances including alcohol, suicidal ideas and intent, presence of depression, irritability, anxiety, anger, 'tension', delusional ideas and perceptual abnormalities.

Most cases of arson are not related to mental illness. A good candidate will acknowledge this in their questioning by investigating whether the fire-setting is likely to lead to financial benefit, perhaps through an insurance pay-out. Pyromania – achieving sexual satisfaction through fire-setting – is a rare condition, but some attempt to explore this would be helpful. If time allows, trying to establish a pattern of fire-setting would be impressive; for example, discussing with the patient about positive and negative reinforcers, such as the relief of tension and the communication of distress to others.

Assess for any social skills deficits, including the ability to communicate distress and any suggestion of learning disability or pervasive developmental disorder (e.g. autism/ Asperger's syndrome). To clarify this, ask about birth problems, developmental milestones, academic achievements and friends at school. Try and gauge the person's level of self-esteem: childhood bullying, peer rejection and social isolation are often seen in patients who set fires.

Discuss past episodes of fire-setting

Ask about past incidents of fire setting, including as a child. Is there a fascination with fire or aspects of fire-setting?

Explore past incidents: what was the context, why did they happen in the man's view and what was his intention?

Discuss each episode systematically, establishing the motivations for the behaviour, any short-term triggers for fire-setting and the outcome.

Take a general forensic history

Take a more general forensic history: evidence of childhood conduct disorder (truanting, bullying, expulsion from school and early age of first contact with the police), previous convictions, age at first conviction, first custodial sentence, previous offences of fire-setting, sexual offences or violent offences. Has the man received treatment in hospital after being convicted of a criminal offence?

FURTHER READING

Burton, P.R., McNiel, D.E. & Binder, R.L. (2012) Firesetting, arson, pyromania and the forensic mental health expert. *J Am Acad Psychiatry Law*, *40*(3), 355–65.

Jackson, H. (1994) Assessment of fire-setters. In: McMurran, M. & Hodge, J. (eds) *The Assessment of Criminal Behaviours in Secure Settings*. London: Jessica Kingsley, pp. 94–126.

Puri, B.K., Baxter, R. & Cordess, C. (1995) Characteristics of fire-setters. A study and proposed multiaxial psychiatric classification. *British Journal of Psychiatry*, *166*, 393–6.

The examiner's mark sheet

Domain/ percentage of marks	Essential points to pass	✓	Extra marks/Comments (make notes here)
1. Communicates appropriately and with empathy 10% of marks	Shows empathy and is non-judgemental Informs patient about the general confidentiality of the interview Demonstrates a good structure in approaching the task		
2. Takes a history of this episode of fire-setting, including precipitants and desired outcome 30% of marks	Takes a history of the current incident Elicits degree of planning involved Determines intention in setting the fire		
3. Explores motivations for setting fire 20% of marks	Assesses the man's mental state at the time of setting the fire Highlights the use of substances, including alcohol Elicits any suicidal ideas and intent Assesses for any social skills deficits		
4. Discusses past episodes of fire-setting 20% of marks	Asks about past incidents of fire setting Explores past incidents Discusses each episode systematically		
5. Takes a general forensic history 20% of marks	Elicits evidence of childhood conduct disorder Discusses previous criminal convictions Highlights any previous offences of fire-setting, sexual offences or violent offences		

⇧ **% SCORE** _____

___ **OVERALL IMPRESSION**
5 (CIRCLE ONE)
Good Pass
Pass
Borderline
Fail
Clear Fail
NOTES/Areas to improve

STATION 7: DISSOCIAL PERSONALITY DISORDER

> **INSTRUCTION TO CANDIDATE**
>
> This patient, aged in her 20s, has attended the emergency clinic complaining of low mood. She claims a long-standing history of 'feeling depressed' since adolescence.
>
> You discover that she has had a row with a neighbour who complained that she was playing music loudly. This led to a physical fight.
>
> You uncover a history of previous damage to property and violence. She admits to having been extremely aggressive towards her ex-partner.
>
> She wants to know what you can do to help her with her regular angry outbursts.
>
> **Take a relevant history to determine the diagnosis.**
>
> **Explain how you intend to assist her.**

ACTOR (ROLE-PLAYER) INSTRUCTIONS

You are nervous about seeing the doctor, being worried about being criticised.

If the doctor is empathetic, offer a candid account of your background.

You are worried about the risk you pose to others.

The situation has reached a crisis because your friends now refuse to socialise with you.

You are curious about the possibilities for treatment.

SUGGESTED APPROACH

Communicate with empathy

The patient has come seeking help, which is a major step, and is likely to need reassurance regarding issues of confidentiality and the types of assistance that mental health services can offer.

Remember to be aware of your own safety during the interview – where are the alarms situated? Are colleagues aware that you are seeing the patient? Is the room set up adequately?

Take a detailed personal and family history

There is little time in the station to establish the diagnosis of a personality disorder. Useful information is likely to come from concentrating on the quality of the patient's relationships. Distinguishing a dissocial personality disorder from an emotionally unstable personality disorder might also be difficult, as both often share common historical features. In reality, comorbidity between 'cluster B' conditions is common.

Family history: exposure to parental violence; parental substance misuse; parental criminality. What was her experience of parental support – was she fearful of her parents? Did she feel able to confide in an adult figure? Did she suffer any abusive experiences?

Personal history: birth trauma; prematurity; developmental milestones. Schooling: oppositional behaviour; relationships with teachers and peers; truancy; detention; suspension; exclusion. Academic progress: evidence of dyslexia or specific learning problems. Occupational history: ability to maintain employment; attitude towards authority figures; any conflict with fellow workers.

Relationship history: pattern of past relationships; promiscuity; experience of cohabiting with others; past violence in relationships. Why have relationships ended? Presence of legal injunctions? Are there any children, and if so, have social services been involved in the care of these children?

In reality, taking a collateral history would be necessary in this case. Asking the patient's permission to speak to someone who knows her well would indicate to the examiner that the candidate is aware of this.

Take a detailed forensic history

Ask about previous criminal offences, cautions, disposal and potential imprisonment. How has she responded to sanctions in the past (e.g. did she comply with the conditions of any community [probation] order or did she reoffend after conviction)? Who have been the past victims of her violence? Has she been aggressive to those who are especially vulnerable (e.g. children, mental health patients or animals)? What have been the circumstances of past violence? Does she display any remorse for past victims or empathy towards them? Eliciting any fantasises of violence or torture would be useful.

Assess for the presence of comorbidity

Assess use of both alcohol and illicit drugs and symptoms of dependence on substances. Has her substance misuse been associated with offending? If so, in what way? Has she offended when intoxicated, when in a state of withdrawal or to pay for substances?

Is there evidence of broader impulsivity (e.g. impulsive deliberate self harm, gambling or risk taking)?

Important aspects of her mental state that require assessment are her mood state (e.g. is her irritability associated with depression, anxiety or hypomania/mania)?

Discuss treatment options

Treatment could be as an out-patient or in-patient, either as a voluntary patient or detained under mental health legislation, dependent on the ongoing risk that she poses to others.

Attempting to build a therapeutic alliance during this initial interview will be important. Validating the effort that she has made will be useful (e.g. 'It's a very important first step that you're here today'). Explore her motivations for attendance.

Try to establish firm boundaries and begin to draw up a treatment contract with the patient, perhaps by suggesting: 'It's often useful if we establish right at the start how we can help you and what you need to do.'

Treat any mental illness or substance misuse.

If out-patient psychological therapy is to be offered, the options include structured problem solving and group or individual anger management. There is limited evidence for the use of medication, but possibilities might include flupenthixol, olanzapine, lithium or fluoxetine. Avoid prescribing benzodiazepines.

Other options for treatment might include attendance at a day hospital or admission to a therapeutic community.

FURTHER READING

Banerjee, P.J.M., Gibbon, S. & Huband, N. (2009) Assessment of personality disorder. *Advances in Psychiatric Treatment, 15*(5), 389–97.

Fagin, L. (2004) Management of personality disorders in acute in-patient settings. Part 2: Less common personality disorders. *Advances in Psychiatric Treatment, 10,* 100–6.

Tyrer, P. & Bateman, A. (2004) Drug treatment of personality disorder. *Advances in Psychiatric Treatment, 10,* 389–98.

The examiner's mark sheet

Domain/ percentage of marks	Essential points to pass	✓	Extra marks/Comments (make notes here)
1. Communicates with empathy 20% of marks	Establishes some rapport Offers reassurance around issues of confidentiality Pays attention to own safety		
2. Takes a detailed personal and family history 20% of marks	Elicits exposure to parental violence/criminality Establishes behaviour at school Discusses occupational history Establishes quality of the patient's relationships		
3. Takes a detailed forensic history 20% of marks	Takes a history of previous offences and cautions Establishes how patient has responded to sanctions Discusses past incidents of violence Elicits any fantasises of violence or torture		
4. Assesses for the presence of comorbidity 20% of marks	Takes history of use of alcohol Takes history of use of illicit drugs Elicits degree of impulsivity Takes history of mood disorder		

⇧ 5. Discusses treatment options | Explores patient's motivation for attendance

20% of marks | Attempts to build a therapeutic alliance

Describes a range of possible psychological treatments

Discusses role of medication

% SCORE _____

___ **OVERALL IMPRESSION**

5 (CIRCLE ONE)

Good Pass

Pass

Borderline

Fail

Clear Fail

NOTES/Areas to improve

STATION 8: MORBID JEALOUSY

INSTRUCTION TO CANDIDATE

You have been asked to see this 30-year-old police officer in your clinic. She was referred by the GP as she had attended A&E on at least six occasions over the last few months with minor injuries. These had included injuries to her hands from punching walls and a laceration to her face from an argument with someone at her partner's place of work.

The police have also been to her home address following calls from the neighbours who were concerned about domestic violence, which she found completely humiliating.

The letter from the GP includes details of a conversation with her brother, setting out her belief that her husband is having an affair and the brother's opinion that this is absolutely not the case.

She has also apparently been misusing both her work time and police information to track her husband's activities.

Elicit the main features of what you believe is the likely diagnosis.

Assess the risk to others and of self-harm/suicide.

ACTOR (ROLE-PLAYER) INSTRUCTIONS

You are angry about your husband's behaviour – you are sure he is having an affair.

You know this because of the way the birds were flying in the sky when he came home from work.

Your belief has led to arguments with your husband.

You have found out the identity of the woman you know your husband is having a relationship with and intend to confront her.

You feel that seeing the doctor is a waste of time but are prepared to sit and discuss the situation if they seem to be interested.

SUGGESTED APPROACH

Introduce self appropriately and establish rapport

One of the key problems with this station is engaging the patient in the assessment; the patient is upset and firmly believes that her husband is committing adultery. The candidate will need to show good communication skills and attempt to show the patient that her own behaviour is causing her distress. Showing empathy without colluding or unfairly supporting the patient's belief about her husband is important.

Establishing how the patient views her attendance at the appointment will be important early on in the interview. In her mind, her husband is to blame for her difficulties, and she is likely to be resistant to the idea that mental health treatment could assist her.

Take a history of the presenting complaint

The patient is suffering from delusional jealousy. The core symptom of her mental disorder is that she believes, on false grounds, that her partner has been sexually unfaithful.

The strength of the patient's belief in her partner's infidelity needs to be established.

The 'evidence' for this belief is important to elicit. How has this been obtained? Often patients will examine their partner's underwear for signs of sexual contact, check mobile phones and e-mails, follow the person, employ a private detective and repeatedly interrogate their partners.

Taking a psychosexual history is important. What has been the quality of the patient's past intimate relationships? Have there been past episodes of similar behaviour? If so, what happened? Were the courts involved?

What is the patient's affect: anger, misery, irritability or apprehension?

Are there any links between the patient's behaviour and the use of alcohol, cocaine or amphetamines? Is there any evidence of an organic cause, such as temporal lobe epilepsy?

Identify and elucidate delusional ideas

Is the delusional belief encapsulated or is it part of another mental disorder, such as depression, schizophrenia or a personality disorder (paranoid or antisocial)?

Assess risk to others

Firstly, consider the risk to the patient's partner and to those whom she perceives to be having an affair with her husband.

We know that she has been violent. Who has she considered attacking? What was the cause of the injuries for which she has attended hospital? If there has been violence, what happened, was there a trigger and why did it stop?

What has been the patient's husband's response? Has this made the situation worse?

The patient in this case is a police officer, which might increase the risk she poses to others. Does she have access to weapons or otherwise confidential information about others, especially her husband's alleged partner?

The risk to others in cases of a delusional disorder can be significant. A good candidate, as well as assessing risk, will make some attempt to consider risk management. Options include detention under mental health legislation or arranging an informal admission to hospital. Treatment with anti-psychotic medication, at the same doses as in schizophrenia, either as an out-patient or in-patient will need to be considered. Psychological treatment in the form of cognitive behavioural therapy, if the patient will allow this, might be useful, as might work in ensuring that the patient's partner does not provoke further conflict with their reaction to the allegations. If the risk to the partner's husband is great, geographically separating the patient from her husband might be necessary.

Assess risk to self

The risk to self also needs to be discussed. The patient is evidently very distressed by her husband's supposed behaviour. Whether she has experienced suicidal ideas and has any intent or plan to harm herself needs to be elicited, as do potential triggers to acting against herself and protective factors against this.

ADDITIONAL POINTS

One cannot guarantee full confidentiality, particularly if other individuals are at risk, and this will need to be established early in the assessment.

FURTHER READING

Fear, C. (2013) Recent developments in the management of delusional disorders. *Advances in Psychiatric Treatment*, 19(3), 212–20.

Kingham, M. & Gordon, H. (2004) Aspects of morbid jealousy. *Advances in Psychiatric Treatment*, 10, 207–15.

The examiner's mark sheet

Domain/ percentage of marks	Essential points to pass	✓	Extra marks/Comments (make notes here)
1. Introduces self appropriately and establish rapport 20% of marks	Shows appropriate empathy without colluding or unfairly supporting the patient's belief about her husband		
	Establishes patients views of her attendance at the appointment		
2. Takes a history of the presenting complaint 20% of marks	Establishes delusional belief of infidelity		
	Elicits patient's evidence for this belief		
	Takes a psychosexual history		
	Enquires about substance use		

3. Identifies and elucidates delusional ideas

   20% of marks

Establishes scope of delusional belief

Briefly assess for symptoms of depression, schizophrenia and paranoid and dissocial personality disorders

4. Assesses risk to others

   20% of marks

Considers the risk to the patient's 'partner' and to those whom she perceives to be having an affair with her husband

Establishes the presence of any violent ideas, intent or plan

Discusses access to weapons

5. Assesses risk to self

   20% of marks

Establishes whether the patient has experienced suicidal ideas and any intent or plan to harm herself

Establishes potential triggers to acting against herself

Assesses protective factors

% SCORE _____

___ **OVERALL IMPRESSION**

5 (CIRCLE ONE)

Good Pass

Pass

Borderline

Fail

Clear Fail

NOTES/Areas to improve

STATION 9: INDECENT EXPOSURE

INSTRUCTION TO CANDIDATE

You are a psychiatry trainee working with out-patients. You are asked to see a 63-year-old man with a history of bipolar affective disorder. The man lives in a housing association flat. His GP has been informed by his housing officer that, whenever she has visited over the past 2 months, the patient has answered the door with his trousers underdone, exposing his penis. He has corrected his attire when told and has appeared embarrassed. The housing officer has noticed pornographic magazines spread openly around the man's living room.

Take a history of the man's behaviour and any other sexually abnormal behaviour and carry out a focussed mental state examination.

ACTOR (ROLE-PLAYER) INSTRUCTIONS

You are distressed and embarrassed.

Unless the doctor shows appropriate empathy, you are unwilling to discuss what has happened.

If interviewed with empathy, explain that you have episodes of confusion.

You have had little interest in sex for many years.

You were ashamed when you released you had inadvertently exposed yourself to the housing officer.

SUGGESTED APPROACH

Demonstrate appropriate communication skills

The patient might well be embarrassed and distressed at coming to the appointment. This should be quickly acknowledged and the overall structure of the assessment should be explained, as should the duty of confidentiality.

Fantasy beliefs, particularly if they concern paraphilic activities, might be difficult to elicit: normalising the issue of sex and being clear with the patient that everyone has sexual ideas could assist with this.

Notwithstanding the difficulty, the situation is potentially serious and a clear assessment of risk needs to be undertaken.

Elicit a description of current behaviour

Whether this is a case of exhibitionism, sheer forgetfulness or a likely prelude to more serious sexual offending needs to be established.

Take an account of the sexually inappropriate behaviour:

What did the patient do? What effect did he believe his actions would have, and what was the effect that he wanted to have (e.g. to make the housing officer fearful, to be caught or as the start of a sexual encounter)? Was the housing officer the intended victim and if so why?

Was exposing himself sexually arousing? Was his penis erect or flaccid? Did he masturbate afterwards?

How much planning was involved? Was the patient intoxicated at the time? What was his mental state: any evidence of mania/hypomania such as an elevated mood, increased energy, quick thoughts, insomnia, lack of fatigue, elevated self-regard, loss of concentration, grandiose ideation, and so forth? Was the man anxious and did exposing himself make him feel less so?

Is there any evidence that the man was confused? Was he taking any disinhibiting medications at the time (e.g. benzodiazepines)? Does he suffer from any physical illnesses, such as diabetes, or a recent head injury that have might have affected his psychological state?

What is his current attitude to what he did: embarrassment, entitlement or pleasure? Does he want treatment?

Take a psychosexual history

The type of pornography in the flat needs to be established. How often does he purchase pornography – is it always of the same type? Does he access Internet pornography?

Taking a psychosexual history will be key. Consider whether he has previously been married or had cohabiting partners.

Is there any evidence of paraphilia as shown by fantasy beliefs, past behaviour or sexual ideas about children? Is the man hypersexual? Discuss the level of his sexual preoccupation as judged by the frequency of masturbation, number of sexual partners and description of 'uncontrollable' urges.

Take a relevant background history

A more wide-ranging forensic history with a view to establishing any general antisocial attitudes will be important. Has he offended in the past? Have there been any sexual offences – past exhibitionism or contact sexual offences (e.g. indecent assault or rape)? Has he undertaken a sex offender treatment programme before?

Also consider his use of alcohol and illicit drugs.

Does he have any regular or predictable access to children?

Assess mood state, including a brief cognitive examination

A mental state examination needs to be focussed on the man's current affective state, symptoms of psychosis and his cognitive functioning, in particular his orientation and his long- and short-term memory.

In view of his age, particularly if this is new behaviour, screen for any cognitive decline. Have there been any episodes of forgetfulness? Has he suffered any form of functional decline: how well does he manage to live independently and complete tasks such as shopping, self-care and travelling around? Has anyone remarked to him about a decline in his memory?

FURTHER READING

Darjee, R. & Russell, K. (2012) What clinicians need to know before assessing risk in sexual offenders. *Advances in Psychiatric Treatment*, 18(6), 467–78.

Russell, K. & Darjee, R. (2013) Practical assessment and management of risk in sexual offenders. *Advances in Psychiatric Treatment*, 19(1), 56–66.

The examiner's mark sheet

Domain/ percentage of marks	Essential points to pass	✓	Extra marks/Comments (make notes here)
1. Demonstrates appropriate communication skills 20% of marks	Uses appropriate techniques to acknowledge patient's distress Establishes duty of confidentiality Attempts to normalise conversation about sexual matters		

2. Elicits a description of current behaviour

20% of marks

- Takes an account of the sexually inappropriate behaviour
- Elicits patient's intention
- Establishes whether patient was sexually arousing
- Notes degree of planning involved
- Describes use of substances and mental state abnormalities, including confusion

3. Takes a psychosexual history

20% of marks

- Considers use of pornography-frequency and type
- Takes a relationship history
- Elicits any evidence of paraphilia as shown by fantasy beliefs and past behaviour
- Establishes sexual drive as judged by the frequency of masturbation, number of sexual partners and description of 'uncontrollable' urges

4. Takes an account of past behaviour

20% of marks

- Takes a forensic history
- Focuses on previous sexual offences
- Elicits history of appropriate treatment, including participation in sex offender treatment programme
- Considers use of alcohol and illicit drugs
- Establishes access to children

5. Assesses mood state, including brief cognitive examination

20% of marks

- Conducts a focussed mental state examination on current affective state
- Elicits any symptoms of psychosis
- Screens for cognitive decline
- Elicits episodes of forgetfulness
- Notes functional decline

% SCORE _____

___ **OVERALL IMPRESSION**

5 (CIRCLE ONE)

Good Pass

Pass

Borderline

Fail

Clear Fail

NOTES/Areas to improve

O LINKED STATIONS

STATION 1(a): BEHAVIOURAL CHANGE – HISTORY TAKING

INSTRUCTION TO CANDIDATE

You are about to see James, a member of staff from a local care home, who is here with Sam, one of the residents with a moderate learning disability who has displayed a marked change in his behaviour recently. He has been withdrawn and banging his head against a wall repeatedly.

Please take a history from James to assist you in coming to a conclusion around the possible explanation for this presentation. You might wish to take notes, since you would be expected to explain your assessment and management at the next station.

ACTOR (ROLE-PLAYER) INSTRUCTIONS

You have been working as a support worker for 3 years in the care home; you have been the key worker for Sam for over a year. You have noticed that over the last 6 weeks, Sam has been moody, not smiling and playful as he used to be. He has lost weight, and at times he is banging his head repeatedly against the wall, at times even causing skin tears to his head. Nothing major has changed at the care home and he usually has a routine that has not changed. However, you know that his mother, who was visiting him every week, has taken ill and is in hospital now.

SUGGESTED APPROACH

Setting the scene

Introduce yourself: 'Hello, my name is Dr_____, I am one of the psychiatrists. How would you like to be addressed?' Greet James and Sam: 'I understand that you have some concerns around a change in Sam's presentation recently. Are you able to explain these in detail for me?'

Completing the tasks

Establish the role of James at the care home: does he do day-to-day caring jobs or managerial jobs, how long has he been working there, how long had he known Sam for, does he work shifts (this may mean he may only get to see Sam during particular shifts), and so forth?

Determine the severity of Sam's learning disability and his developmental age in order to help tailor your communication accordingly. 'What can Sam do, with respect to daily activities? What about budgeting or using computers? What about his language skills? Can he manage his daily routine?'

Elicit an accurate history demonstrating the events leading up to the change in behaviour.

Obtain a description of the behaviour: 'How has Sam changed? How withdrawn is he – how is this different from his usual behaviour? How often does he seem to be like this? Is there a pattern to this? Is he worse at any particular time of the day? Describe the head banging and how severe is it?'

Obtain a chronology and progression of the events: 'When did it start? What makes it worse? Were there any possible triggers?'

Possible causes: these could be psycho-social or physical health-related. Has there been a change in close relationships? Have there been any changes in the patient's personal circumstances or the environment? (In this case, the separation from his mother who was visiting him until recently could be a trigger.) Assess the patient's interests and hobbies and whether he is able to access them as before.

Does Sam have any physical or sensory impairment or other health conditions? Have the staff contacted the GP and dentist to rule out any physical health causes? Rule out iatrogenic causes: has any medication been started/stopped recently, or the dose changed?

Past history: how long have the staff known the patient? Are there records of his previous functioning and behaviour? Have any behavioural strategies worked for him in similar situations before?

Current management: is there a behaviour plan in place at present? If so, the details are to be clarified. Are staff aware of ABC charts (antecedent, behaviour, consequence)? Ask the care staff about the resources at the home and whether these are appropriate to the patient's needs.

Ask about withdrawal, poor sleep, loss of interest, lack of appetite and tearfulness as symptoms of depression. Ask about any crying episodes, increases in irritability and anything he might have said to suggest hopelessness. Does he think that he has been bad (feelings of guilt)? Has he expressed anything about feeling threatened by someone (persecutory ideas)?

You may say, 'Have you noted any changes to Sam's routine? Have his patterns of eating, sleeping and activities changed recently? Does he look worried? Does he look suspicious? Does he talk when there is no one around? Does he see things others cannot see?'

Risks

A risk assessment, including risk to self (suicidal ideation, self-harm and self-injury), risk of harm to others (physical aggression and hurting others), self-neglect, risk of exploitation (ask whether he is frightened of someone and whether he has experienced inappropriate behaviour) and risk of placement breaking down, is to be completed.

Aetiology

Consider:

- Social/environmental changes/changes to routine.
- Physical health.
- Psychiatric: rule out depression. Are biological symptoms of depression elicited (e.g. changes in appetite, sleep, anhedonia, withdrawal, tearfulness and diurnal variation in symptoms)?
- Risk: ask about death wishes, suicidal thoughts/active plans for suicide and self-harming, as well as clarifying risk of self-neglect and risk to others.

Points to consider

Rapport with carer and being sensitive.

Establishing baseline functioning of patient.

Obtaining a past and family psychiatry history of psychiatric disorder.

Demonstrating precipitating factor.

Ruling out physical/environmental and social causes systematically before considering a psychiatric explanation.

Thorough risk assessment. Psychiatric illness is four times more common in individuals with learning disability (LD) compared to the general population.

FURTHER READING

Challenging behaviour and learning disabilities: NICE Guidance. http://www.nice.org.uk/guidance/ng11

The examiner's mark sheet

Domain/ percentage of marks	Essential points to pass	✓	Extra marks/comments (make notes here)
1. Rapport and communication 20% of marks	Establishes rapport with carer Empathy Appropriate use of open and closed questions		
2. Takes a history of changes in behaviour 20% of marks	Description of behaviours Chronology of events Any triggers, patterns		
3. History of possible causes 20% of marks	Considers psychological, social, environmental and medical causes of change in behaviour		
4. Depression as a likely cause 20% of marks	Identifies depression as a likely cause of behavioural change Explores detailed symptoms of mood disorder Explores other psychiatric symptoms such as delusions and hallucinations		
5. Risk assessment 20% of marks	Demonstrates thorough risk assessment – to self, any aggression to others, self-neglect and exploitation		

⇑ **% SCORE** _____

___ **OVERALL IMPRESSION**

5 (CIRCLE ONE)

Good Pass

Pass

Borderline

Fail

Clear Fail

NOTES/Areas to improve

STATION 1(b): BEHAVIOURAL CHANGE – DISCUSSION

> ## INSTRUCTION TO CANDIDATE
>
> You have just spoken to care worker James, who looks after Sam, in the previous station. The care home manager is worried about Sam and asks what is going on with him. He is anxious how to manage Sam in his care home and would appreciate some help.
>
> **Please explain the findings of your assessment and the management plan to the manager. Address any concerns that he might have.**

ACTOR (ROLE-PLAYER) INSTRUCTIONS

You are the manager of the care home where Sam lives. You are worried about his recent change in behaviour and are anxious regarding how to manage him at the care home. You want to know if the mental health team can help and what the care home staff can do to help the situation. You ask the doctor to explain further if you do not understand. You want to know how to keep Sam safe.

SUGGESTED APPROACH

Setting the scene

Introduce yourself: 'Hello, my name is Dr_____, I am one of the psychiatrists. How would you like to be addressed? I gather you are concerned about Sam. I have spoken to James and I shall be explaining to you my understanding of the recent change in Sam's behaviour. We shall then discuss ways to manage it. I shall also address any concerns that you may have.'

Completing the task

In this task, you will have to allow the manager to express his concerns first. After listening to him, you will have to explain what you think is the likely scenario here: Sam is probably suffering from depression following separation from his mother. You then inform him that you will be arranging to see Sam at the care home very soon to complete your assessment. 'Mr_____, I am sure you are worried about Sam and his recent change in behaviour. I have spoken to James at length and, from what I gathered, I think Sam is probably experiencing depression. This is probably because he is missing his mum.'

M: Doctor, are you sure? Why do you think so?

C: It seems in the past few weeks Sam has seemed withdrawn, experiencing poor sleep and appetite, not being his usual happy self and banging his head – these could be his way of expressing his psychological distress.

- Give the diagnosis of depression and its comorbidity with learning disability.
- Explain the diagnosis.
- Check understanding and explain the reasons behind your conclusion.

M: Is there anything you can do to help Sam?

C: I shall first come and see him and complete my assessment. There are various treatment options to address the depressive symptoms. Medical management will be to consider antidepressants and, for acutely disturbed behaviour, some anxiety-alleviating medication.

M: Is there anything the care home can do?

C: Certainly. We know that depressive symptoms improve by incorporating activities that brings pleasure and a sense of achievement in daily life. We need to think about what Sam usually enjoys and what gives him a sense of achievement. This could be watching his favourite movies, listening to music or playing his favourite sport. In the meantime, it may help to arrange for him to visit his mother in the hospital too, if possible.

- Ask if there are any questions before moving on to discuss treatment options.
- Management options – bio-psycho-social approach.
- Address the carer's concerns and provide reassurance.

Points to consider

- Do not forget to mention regular cardiovascular exercise, activity scheduling and sleep hygiene.
- Cognitive behavioural therapy: this is an evidence-based psychological therapy, but one would need to ascertain Sam's level of learning disability to engage in this.
- Antidepressant medication.
- Mention patient choice and capacity.
- Risk management and safety advice: ask about keeping Sam safe and allocating more one-to-one time with his care worker in order to prevent him from head banging and to respond quickly if he does so.

FURTHER READING

http://www.mentalhealth.org.uk/publications/learning-disabilities-iapt-positive-practice-guide

Hurley, A.D. (2008) Depression in adults with intellectual disability: Symptoms and challenging behaviour. *Journal of Intellectual Disability Research*, 52(11), 905–16.

Jennings, C. & Hewitt, O. (2015) The use of cognitive behaviour therapy to treat depression in people with learning disabilities: A systematic review. *Tizard Learning Disability Review*, 20(2), 54–64.

The examiner's mark sheet

Domain/ percentage of marks	Essential points to pass	✓	Extra marks/comments (make notes here)
1. Rapport and communication 20% of marks	Establishes rapport with care manager Empathy and acknowledges his anxiety Appropriate use of jargon-free language		
2. Explains possible diagnosis 20% of marks	Explains likely diagnosis of depression Details the rationale for this diagnosis		
3. Addressing concerns 20% of marks	Listens to the manager Acknowledges his worries and alleviates his anxiety		
4. Treatment options 20% of marks	Explores bio-psycho-social approach in dealing with depression Demonstrates knowledge of treatment of depression in LD patients		
5. Risk assessment 20% of marks	Demonstrates awareness of risks associated and discusses strategies to minimise risks		

% SCORE _____

OVERALL IMPRESSION

___ **5** (CIRCLE ONE)

Good Pass

Pass

Borderline

Fail

Clear Fail

NOTES/Areas to improve

O SINGLE STATIONS

STATION 2: LEARNING DISABILITY AND CAPACITY TO CONSENT

INSTRUCTION TO CANDIDATE

You are about to meet Jen, a woman with learning disabilities who lives in supported accommodation and has been brought to accident and emergency

(A&E) by a support staff member, Sarah, presenting with haematemesis. The A&E medics would like to perform more investigations, including blood tests, chest x-ray and endoscopy and ultrasound of the abdomen and are unsure whether she has the capacity to consent to these.

Please assess Jen's capacity to consent to the investigations. There is no need to perform a mental state examination. Address Sarah's concerns.

ACTOR (ROLE-PLAYER) INSTRUCTIONS

You are Jen; you have been vomiting blood since morning. You live in supported accommodation but you have your own flat where you independently carry out most of your daily activities. You are very anxious about the hospital environment and want to go home, as you are out of your usual comfort zone. You trust your support worker Sarah more than anybody else. You tell the doctor that you do not want any more treatment as you are scared in the hospital and want to go home. You appear anxious and reluctant to speak, but if the doctor is empathic and involves Sarah in explaining matter to you, you trust him or her.

SUGGESTED APPROACH

Setting the scene

Introduce yourself: 'Hello, my name is Dr_____, one of the psychiatrists. How would you like to be called?' Explain your role to the patient and the staff. Explore the patient's understanding of the situation: 'I gather you have been unwell. Can you tell me what happened?'

Completing the tasks

Ask the patient to explain their reason for attending A&E: 'Are you able to tell me why you are here?' Clarify the information provided by the A&E medics: 'What did the doctors say?' Cross-check with the staff member to corroborate this information. Once you have assessed the patient's understanding of the current situation, proceed to enquire about the actual procedure which is proposed. Check the patient's level of knowledge and understanding first: 'Do you know what an endoscopy means?' If the patient is reluctant to talk to you, ask for the help of her support worker to explain what you are saying to Jen. Remember that Jen is out of her usual surroundings and she will respond better to familiar faces.

Provide information again regarding investigations (indications, risks and benefits and the procedure itself). You may have to mention that you will check with your medical colleagues about any aspect of the procedure you are unsure of. Then ask the patient to repeat the information to you. Then ask whether she has decided to undergo the investigations: 'Now that we have discussed a lot about endoscopy, what do you think? Do you consider that this is a good treatment option for you right now?'

Ask her to explain her decision to consent/not consent to the procedures. If she still refuses, ask her what her reasons are for refusing. Conduct a cognitive examination (orientation to time, place and person and digit span for working memory should be sufficient for a gross estimate of cognition).

A brief mental state examination in order to rule out mental health disorders affecting Jen's capacity should be completed. For example, depressive symptoms like hopelessness or death wishes could influence her decision to refuse investigations, or psychotic symptoms like persecutory delusions could affect her capacity and should be explored. Remember that capacity is decision specific and time specific.

Addressing staff's concerns

The support worker may ask questions such as, 'How should I go about managing the situation?' Reassure her that the medical team are looking to investigate further, and you will liaise with them regarding how urgent this situation is. If Jen is stabilised with supportive measures, then these can be arranged as out-patient care. However, if her condition deteriorates, they will probably want to observe her in the hospital and arrange for further treatment. Offer to arrange a meeting with the medical team to discuss these options.

Points to consider

- Clarify the extent of learning disability.
- Clarify dementia/delirium/other factors which could impact on the decision-making process.
- Awareness of the impact of current mental health and belief decisions on decision making.
- Making an unwise decision does not by itself imply a lack of capacity.
- Facilitate information giving/support for making decisions.

ADDITIONAL POINTS

- Remember that treatment is in the patient's best interests.
- Advance directives.
- Independent Mental Capacity Advocate.

FURTHER READING

Making Decisions – The Independent Mental Capacity (IMCA) Service (2009) *Department of Health and Office of the Public Guardian*. https://www.gov.uk/govern-ment/uploads/system/uploads/attachment_data/file/365629/making-decisions-opg606-1207.pdf

The examiner's mark sheet

Domain/ percentage of marks	Essential points to pass	✓	Extra marks/comments (make notes here)
1. Rapport and communication 20% of marks	Establishes rapport with anxious patient		
	Shows empathy and acknowledges patient's anxiety		
	Appropriate use of jargon-free language		
2. Demonstrates understanding of the principles of the Mental Capacity Act 30% of marks	Understanding relevant information and alternatives		
	Weighing the pros and cons of options		
	Arriving at a decision		
	Able to communicate the decision		

⇧ 3. Addressing concerns

20% of marks

Listens to the support worker

Acknowledges her worries and alleviates her anxiety

4. Able to assess Jen's capacity

20% of marks

Able to explore factors affecting mental capacity – level of LD

Rules out other psychiatric conditions and cognitive impairment as possible causes affecting mental capacity

5. Aware of limitations

10% of marks

Is mindful that this situation warrants complex discussions about medical complications – this will necessitate involving the medical colleagues in further discussion

% SCORE _____

___ **OVERALL IMPRESSION**

5 (CIRCLE ONE)

Good Pass

Pass

Borderline

Fail

Clear Fail

NOTES/Areas to improve

STATION 3: BEHAVIOURAL DISTURBANCE IN LD

INSTRUCTION TO CANDIDATE

This is Michael Stern. He is 18 years old, has a learning disability and lives at home with his parents. His mother is his main carer. He also attends a special school. Over the last few weeks, he has become significantly more aggressive. This is mainly focussed towards himself. He will bang his head repeatedly against the wall at home and he has been picking at his arms so that he has multiple skin lesions.

Assess this man and consider the important aetiological factors.

ACTOR (ROLE-PLAYER) INSTRUCTIONS

You are seeing the psychiatrist, whom you have never met. You are very reluctant to talk to him or her, but if they are empathic and allows you to speak slowly, you trust them. You have been feeling rough for a few weeks because other boys at school are making fun of your stuttering. You tend to stutter when anxious. You do not feel like talking about this to anyone, but when frustrated, you bang your head against the wall.

SUGGESTED APPROACH

Setting the scene

Introduce yourself normally – do not treat the patient like a child. 'Hello, I am Dr_____, nice to meet you. I have come to talk to you in order to understand if I can be of any help.' Do not appear patronising or be over-familiar with him. Treat him with respect and, if communication is difficult, adjust your style accordingly. Explain the assessment and inform him that his parents are worried about him. Allow him to speak and build a rapport.

Completing the tasks

History taking: ask simple questions, preferably short ones. Start with open-ended questions and progress on to more closed questions. Clarify what he understands about the situation: 'Your mum is worried about you – do you know why? How have things been recently? What happened to your arms? Why have you done this?'

Consider the aetiology using a bio-psycho-social approach and enquire about the following in a way that the patient can understand:

Psychiatric comorbidity (e.g. depression, bipolar disorder or psychosis). 'How have you been feeling lately? Have you had any ups and downs in your mood? Have you felt threatened? Have you felt suspicious? Do you feel safe? Have you heard anyone talk to you when there is nobody around?'

An organic disorder (e.g. epilepsy, hypothyroidism or urinary tract infection [UTI]). 'How is your health? Have you had any fits? Have you had any fevers or been unwell?'

Physical conditions (e.g. constipation, oesophagitis/gastritis, dental caries [with or without pain] or worsening sensory impairment [hearing/vision]). 'Are you in any pain? Are you in any discomfort at all? What about your eyesight? Do you hear well?'

Iatrogenic: medication – adverse effects (paradoxical agitation). 'Have you started taking any new medications?'

Substance misuse: alcohol, amphetamines, solvents and withdrawal states. 'Have you experimented with any drugs?'

Related to the disability itself: specific conditions are known to have an association with behavioural disturbance (e.g. Lesch–Nyhan syndrome, phenylketonuria, Cornelia de Lange syndrome, etc.); you may want to clarify this with the patient's GP.

Psychological

Look for evidence of emotional stress. Ask about familial relationships and recent stressors. Have there been arguments at home or school? Consider any behavioural component to the self-harm and any positive gain. This should not be assumed to be 'attention-seeking behaviour', but rather a way of communicating distress or unpleasant feelings. More appropriate ways of communicating are aspects that a psychologist could assist with. What about the work or school setting: is he being bullied or is he having any relationship difficulties?

Social

Enquire about close relationships. Has anyone close to the family or friend/staff member from school moved away? Has the daily routine changed? Has the patient recently moved home or has something changed at home?

Problem solving

This is a challenging station as you are attempting to take a history in a short period of time from someone who might not be forthcoming or who will be disturbed. The actor may be instructed to have slow or delayed answers to your questions, so patience is key, despite time pressures.

To help with communication, you should:

Use simply phrased questions and concepts

Use clear and direct language

Keep reassuring the patient throughout

Do not appear hurried or intimidating

Allow time for answers – do not worry about silence

Avoid jargon

Use an age-appropriate style and terminology

Use body language/gesturing as well as speech if necessary

Repeat questions if necessary

ADDITIONAL POINTS

Risk assessment: always consider the possibility of physical, emotional or sexual abuse in vulnerable individuals. Ask about the self-harm and head banging. Although such behaviours are likely to be related to frustration or distress, you need to enquire about suicidality and homicidal thoughts. Psychiatric illness is four-times as common in LD compared to the general population.

FURTHER READING

Emerson, E. (2001) *Challenging Behaviour: Analysis and Intervention in People with Severe Intellectual Disabilities*. 2nd edn. Cambridge: Cambridge University Press.

http://www.challengingbehaviour.org.uk

The Challenging Behaviour Foundation provides information and support to parents and carers of individuals with severe learning disabilities.

The examiner's mark sheet

Domain/ percentage of marks	Essential points to pass	✓	Extra marks/comments (make notes here)
1. Rapport and communication	Establishes rapport with LD patient		
20% of marks	Shows empathy and acknowledges patient's reluctance to speak		
	Appropriate use of jargon-free language		⇩

⇑ 2. History taking — Explores the chronology of events

    25% of marks — Elicits changes in behaviour

3. Aetiology – psychiatric conditions — Explores psychological causes of behavioural changes – anxiety, depression or psychosis

    25% of marks

4. Environmental and medical causes — Rules out other causes – pain, change in routine or changes in environment

    20% of marks

5. Risk assessment — Explores risk to self and risk of aggression to others

    10% of marks

% SCORE _____

___ **OVERALL IMPRESSION**

5 (CIRCLE ONE)

Good Pass

Pass

Borderline

Fail

Clear Fail

NOTES/Areas to improve

STATION 4: FRAGILE X SYNDROME

> ### INSTRUCTION TO CANDIDATE
>
> Mr Roberts and his wife have come to see you. They have noticed that their son, now 4, had been slow to speak compared to his peers. He seems to be clumsy and slower to learn in new situations. He was seen by the paediatricians and diagnosed with fragile X syndrome (FXS) following genetic testing. The parents have been referred to your unit for advice regarding his recent change in behaviour. They also want to know the risks of further children being born with this condition.
>
> **Meet them and address their queries.**

SUGGESTED APPROACH

Set the scene

Introduce yourself: 'Hello, my name is Dr_____, I'm one of the psychiatrists. Thank you for coming to see me today about your son. Can I ask his name?' Establish the purpose of this meeting: 'I understand that you've seen the paediatric doctors recently. Is that correct? Did they talk to you about his diagnosis?' Empathise with their difficult situation: 'It must be a worrying time for you since you found out about the diagnosis. Can I ask what you already know about fragile X syndrome?'

Completing the tasks

Remember to talk in lay terms and avoid medical jargon. You could briefly demonstrate to the examiner your understanding of the condition by asking when the parents first became concerned. Had they noticed any unusual physical characteristics? 'Sometimes parents are concerned that their children's ears seem bigger than expected or their child's face is large or longer. Are these things that you've noticed?'

In FXS, there is a problem with connective tissue development. Those with FXS can have double-jointedness or lax joints. The skin may be soft, with a velvety texture. Testicular enlargement in men after puberty can be striking. Explain that these physical changes occur with FXS, particularly in boys (up to 80%). The parents may be worried about his intelligence. You will have to explain that intelligence may be impaired, and 80% of boys will have an IQ of <70, which is the cut-off point for normal IQ.

Behaviour

The parents will be worried about his behavioural disturbances. Ask about his current behaviour. Take a history of what is happening, frequency, triggers, how long it lasts and what seems to settle him, if anything. Behaviour is often the presenting feature prior to a formal diagnosis. Enquire about the following:

Speech disturbance (FXS speech has been described as jocular or cluttered): 'Have you noticed anything unusual with his way of speaking?'

Attentional deficit: 'Is he able to concentrate on tasks for prolonged periods?'

Mannerisms (commonly involving the hands and flapping): 'Does he engage in any actions or mannerisms repeatedly?'

Autistic-like behaviour (accounts for perhaps 2%–3% of autism): 'Does he seem to be lost in his own world quite often? How does he interact with other children? What would you say about his social skills?'

Sensory defensiveness (avoids loud noises, bright lighting, touch and strong smells): 'Is he overly sensitive to loud noise, touch, brightness or strong smells?'

Emotional instability: 'Are there sudden periods of crying or emotional outbursts?'

Anxiety: 'How does he cope in unfamiliar situations?'

Management advice

A multidisciplinary approach (mental health services, school, social workers and voluntary agencies) is advised, and engagement with LD services is recommended.

Speech and language therapy

This can help with language development, impaired pronunciation and rate of speech. If speech is delayed, they can help teach non-verbal ways of communicating.

Occupational therapy

This can help to adjust tasks and conditions to match his needs and abilities. It can also help with sensory defensiveness by using appropriate stimulatory or calming activities in order to alter his responses to sensations.

Physiotherapy

This can help to improve motor control, posture and balance. At school, it can help a child who is easily overstimulated or who avoids body contact to take part in sports.

Psychology

Psychologists can assist by teaching parents or teachers to identify why a child acts in certain ways and how to prevent distressing situations, as well as teaching the child to cope with the distress.

Education

Psycho-education is for both the child and family. It is also important that the school understands that the child may have problems with auditory processing, concentration and abstract concepts.

Medication

Medication is used for behaviour when other interventions have been ineffective. Medication is not without risk of side effects and should be used cautiously. A proportion of children will need anticonvulsants for epilepsy, and these drugs can also help with behavioural and mood instability. Sometimes, different doses or combinations of medications are needed for maximum benefit. Stimulants such as methylphenidate can be of benefit where attention deficit or hyperactivity is pronounced. Similarly, aggression can be treated with mood stabilisers or antidepressants.

Risk to further child

FXS is the most common form of inherited intellectual disability. Although called FXS, the affected area is not fragile at all. It is an area where there is an abnormal expansion of DNA material on the long arm of the X chromosome. Men have one X chromosome and women have two X chromosomes. As such, this condition can affect both boys and girls.

As their son has the condition, he will have inherited the condition from his mother, as she has passed on her X chromosome. As the mother has the pre-mutation, she will have a 50% chance of passing it on to future sons and daughters.

You might suggest that formal genetic counselling is advisable if they are seriously considering more children. This service would be better able to advise on the chances of passing on the pre-mutation or full mutation. Without the results of the parental genetic tests, you would be unable to accurately predict this. Should their son have children in the future, he will pass on the mutation to all of his daughters, but to none of his sons.

Problem solving

It is important to consider the timescale of behavioural change. Enquire about other causes of this; for example, an underlying physical illness (UTI/pain), organic disorder (e.g. epilepsy) or concurrent mental illness.

Testing eyesight and hearing is essential. FXS is associated with short- and long-sightedness, squints and glue ear. These can aggravate speech and language problems and cause frustration.

ADDITIONAL POINTS

Follow-up and engagement with services is important in order to help the child as they develop. Epilepsy (20%), challenging behaviour and mood disorders occur more frequently after puberty.

FXS usually occurs with an expansion of the *FMR1* gene on the X chromosome through CGG trinucleotide repeats. In the full mutation, there are more than 200 repeats (normal <54).

The Fragile X Society (www.fragilex.org.uk) is a UK registered charity providing support, information and friendship to families whose children and relatives have fragile X syndrome.

FURTHER READING

Hagerman, R.J. & Hagerman, P.J. (eds) (2002) *Fragile X Syndrome – Diagnosis, Treatment and Research*. 3rd edn. Baltimore, MD: John Hopkins University Press.

The examiner's mark sheet

Domain/ percentage of marks	Essential points to pass	✓	Extra marks/comments (make notes here)
1. Rapport and communication 20% of marks	Establishes rapport with worried parents		
	Shows empathy and acknowledges their anxiety		
	Appropriate use of jargon-free language		
2. History taking 25% of marks	Explores the behavioural issues		
	Elicits the changes in behaviour		
3. Addressing concerns 30% of marks	Able to demonstrate knowledge of fragile X syndrome		
	Aetiology		
	Symptoms		
	Management		
4. Explores relevant concerns 25% of marks	Allows parents to ask their questions		
	Checks if they have understood the information		
	Seeks clarification		
	Offers written information and self-help strategies		
	Explains in simple terms		

% SCORE _____

OVERALL IMPRESSION

4 (CIRCLE ONE)

Good Pass

Pass

Borderline

Fail

Clear Fail

NOTES/Areas to improve

Chapter 8

Liaison psychiatry
Babu Mani

O LINKED STATIONS

STATION 1(a): PSYCHIATRIC LUPUS

INSTRUCTIONS TO CANDIDATE

You are a liaison psychiatrist. The rheumatologist has asked you to see a lady who has been diagnosed with Systemic Lupus Erythematosus (SLE) and antiphospholipid syndrome. Recent investigations including a magnetic resonance imaging (MRI) scan have indicated secondary small vessel disease.

She has been referred to you as she has become increasingly forgetful and reports that she frequently forgets where she was meant to be going when out driving her car.

Assess this lady's difficulties, carrying out any relevant brief cognitive testing.

ACTOR (ROLE-PLAYER) INSTRUCTIONS

You are Mrs Norah Jones and you are 62 years old.

You were diagnosed with SLE and antiphospholipid syndrome a year ago and you attend the rheumatology clinic regularly.

You have become forgetful in the last 6 months and you had a MRI scan done 3 weeks ago.

You have been driving for more than 40 years and you drive to the local supermarket every week to do your shopping. Your daughter lives 20 miles away and you drive every other weekend to see your grandchildren.

You have lost your way a few times and you are becoming more anxious about losing your way.

SUGGESTED APPROACH

Setting the scene

Begin the station by introducing yourself to the patient: 'Hello, Mrs_____, I am Dr_____, the psychiatrist. I have been asked by my colleagues to have a brief discussion with you about your difficulties. What is your understanding of this assessment?'

The candidate should make it clear that they are a psychiatrist and that the rheumatologists have asked for a second opinion. The candidate can begin the interview by informing the patient that they would like to ask her a few questions around her difficulties, including a few questions specifically testing her memory.

Completing the task

1. Take a brief history about:
   - Onset of difficulties, nature of difficulties and progression in the context of SLE. Other exacerbating factors – adjusting to diagnosis, stressful life events, financial concerns (e.g. secondary to loss of job).
   'Can you tell me a bit about your forgetfulness? How long you have noticed this? Has anyone else observed this? How has your memory changed?'
   - How have memory problems impacted on her functioning, including driving (e.g. does she need extra help with any activities of daily living and has she stopped work as a result)?
   'Have your daily activities changed due to changes in memory? Do you find yourself relying on others more than before?'
   - Screen for mood and anxiety disorders, psychotic symptoms, drug and alcohol use and other previous psychiatric history. Current medications – is she taking an antidepressant?
   'How do you generally feel in yourself? Have you been worrying lately?'

2. Brief risk assessment – including risk to self and driving. Communicate concerns regarding driving to patient. 'Have things ever been so bad that you considered ending your life? Have you noted any difficulties in driving? Have you had any accidents or near-misses?'

3. Perform brief cognitive testing.
   - Mini-mental state examination (MMSE) plus frontal lobe tests
   - If time permits, tailor to history: additional simple questions (e.g. knowledge of recent news events/current affairs, drawing a clock face, parietal lobe tests, etc.)

4. Thank the patient and conclude the station. 'I am pleased we could meet and discuss these issues. I have tried to assess your memory changes today and hopefully we can meet soon to discuss how we can go about helping you further. Until then, I think it is safest for you not to drive.' If there are any positive findings from cognitive assessment, explain them to the patient and advise on further neuropsychological tests.

ADDITIONAL POINTS

1. This station should be handled in the same way as assessing memory problems in any other context (e.g. old age psychiatry). It is important to ensure that a functional psychiatric illness, such as depression, is not masquerading as memory disturbance. Underlying vascular disease in the brain may also predispose to secondary mood and psychotic disorders.

2. The Driver and Vehicle Licensing Agency (DVLA) has issued fairly clear guidelines on driving for a number of conditions. https://www.gov.uk/guidance/assessing-fitness-to-drive-a-guide-for-medical-professionals

The examiner's mark sheet

Domain/ percentage of marks	Essential points to pass	✓	Extra marks/comments (make notes here)
1. Rapport and communication 20% of marks	Clear communication		
	Open and closed questions		
	Empathy		
	Demonstrating patience		

⇧ 2. History taking   Elicits history relating to
    20% of marks   cognitive domain dysfunction

3. Cognitive tests   Able to perform relevant
   20% of marks   cognitive tests

4. Conclusion   Able to provide feedback to
   20% of marks   patient following assessment
                         and offer reassurance

5. Risk assessment   Identifies risk of driving and gives
   20% of marks   appropriate advice on driving

% SCORE _____   ___ **OVERALL IMPRESSION**

                                   5   (CIRCLE ONE)

                                        Good Pass

                                        Pass

                                        Borderline

                                        Fail

                                        Clear Fail

                                        NOTES/Areas to improve

STATION 1(b): SLE – DISCUSSION WITH RHEUMATOLOGIST

INSTRUCTION TO CANDIDATE

You have spoken to Mrs Jones in a previous task. The rheumatologist is interested to know your thoughts following your assessment.

Discuss this case with the referring practitioner and discuss how you think this lady should be managed from a psychiatric point of view.

ACTOR (ROLE-PLAYER) INSTRUCTIONS

You are a consultant rheumatologist and you have been following up Mrs Norah Jones in your clinic.

You have recently reviewed Mrs Jones in your clinic and you are satisfied that her SLE is under control.

You are concerned about her memory difficulties and worried that she may be developing dementia.

You would like to know what further investigations are required and want to know the management plan.

You feel that she should be prescribed anti-dementia medication and would like to know the psychiatrist's thoughts.

SUGGESTED APPROACH

Setting the scene

Introduce yourself: 'Hello, Dr_____, I am Dr_____, the psychiatrist. I have seen your patient Mrs Jones; as you know, she has been worried about her memory. Shall we discuss about how we proceed?'

Completing the task

1. Discuss your main findings and likely differential diagnosis for memory changes (depression, medication-related, organic hypothyroidism or vascular changes in brain).

2. Discuss management and further investigations.

3. Discuss the issue of driving and the DVLA.

Further investigations to be considered include:

Biological investigations: urine drug screen (if not already carried out by referrer), dementia screen-B12/folate/ thyroid function tests (TFTs), other vascular risk factors and relevant neuroimaging.

Psychological investigations: formal neuropsychological assessment/testing. Objective rating scales for mood (e.g. Beck's Depressive Inventory both pre- and post-treatment with an antidepressant).

Social investigations: collateral history from a family member or friend would be extremely important to obtain. Consider occupational therapy assessment. Objective rating scales (e.g. Global Assessment of Functioning) might also be used.

Management:

Rh: What do you suggest as further course of action?

C: The history and examination suggest that this lady may be suffering from comorbid depression. I would like to treat the depression, and suggest that she should have her memory and mood reassessed at a suitable time point (e.g. 2–3 months). I would like to follow this patient up frequently in the initial stages of treatment.

Suitable treatment might include a selective serotonin reuptake inhibitor (SSRI; although note contraindications with increased risk of gastrointestinal bleed if prescribed aspirin for pro-thrombotic tendencies) or other antidepressants such as mirtazapine or venlafaxine. Other possibilities might include psychological interventions (cognitive behavioural therapy [CBT]), although underlying cognitive impairment may limit how far the patient is able to take part in this therapy. She may benefit from supportive counselling if she is finding it difficult to adjust to the diagnosis. Simple aids could be suggested to help with her memory problems (e.g. dosette box for medications, a diary and wall clock with date for appointments, calendars and alarms).

As this is a liaison psychiatry station, how the candidate discusses these possibilities with the referrer will be assessed.

Rh: What about her driving?

C: I am concerned about this lady continuing to drive at this point in time, as she appears to have greatly impaired recent memory, and this could impact on her judgement. I would suggest that she stops driving for now, and that she could be referred for further neuropsychological testing, which may inform medical recommendations to the DVLA. She should also inform her insurers. The issue of driving could be revisited after her depressive illness has been adequately treated and her memory problems have been reassessed. If she can demonstrate that her skills are sufficiently retained and that the progression of the underlying brain impairment is slow, she may be able to drive subject to annual review/a formal driving assessment.

FURTHER READING

DVLA (2007) For medical practitioners: At a glance guide to the current medical standards of fitness to drive. http://www.dvla.gov.uk/media/pdf/medical/aagv1.pdf

Taylor, D., Paton, C. & Kerwin, R. (2007) *The Maudsley Prescribing Guidelines*, 9th edn. London: Informa Health Care.

The examiner's mark sheet

Domain/ percentage of marks	Essential points to pass	✓	Extra marks/comments (make notes here)
1. Rapport and communication 20% of marks	Clear communication Being professional to the colleague Being focussed and effectively communicating		
2. Explaining diagnosis and differentials 20% of marks	Demonstrates knowledge of common causes of memory loss		
3. Investigations 20% of marks	Demonstrates knowledge of wide variety of aetiologies of memory loss and considers relevant investigations		
4. Management 20% of marks	Demonstrates knowledge of treatment of pseudo-dementia and memory loss		
5. Driving and DVLA 20% of marks	Able to recognise risks of driving, refers to DVLA guidance and makes appropriate risk management plan		

% SCORE _____

___

5

OVERALL IMPRESSION

(CIRCLE ONE)

Good Pass

Pass

Borderline

Fail

Clear Fail

NOTES/Areas to improve

STATION 2(a): CAPACITY TO CONSENT

INSTRUCTION TO CANDIDATE

You are asked to urgently see a young man who has stabbed himself and is refusing surgical treatment. The wound has been bandaged; however, the surgeons wish to take him to theatre and perform life-saving surgery, without which they feel he might die. His mother reports that over the last year he has become more reclusive and withdrawn. In accident and emergency (A&E), he is mute and does not answer any of your questions.

Take a history from this gentleman's mother and assess his capacity regarding consent to medical treatment.

You may wish to take notes as you will be asked to discuss his likely differential diagnosis and management with his brother at the next station.

ACTOR (ROLE-PLAYER) INSTRUCTIONS

You are the mother of Adam Smith who has been brought to hospital after he stabbed himself.

You are worried that he is refusing treatment and the surgeon has told you that without treatment, he will die.

You want him to have the surgery and want the surgical team to proceed.

Your son had been quiet and reclusive over the past year and he hardly goes out of the house.

You have been trying to get him to be seen by the mental health team.

Your son had become 'mute' over the last week and has not been eating and drinking properly.

Your son went through a divorce a year ago and his ex-wife has moved to Australia with their 6-year-old son – Adam was very close to his son.

SUGGESTED APPROACH

Setting the scene

Introduce yourself and explain the purpose of your visit: 'Hello, Mrs＿＿＿, I am Dr＿＿＿, the psychiatrist. I can imagine how difficult this situation is for you. I have seen your son and he is mute. I would appreciate it if I can gather some information from you about him.'

This is a difficult situation, and you can say so as part of your opening introduction. Make attempts to establish rapport with the patient and the mother. Despite the gravity of the situation, you should assume that the patient has capacity unless you are able to prove otherwise.

Completing the task

1. Take a brief history about what happened. As the patient is not communicating at this stage, this should be done through the family member.
   • Clarify age of patient.
   • Circumstances leading to the current presentation: 'How was your son found, what events preceded him stabbing himself?'

- Onset and nature of any mental health difficulties preceding the attempt by the patient to stab himself: 'Was there a clear change in his mental state or routine functioning noted over the preceding days/months?'
- Is there a preceding history of potential prodromal features to a psychotic episode (e.g. social withdrawal, decline in functioning, apathy/loss of drive or odd behaviour)?
- Is there a possible preceding history of a mood disorder (stressful life events or history of affective symptoms/biological features of depression) noted by mother?
- History of previous bizarre behaviour or bizarre beliefs expressed to/noted by mother: is there a possible prior history of auditory hallucinations?
- Is there a previous psychiatric history, including previous attempts to harm self? Concerns by family member as to his self-harm/suicide risk?
- Is there a family history of psychosis, suicide or depression?
- Is there a history of illicit substance misuse/dependency (cannabis, cocaine, etc.) or alcohol misuse or dependency?
- Is there any forensic history of note?

2. Assess the patient's mental state and capacity to accept or decline treatment.
   - Mental state examination in this station will be merely an observation as you will not be able to communicate with the patient. It may be worth noting if he appears to be responding to internal stimuli (e.g. auditory or visual hallucinations) and you may wish to examine him, if appropriate, for associated catatonic features.
   - In this station, the patient is mute and will not be able to communicate with you either verbally or otherwise; however, you must show that you have made attempts to adequately communicate with the patient, and you may wish to check this with his relative.
   - You may wish to check with his mother if her son has any pre-existing religious or cultural beliefs which might have affected his decision (e.g. Jehovah's witness/blood products, etc.).

3. Turn to the patient's mother and summarise your findings and likely diagnosis.
   - Given the history and the patient's presentation (which represents a clear change in mental state indicative of an underlying mental disorder, which you will elaborate upon in the next station), it is likely that on *balance of probabilities*, this patient lacks the capacity to consent to treatment for his injury.
   - You should explain to his mother that, given the urgency of the situation (life threatening), the medical team should be advised to act in his best interests; however, his capacity will need to be reassessed once his medical condition has been adequately managed.

ADDITIONAL POINTS

1. Candidate should explain that as this is a life-threatening situation, measures should be taken to act in the patient's best interests; however, his capacity for any further interventions should be reassessed when he has had treatment for the injury.

2. The history and clinical presentation noted in this station should allow you to summarise the likely differential diagnosis and likely management to the examiner in the next station. The marks awarded in this station are mostly for history taking, brief risk assessment, difficult communication and brief case discussion (with the patient's mother).

3. The general principles regarding the assessment of capacity still apply.[1] Based on the history, it seems likely that the gentleman has an impairment or disturbance of the mind which, at present, makes him unable to make a decision regarding surgical treatment and may

be affecting his ability to weigh up and use information as part of the decision-making process. However, he is unable to communicate directly with you, and so you have been unable to directly assess whether he has fulfilled the basic functional tests of capacity: (a) does he understand all of the relevant information; (b) can he retain that information; (c) can he use or weigh up that information as part of the decision-making process; and (d) can he communicate his decision? Based on a balance of probabilities, you may argue that this gentleman at present lacks capacity regarding potential surgical treatment, and that a decision will need to be taken in his best interests.

REFERENCE

1. Booklets on all aspects of the Mental Capacity Act can be downloaded from http://www.dca.gov.uk/legal-policy/mental-capacity/publications.htm#mental

The examiner's mark sheet

Domain/ percentage of marks	Essential points to pass	✓	Extra marks/comments (make notes here)
1. Rapport and communication 25% of marks	Clear communication Open and closed questions Empathy towards mother Demonstrating patience and attempting to establish rapport with mute patient		
2. History taking 25% of marks	Elicits relevant collateral history from mother regarding any underlying mental illness		
3. Capacity assessment 25% of marks	Demonstrates the principles of MCA		
4. Feedback to mother 25% of marks	Concludes the findings to mother, summarises action plan and explains the rationale		

% SCORE _____

___ **OVERALL IMPRESSION**

4 (CIRCLE ONE)

Good Pass

Pass

Borderline

Fail

Clear Fail

NOTES/Areas to improve

STATION 2(b): DISCUSSION WITH RELATIVE

INSTRUCTION TO CANDIDATE

The patient, Adam Smith, whom you assessed, has been admitted to the surgical ward. His brother has come from Spain and would like to talk to you about Adam's likely psychiatric diagnosis and treatment. He is worried about the risk to him if he were to go home from the surgical ward.

Assume that the gentleman is happy for you to communicate with his brother. You do not need to assess his capacity to consent to psychiatric treatment. Speak to patient's brother and address his concerns.

ACTOR (ROLE-PLAYER) INSTRUCTIONS

You are Gavin Smith and you are the brother of Adam.

You live in Spain with your wife and two daughters. You have been concerned about your brother for the past year ever since his divorce.

Adam is a very outgoing person, but in the last 6 months, he has not been going out at all.

Adam used to ring you every week, but you have not heard from him for the past 6 months.

You have heard from your mother that he has lost 4 stone of weight. He has not been sleeping and has been neglecting himself.

You are grateful to the psychiatrist for his/her help with surgical treatment. You would like to know what is going to happen next.

SUGGESTED APPROACH

Setting the scene

Introduce yourself again to the patient's brother: 'Hello, I am Dr_____, glad we could meet. Hopefully I can be of help regarding your brother.' The actor playing the role of the mother may initiate the discussion by explaining her concerns. You may therefore wish to start this station with a fairly open statement.

Completing the task

1. Discuss the likely differential diagnosis (e.g. first episode psychosis/paranoid schizophrenia, depression or drug-induced psychosis): 'There are quite a few conditions that may be underlying his presentation. He could be having a psychotic episode, depressive disorder or there is a possibility that his presentation could be related to illicit drugs.'

2. Further investigations might include:
   - Biological – urine drug screen (note recent NICE[1] recommendations which have concluded that neuroimaging should not be a routine investigation in psychosis unless other organic causes are suspected), basic bloods including thyroid function tests and assessment of alcohol withdrawal if appropriate.
   - Psychological – objective rating scales (e.g. Brief Psychiatric Rating Scale [BPRS]/Beck Depression Inventory [BDI] if communicative).

- Social – further collateral history from other relatives/partner/other agencies (e.g. if has children).

3. Risk: the brother may be worried about further discharge plans from hospital. Obtain further history from the brother regarding relevant risk areas (risk to self, risk of self-neglect and risk of aggression) and elicit whether he has any other concerns around his risk and why he is concerned about him if he were to go home.
   - Risk to self (self-harm) – previous self-harm or suicide attempts. Did he express his wish to harm himself to anyone beforehand, or was he secretive/attempted to avoid being found after he stabbed himself?
   - Risk to self (self-neglect) – had he been eating and drinking adequately/any concerns about oral intake and weight loss? Any concerns over his personal care?
   - Risk from others – had his brother been concerned about his vulnerability of exploitation from others?
   - Risk to others – any associated forensic history. Has he ever attempted to harm anyone else? Has he ever expressed a wish to harm others? Does he have children? Are the children on the child protection register?

4. Management:
   - You should explain that once he is medically stable, you will want to reassess his mental state and consent to psychiatric treatment. You may have to consider an assessment under the Mental Health Act, with a view to an admission for a period of assessment. However, you would need to check if he is willing to accept treatment informally first.
   - Management (in short term): you may wish to consider medication (e.g. commencing an atypical neuroleptic at the doses recommended by NICE guidelines)[2]; one-to-one registered mental health nurse (RMN) input on surgical ward, given ongoing concerns regarding possible harm to himself; possibly suggest assessment under Section 5(2) of the Mental Health Act to surgical team if he attempts to leave and they are concerned about his risk to himself or his safety.
   - Management (in longer term)[2]: referral to first onset psychosis team or community mental health team and consider Care Programme Approach. Monitor response to medication/side effects and titrate dose accordingly, provide support/referral to services for any substance misuse issues if appropriate, family therapy (if family agreeable), CBT or other psychological approaches if it was felt that he would be able to work with this model of therapy. Consider longer-term support for social skills – assistance with employment, further education goals, housing and benefits, etc.

ADDITIONAL POINTS

1. The vignette indicates that risk assessment is an important part of this station and will influence your subsequent management plan.

2. Biological, psychological and social approaches should be considered when thinking about the investigation and management of this patient.

REFERENCES

1. NICE (2008) Structural neuro-imaging in first episode psychosis. http://www.nice.nhs.uk/nicemedia/pdf/TA136Guidance.pdf

2. NICE (2002) Schizophrenia: Core interventions in the treatment and management of schizophrenia in primary and secondary care. Clinical guideline 1. http://www.nice.nhs.uk/nicemedia/pdf/CG1NICEguideline.pdf

The examiner's mark sheet

Domain/ percentage of marks	Essential points to pass	✓	Extra marks/comments (make notes here)
1. Rapport and communication 20% of marks	Clear communication Open and closed questions Empathy Demonstrating patience with worried relative		
2. History taking 20% of marks	Elicits necessary collateral history to ascertain mental health condition		
3. Risk assessment 20% of marks	Performs adequate risk assessment on relevant topics		
4. Management 20% of marks	Demonstrates bio-psycho-social approach to further investigations and management		
5. Addressing concerns 20% of marks	Able to offer advice and address the questions of worried relative		

% SCORE _____

___
5

OVERALL IMPRESSION
(CIRCLE ONE)

Good Pass

Pass

Borderline

Fail

Clear Fail

NOTES/Areas to improve

STATION 3(a): CONVERSION DISORDER – HISTORY TAKING

INSTRUCTION TO CANDIDATE

You are asked to provide an opinion on 25-year-old Jane Smith, referred by the neurologists as she has become wheelchair bound and is no longer able to walk over the last 6 months. All neurological investigations, including detailed neuroimaging, have been reported as normal. She was the passenger in a tragic car accident 6 months previously in which her mother, who was the passenger, was killed.

> **Take a history from this lady. Conduct a mental state examination of this lady, eliciting any abnormal psychopathology.**
>
> **You may wish to take notes as you will be asked to discuss this case in the next station.**

ACTOR (ROLE-PLAYER) INSTRUCTIONS

You are Ms Jane Smith and you have 'not been able to walk' for the past 6 months.

You were involved in a car accident 6 months ago – you lost control of the car and the car hit a tree at a high speed.

Your mother was killed in the accident.

You developed 'paralysis' of the lower limbs following the accident – you had to miss the funeral of your mother as you were in the hospital because of 'paralysis'.

You are frustrated with the neurologist as they have not been able to find the 'cause'.

You are upset that you have to see a psychiatrist – people can clearly see that you 'cannot walk' and you are disappointed that there is a suggestion that 'it is all in your mind'.

Your father is very supportive.

You are depressed that you are not getting better and you are hoping that the neurologist will soon be able to find out the cause of the problem.

SUGGESTED APPROACH

Setting the scene

Begin the station by explaining that you have been asked by your neurology colleagues to provide an opinion on this lady's difficulties. Introduce yourself: 'Hello, Ms_____, I am Dr_____, the psychiatrist. I am here to see you at the request of neurologists to see if I can be of any help.' Start off by asking her what her difficulties are and why she believes she has been referred to see you.

The candidate should make it clear that they are a psychiatrist and that the neurologists have asked for a second opinion. The candidate can begin the interview by informing the patient that they would like to ask her a few questions around her difficulties.

Completing the task

1. Take a brief history
   - Demonstrate an empathic and sensitive approach to the patient, especially when exploring aspects of the accident with her. Elicit from the patient and her father whether they were in agreement with the referral or whether they feel that there is an underlying undiagnosed physical cause. 'What do you think about seeing a psychiatrist?'
   - Nature of difficulties and onset and chronology with respect to the accident. 'How did your problems with walking begin?'
   - Other aspects of history: previous psychiatric or medical history, drug and alcohol use, prior premorbid functioning, previous childhood abuse, previous medical illnesses in childhood/time off school, illnesses in parents, long periods of sickness, current familial/social support, pending litigation, potential secondary gain from

disability/the consequences of recovery versus ongoing disability and current input (e.g. physiotherapy) for her difficulties. 'Have you suffered period of ill health before? What was going on then? How do you see your situation now? Is there anything else worrying you?'

- Her view of the difficulties. What does she think is causing her mobility problems? What is her view on treatment; specifically, what is her view on psychological therapies? What is her view for the future? Does she think she can ever get better or does she view herself as permanently disabled?
- What has she been told by other medical practitioners? Has she had all of the results of investigations explained to her? Does she feel reassured that neuroimaging and other investigations have been reported as normal?
- Mental state examination: ensure that no abnormal or psychotic beliefs are apparent. Exclude depressive and anxiety symptomatology. Ensure that no symptoms that are indicative of an atypical grief reaction are present.

2. Thank the lady and conclude the discussion by briefly summarising your findings to her and her father. Address any concerns which she or her father may have. 'From the discussion we have had, I understand your walking became affected rather suddenly after the tragic accident. Sometimes extreme shock can put a lot of stress on our mind, and this can get "converted" into physical health symptoms. Have you considered that this could be related to your mind?'

ADDITIONAL POINTS

Dissociative motor disorders are classically associated 'with traumatic events, insoluble and intolerable problems, or disturbed relationships', and have a psychogenic origin.[1] Patients may show a 'striking denial' of obvious problems or difficulties, despite these being fairly apparent to observers, and may attribute distress to the resulting disability instead.[1] Calm acceptance of disability ('la *belle indifference*') may also be apparent,[1] although is not necessary for diagnosis and may be present in only 6%–41% of patients.[2] For a diagnosis of a dissociative motor disorder, it should be possible to make a clear psychological formulation of why the patient is presenting in this way at this time.[1]

Dissociative disorders frequently present with other comorbid psychiatric conditions, with comorbid mood and anxiety disorders reported in up to 80% and comorbid personality disorders also frequently reported.[3] Candidates should ensure that they have screened for other functional comorbidities, as the presence of these will influence management decisions, as discussed in the next station.

Explaining your thoughts to the patient and her father may on the surface appear difficult. However, a collaborative and flexible approach (suggested by Bass & May, 2002) when assessing patients with multiple functional somatic symptoms may also be relevant here[4]; for example, interview cues such as 'I wonder if you've thought of it like this?'[4] or making tentative 'reframing' links between the trauma and the onset/temporal sequence of the symptoms may be helpful to the patient.[4]

In an ideal situation, you would have at least an hour (and possibly further interviews) when seeing a patient like this, so you may also wish to conclude the interview by indicating that you would like to see them again, with more time in hand to explore some of the difficult issues touched upon in this very brief review.

REFERENCES

1. WHO (1992) *The ICD-10 Classification of Mental and Behavioural Disorders: Clinical Descriptions and Diagnostic Guidelines*. Geneva: WHO Press.

2. Brown, R.J. (2006) Dissociation and conversion in psychogenic illness. In: Hallett, M., Fahn, S., Jankovic, J., Lang, A.E., Cloninger, C.R. & Yudofsky, S.C. (eds) *Psychogenic Movement Disorders: Neurology and Neuropsychiatry*. Philadelphia, PA: AAN Press.

3. Ovsiew, F. (2006) An overview of the psychiatric approach to conversions disorder. In: Hallett, M., Fahn, S., Jankovic, J., Lang, A.E., Cloninger, C.R. & Yudofsky, S.C. (eds) *Psychogenic Movement Disorders: Neurology and Neuropsychiatry*. Philadelphia, PA: AAN Press.

4. Bass, C. & May, S. (2002) Clinical review: ABC of psychological medicine. Chronic multiple functional somatic symptoms. *BMJ, 325*, 323–6.

The examiner's mark sheet

Domain/ percentage of marks	Essential points to pass	✓	Extra marks/comments (make notes here)
1. Rapport and communication 25% of marks	Clear communication Open and closed questions Empathy Demonstrating patience		
2. History taking 25% of marks	Chronology of symptoms Denial Previous psycho-social stressors during childhood Any chronic illness in family Perception of illness Any secondary gain		
3. Comorbidities 25% of marks	Explores coexisting depression, anxiety or psychosis		
4. Feedback 25% of marks	Able to conclude sensitively the findings and likely dissociative motor disorder and explain diagnosis to patient		

% SCORE _____

_____ **OVERALL IMPRESSION**

4 (CIRCLE ONE)

Good Pass

Pass

Borderline

Fail

Clear Fail

NOTES/Areas to improve

STATION 3(b): CONVERSION DISORDER – EXPLANATION

INSTRUCTION TO CANDIDATE

You are going to see Mr Edward Smith, father of Jane Smith. He would like to know what is going on with his daughter. He would like to discuss possible treatment and future prognosis with you.

Discuss your findings with him and outline the investigations, treatments and prognosis for this lady.

ACTOR (ROLE-PLAYER) INSTRUCTIONS

You are Edward Smith and you are the father of Jane Smith who has been 'paralysed' from the waist down since the car accident 6 months ago in which your wife was killed.

The neurologist has told you that all of the investigations are normal and that the cause of the problem is 'psychological'.

You cannot understand that such a serious problem could all be 'in her mind'.

You are trying to support your daughter as much as you can.

You are worried that your daughter is depressed and that she feels responsible for your wife's death.

You would like to know what your daughter is suffering from and the treatment options.

SUGGESTED APPROACH

Setting the scene

Begin this station by introducing yourself to the father. You may want to acknowledge the difficulties that Jane and her father have been going through in the last 6 months. 'Hello, Mr_____, I am Dr_____, I gather you would like to discuss your daughter's health problems with me.'

Completing the task

1. Discuss your main findings and likely differential diagnosis.
   - The history and examination suggest that this lady is suffering from a fairly clear dissociative motor disorder. 'I think Jane is suffering from what we call dissociative motor disorder. It is a condition in which, following severe psychological trauma, the mental distress can present as physical symptoms, in this case, as paralysis of limbs.'[1]
   - You should highlight whether or not you thought there was any other psychiatric comorbidity present, such as major depression, anxiety or substance misuse.
   - You may inform aspects of the history in support of this diagnosis.

2. Discuss further investigations and management.
   'Ideally, I would like to gather more information from you and Jane, following which I shall be looking at certain routine investigations.'
   - You may inform the father that this is a complicated presentation and you would usually want more time to conduct the assessment, and that part of your plan might be to review this lady and her father again in order to gain further information.

- You should discuss management with him in the same way as for other stations:

Biological investigations: obtain confirmation that there is no comorbid history of illicit substance misuse, possibly by obtaining a urine drug screen, and check routine blood tests, including vitamin levels, and ensure that these are normal. You may want to specify thyroid function tests to exclude underlying endocrine abnormalities.

Psychological investigations: psychological rating scales such as the BDI[2] or the Hospital Anxiety and Depression Rating Scale[3] are useful for objective measures of depression or anxiety. If she is clinically depressed, the BDI can also be used to monitor response to treatment.

Social investigations: suggest that you would like to obtain further collateral medical and social history from this lady's GP. You may want to explore this lady's social network and premorbid role/social functioning in further detail at the next review (this may provide clues of other unconscious motives).

Management: 'The management of this condition is a combination of medications and psychological help. Psychotropic medications are indicated if Jane is depressed or anxious. Psychological therapies will address any unhelpful thinking patterns that Jane may have regarding her situation, and will help her to modify some of this thinking and these behavioural patterns. We will try to help her social situation, and if she wishes, we shall liaise with her employer.'

Medical: treat a depressive/anxiety disorder if there is evidence of this on mental status examination and suggest an SSRI as appropriate. She may need a referral to physiotherapy if there is evidence of atrophy of leg muscles, and input from the physiotherapist may also include a programme of graded exercise.[4]

Psychological: cognitive behavioural therapy may be appropriate if she can demonstrate the ability to fruitfully use this approach and is keen to consider this. Bereavement counselling may be appropriate if there are unresolved grief issues related to the accident. You may also want to suggest suitable literature or self-help books, and suggest patient/user groups for added support.[4] It may be important to involve the patient's father/social network in any programme of psychological therapy, especially if secondary gain has become prominent (e.g. in supporting the family to allow the patient to become independent of maintaining a passive/dependent role).[4]

Social: this should be tailored to her social circumstances. If at all possible, return to work/education, which may play an important part in longer-term rehabilitation, although in some cases work may be another form of stress to the patient and could impede rehabilitation.[4]

3. Give an indication of longer-term follow-up and prognosis.
   'Usually, dissociative disorders can be difficult to manage, although positive factors relating to her prognosis include clear onset following a psychological stressor, good premorbid functioning and family/social support networks, as well as a recent onset with short associated history.'[4]

ADDITIONAL POINTS

As this section focusses on management, it may be fruitful to divide up aetiology into 'predisposing', 'precipitating' and 'maintaining' factors and suggest strategies to deal with each using a bio-psycho-social framework.

REFERENCES

1. Bass, C. & May, S. (2002) Clinical review: ABC of psychological medicine. Chronic multiple functional somatic symptoms. *BMJ*, 325, 323–6.

2. Beck, A.T., Ward, C.H., Mendelson, M., Mock, J. & Erbaugh, J. (1961) An inventory for measuring depression. *Archives of General Psychiatry, 4*(6), 561–571.

3. Zigmond, A.S. & Snaith, R.P. (1983) The Hospital Anxiety and Depression Rating Scale. *Acta Psychiatrica Scandinavica, 67*, 361–70.

4. Gill, D. & Bass, C. (1997) Somatoform and dissociative disorders: Assessment and treatment. *Advances in Psychiatric Treatment, 3*, 9–16.

The examiner's mark sheet

Domain/ percentage of marks	Essential points to pass	✓	Extra marks/comments (make notes here)
1. Rapport and communication 25% of marks	Clear communication Open and closed questions Empathy Demonstrating patience with distressed relative		
2. Explanation 25% of marks	Able to explain complex psychological condition to non-medical person		
3. Management 25% of marks	Demonstrates knowledge of management of conversion disorder Uses a bio-psycho-social approach		
4. Addressing concerns 25% of marks	Able to have discussion about prognosis Addresses concerns of relative		

% SCORE _____

___   **OVERALL IMPRESSION**

4   (CIRCLE ONE)

Good Pass

Pass

Borderline

Fail

Clear Fail

NOTES/Areas to improve

STATION 4(a): ALCOHOL WITHDRAWAL – COLLATERAL HISTORY

INSTRUCTION TO CANDIDATE

You are a liaison psychiatrist. The surgical team asks you to come and see an elderly gentleman who was admitted 2 days ago with a fractured right femur. He underwent an emergency surgery. Post-operatively, he has presented as 'confused' and uncooperative. His wife is by his bedside and is fairly concerned; she reports that he has a significant history of alcohol use. He has not yet been commenced on any treatment, as the surgical team were not aware of his alcohol use.

Take a history from the gentleman's wife. You may want to take notes as in the next station you will be asked to discuss your findings and management.

ACTOR (ROLE-PLAYER) INSTRUCTIONS

You are Mrs Mary Stuart and your husband Mr John Stuart was admitted following a fall and sustaining right-sided hip fracture. He had to undergo an emergency surgery.

You are concerned that he has been confused since the admission to hospital.

You are concerned that his condition is going to deteriorate unless he cooperates with the treatment.

Your husband did not have any memory problems prior to the admission.

Mr Stuart 'likes his drink' and drinks a bottle of wine every day.

You want her husband to get better soon and get back home as soon as possible.

SUGGESTED APPROACH

Setting the scene

Introduce yourself to the patient's wife. Begin by explaining that you have been asked by the surgical team to provide an opinion on her husband's confusion. 'Hello, Mrs_____, I am Dr_____, the psychiatrist. I have been asked to see your husband. I gather he had an unfortunate fall and underwent surgery.'

Completing the task

The task here is to take a collateral history from the wife to ascertain the most likely diagnosis. You know that the patient is a regular drinker. So, aside from focussing on alcohol use, you should also enquire after other possible causes of her husband's confusional state. Clues to the diagnosis will be apparent by getting a clear picture of his premorbid functioning, as well as onset of the current presentation and reported psychopathology. The vignette suggests that alcohol use is an important part of the presentation and so you should ensure that you leave enough time to take an adequate alcohol history.

History taking

1. Take a corroborative history from the gentleman's wife.
   - When did she first notice that he was more confused? Was his confusional state fairly sudden/acute in onset (onset pre- or post-operative)?
   - Clarify from his wife in what way is he 'confused' (e.g. disorientated, paranoid, not recognising her, memory difficulties or confabulation). Is there evidence of nighttime confusion or of agitation? Is there evidence of clouding of consciousness/sensorium? Are there tactile disturbances?[1]

- Has he been hallucinating (visual [e.g. Lilliputian or insects] or auditory hallucinations)? Have there been any concerns regarding his behaviour (e.g. agitation or anxiety)? Is there a tremor? Is he sweating?[1]
- Is there a previous history of medical or psychiatric comorbidity? Is he prescribed any medication? Is there a previous history of admission for alcohol detoxification/input from alcohol detoxification services? Is there a history of psychiatric service involvement? Is there a previous history of delirium tremens or severe alcohol withdrawal/alcohol withdrawal-related seizures? Is there a history of (other) illicit substance misuse?
- Premorbid functioning: is there a pre-existing history of memory problems/cognitive impairment? What was his level of functioning prior to admission – was this affected by his alcohol use and/or memory problems? Was there a premorbid history of apathy, increased dependency on wife for activities of daily living, etc., prior to admission?

Alcohol history

- When was his last drink (NB signs of alcohol withdrawal peak within 24–48 hours)?[2]
- Current (pre-admission) alcohol use (drinks every day or days off from alcohol use?); what is his current pattern of use, what time does he usually have his first drink and how much is his average daily intake (units)? Has there been evidence of narrowing of drinking repertoire?[3]
- Does she think he has problems controlling onset, levels and termination of use? Does he crave alcohol? Does he ever drink to blackout? At home, is he secretive with respect to his alcohol use? Does he drink to the detriment of other interests/activities? Have there been any medical, psychological or social consequences to him from alcohol use? Does he continue to drink despite this? Is there evidence of tolerance? Has his wife ever noted features of alcohol withdrawal?
- Does she know how old he was when he first started to drink and when his alcohol use first started to escalate? Has he had any periods of abstinence or input from Alcoholics Anonymous?

ADDITIONAL POINTS

1. The primary diagnosis should be severe alcohol withdrawal or alcohol withdrawal-associated confusional state ('delirium tremens') on a background of alcohol dependence.[2] This is a life-threatening condition associated with convulsions.[1] Delirium tremens is characterised by clouding of sensorium or acute confusional state, tactile disturbances, auditory and visual hallucinations, agitation and severe tremor.[1] Also be vigilant for a possible diagnosis of Wernicke's encephalopathy, characterised by a classic triad of confusion, ataxia and ophthalmoplegia.[4] It is more common than is usually thought and is frequently missed or undertreated.[4] All patients presenting with severe alcohol withdrawal should always be treated with parenteral thiamine.[1,2]

2. For a diagnosis of alcohol dependence (F10.2) according to ICD-10, there should be evidence of the presence of a 'cluster of behavioural, cognitive, and physiological phenomena that develop after repeated substance use and that typically include a strong desire to take the drug, difficulties in controlling its use, persisting in its use despite harmful consequences, a higher priority given to drug use than to other activities and obligations, increased tolerance, and sometimes a physical withdrawal state.'[2]

REFERENCES

1. Kosten, T.R. & O'Connor, P.G. (2003) Management of drug and alcohol withdrawal. *New England Journal of Medicine, 348*, 1786–95.

2. Taylor, D., Paton, C. & Kerwin, R. (2007) *The Maudsley Prescribing Guidelines*, 9th edn. London: Informa Healthcare, p.465.

3. WHO (1992) *The ICD-10 Classification of Mental and Behavioural Disorders: Clinical Descriptions and Diagnostic Guidelines*. Geneva: WHO Press.

4. Thomson, A.D., Cook, C.H.C., Touquet, R. & Henry. J.A. (2002) Invited special article: The Royal College of Physicians Report on Alcohol: Guidelines for managing Wernicke's encephalopathy in the accident and emergency department. *Alcohol and Alcoholism, 37*(6), 513–21.

The examiner's mark sheet

Domain/ percentage of marks	Essential points to pass	✓	Extra marks/comments (make notes here)
1. Rapport and communication 25% of marks	Clear communication Open and closed questions Empathy Demonstrating patience with anxious relative		
2. History of alcohol withdrawal 25% of marks	Demonstrates knowledge on symptoms of alcohol withdrawal/delirium tremens (DT)		
3. Differentials 25% of marks	Explores other possible causes of confusion, dementia, head injury, systemic illness and drugs		
4. Alcohol history 25% of marks	After identifying alcohol withdrawal as likely cause of confusion, proceeds to obtain alcohol dependence history		

% SCORE _____

____

4

OVERALL IMPRESSION

(CIRCLE ONE)

Good Pass

Pass

Borderline

Fail

Clear Fail

NOTES/Areas to improve

STATION 4(b): ALCOHOL WITHDRAWAL – MANAGEMENT

> **INSTRUCTION TO CANDIDATE**
>
> You have met with Mrs Stuart and later seen the patient. Now, discuss your findings with the surgical registrar.
>
> **You should discuss the likely differential diagnosis and advise them of further management.**

ACTOR (ROLE-PLAYER) INSTRUCTIONS

You are the surgical registrar.

You and your consultant operated on this gentleman 2 days ago and Mr Stuart had a successful surgery.

You are concerned that Mr Stuart is very confused and not cooperative with the treatment.

Mr Stuart had reported that he was a 'social drinker' at the time of admission – you were not aware that he was a heavy drinker.

You would like some advice on how to manage the gentleman.

SUGGESTED APPROACH

Setting the scene

Introduce yourself to the surgical registrar: 'Hello, Dr_____, I am Dr_____, the psychiatrist. I have seen Mr Stuart – he seems confused, as you are aware. Hopefully we can discuss what is going on and formulate a management plan.'

Completing the task

1. Begin by summarising your findings: focus on salient points gleaned from the previous station. 'Mr Stuart seems to have been a regular drinker, and from his wife's history, I think he has alcohol dependence syndrome. Following the surgery, he is very confused and disorientated with reduced alertness. He is very likely to be experiencing symptoms of alcohol withdrawal.'

2. Discuss the likely differential diagnosis (acute confusional state secondary to alcohol withdrawal/delirium tremens, acute confusional state secondary to other causes or Wernicke's encephalopathy): 'There could be other possible reasons for this confusion; for example, any head injury sustained during the fall, medication-related or Wernicke's encephalopathy.'

3. Explain that you would want further information prior to confirming the diagnosis.
   - This should include interview and examination of the patient (MMSE, other tests of cognition and clinical examination [signs of alcohol withdrawal[1]] and neurological examination). If there was a premorbid history of memory problems with acute-onset confusional state, then also consider causes of acute-on-chronic confusional states (e.g. superimposed on a possible dementia).
   - Further investigations: basic bloods, including full blood count (FBC), urea and electrolytes (U&Es), liver function tests (LFTs), septic screen, urine drug screen,

breathalyser (for blood alcohol concentration). Consider a computed tomography/ MRI brain scan if neurological features are evident or a history of premorbid memory problems is present.

4. Discuss the management (acute/immediate management): remember you are discussing with a medical colleague and you can/should use technical terms and names of specific drugs and dosages.
   - If severe withdrawal from alcohol is suspected, suggest intravenous diazepam. As seizures may be a feature of severe withdrawal/delirium tremens, the candidate may also be inclined to suggest an opinion from the medical team, particularly as electrolyte abnormalities may occur and parenteral fluid support may be needed.[1,2]
   - If less severe, commence on regime of chlordiazepoxide or diazepam. Consider oxazepam if there are concerns regarding the patient's liver function (be familiar with an appropriate treatment regime with example dosing).[1]
   - 'Stat' dose of benzodiazepine, depending on blood alcohol concentration and withdrawal features.[1]
   - Titrate dose to alcohol withdrawal symptoms (candidate could suggest the use of objective rating scales for surgical nursing staff to use on the ward; e.g. Clinical Institute Withdrawal Assessment of Alcohol Scale, Revised [CIWA-Ar]).[3] In addition, pulse and blood pressure should be monitored. In severe withdrawal, institute frequent (1–2 hourly) monitoring of observations.[2]
   - Commence dose reduction of benzodiazepine after initial period of assessment (24 hours); this should be tailored to patient's withdrawal symptoms. The general rule of thumb is to reduce by 20% of baseline dose each day.[1] The candidate may also suggest as required (*prn*) benzodiazepine for 'breakthrough' symptoms.
   - All patients presenting with features of alcohol dependence should also be commenced on intramuscular thiamine in order to prevent the development of Wernicke's encephalopathy.[1,4] Intravenous thiamine is preferred if a diagnosis of Wernicke – Korsakoff syndrome is suspected.[1,4] Give for 5 days, followed by oral thiamine supplementation.[1,4]

5. Discuss the medium/longer-term management.
   - You should suggest that you will return to review the patient's mental state post-detoxification for signs of cognitive impairment or psychopathology.
   - You may suggest assessing the patient's motivation at this time in order to address his alcohol use.
   - Following successful detoxification, the patient should be given details of self-referral to local alcohol services or hospital liaison alcohol services (if available). Psycho-social measures will be needed to maintain long-term abstinence (individual/motivational input, group psychological input, etc.).
   - If there is evidence of cognitive impairment, you may suggest neuroimaging and referral to older adult services for follow-up (especially if there is evidence of impact on functioning and the possibility of underlying cognitive impairment). Suggest occupational therapist (OT) assessment if there are related concerns over functioning at home.
   - You should recommend to the surgical team that the patient is discharged with thiamine supplements.

ADDITIONAL POINTS

1. As this is a diagnosis and management station, a helpful structure would be:
- Present the likely differential diagnosis (suggest most likely diagnosis first). Support the differential diagnoses by salient findings gleaned from the history which you gathered in the first station.
- List any further investigations or assessments that had not been done yet. Discuss the management: acute management should be followed by

medium- to longer-term management. Consider the 'bio-psycho-social' model for this section of the station.

2. The CIWA-Ar is a ten-item scale measuring features of alcohol withdrawal over a variety of domains. Each section is scored from 0 to 7. For severe withdrawal, patients score >15. For moderate withdrawal, patients score 8–15. In mild withdrawal, patients score <8.[1] High-scoring patients are at an increased risk of convulsions and delirium.[2]

3. Wernicke's encephalopathy is a frequently underdiagnosed condition that is associated with high levels of morbidity and mortality.[4] The classic clinical triad of confusion, ataxia and ophthalmoplegia is in fact seen in less than a third of cases.[4] Untreated, Wernicke's encephalopathy proceeds to Korsakoff's psychosis, with high personal and social costs.[4] Malnutrition with chronic alcohol use is a risk factor for the development of Wernicke's encephalopathy.[4] Current treatment recommendations suggest 'one pair intramuscular/intravenous ampoules high potency B-complex vitamins daily over 3–5 days,'[1] as oral thiamine is poorly absorbed.[4] Glucose should not be given without thiamine as this may precipitate Wernicke's encephalopathy.[1,4]

REFERENCES

1. Taylor, D., Paton, C. & Kerwin, R. (2007) *The Maudsley Prescribing Guidelines*, 9th edn. London: Informa Healthcare, p.465.

2. Kosten, T.R. & O'Connor, P.G. (2003) Management of drug and alcohol withdrawal. *New England Journal of Medicine, 348,* 1786–95.

3. Sullivan, J.T., Sykora, K., Schneiderman, J., Naranjo, C.A. & Sellers, E.M. (1989) Assessment of alcohol withdrawal: The revised clinical institute withdrawal assessment for alcohol scale (CIWA-Ar). *British Journal of Addiction, 84,* 1353–7.

4. Thomson, A.D., Cook, C.H.C., Touquet, R. & Henry, J.A. (2002) Invited special article: The Royal College of Physicians Report on Alcohol: Guidelines for managing Wernicke's encephalopathy in the accident and emergency department. *Alcohol and Alcoholism, 37*(6), 513–21.

The examiner's mark sheet

Domain/ percentage of marks	Essential points to pass	✓	Extra marks/comments (make notes here)
1. Rapport and communication 25% of marks	Clear communication Open and closed questions Empathy Demonstrating professional behaviour		
2. Diagnosis 25% of marks	Able to explain relevant diagnosis and the rationale		
3. Differentials 15% of marks	Gives consideration to other possible causes of confusion and explains why		

⇧ 4. Management

    35% of marks

Advises appropriate bio-psycho-social approach towards management

Gives consideration to nursing care

Discusses long-term management and follow-up

% SCORE _____

    ___ **OVERALL IMPRESSION**

4   (CIRCLE ONE)

Good Pass

Pass

Borderline

Fail

Clear Fail

NOTES/Areas to improve

○ SINGLE STATIONS

STATION 5: DELIRIUM – HISTORY TAKING

> **INSTRUCTION TO CANDIDATE**
>
> You are a liaison psychiatrist. The medical team call you to review 86-year-old Mr Arthur Williams on a medical ward, who is being managed for an infective exacerbation of chronic obstructive pulmonary disease (COPD). The medical house officer reports that he has become 'acutely paranoid' and confused, frequently not knowing where he is. He believes that staff are trying to poison him and he refuses to eat or drink. The house officer has spoken to the daughter of Mr Williams and has gathered collateral information.
>
> **See Mr Williams and also speak to the house officer and take a relevant history to arrive at a diagnosis.**

ACTOR (ROLE-PLAYER) INSTRUCTIONS

You are the house officer on the medical ward.

Your team is looking after Mr Williams, who was admitted with a chest infection.

You are concerned that Mr Williams is very paranoid and is 'psychotic'.

He has not slept well in the last few days and has been agitated on the ward, accusing the staff of trying to poison him.

The medical team feel that he is psychotic and want him transferred to a psychiatric hospital.

You have spoken to his daughter, who has reported that Mr Williams did not have any memory problems or paranoid symptoms prior to this admission.

Mr Williams is compliant with his medication and his COPD is getting better.

SUGGESTED APPROACH

Setting the scene

Introduce yourself to the patient and to the medical house officer. Begin by explaining to the patient that you have been asked by the medical team to provide an opinion regarding current difficulties. Given the vignette, you should already be considering possible organic causes of the presentation, so you may wish to make apparent at this stage that you will want to ask the patient questions regarding his orientation, as well as review the history and recent medical management/medications with the house officer. 'Hello, Mr_____, I am Dr_____, a psychiatrist. I am here to talk to you and understand your situation to see if I can be of any help. I will be assessing your memory as well, if that is OK?'

Completing the task

1. Take a brief history and mental state examination from the patient.
   - Clarify with the patient why he has not been eating and drinking. Does he have any other abnormal or delusional beliefs?
   - Check for affective and anxiety symptoms.
   - Is there a current or previous history of alcohol or substance misuse?
   - Mental state examination and brief cognitive assessment (abbreviated mental test due to limited time or confusion assessment method): is the patient orientated and lucid?

2. Brief history from the medical house officer/Foundation year 1 (FY1) (tell the patient that you are going to speak to the doctor and get some medical information about him).
   - How long has he been an in-patient and when did the team first notice the problems? Did the change in mental state come on abruptly or gradually? Has there been an associated history of fluctuating lucidity/disorientation/changes to consciousness and attention? Is there an associated history of visual hallucinations? Are there any obvious changes to the patient's sleep – wake cycle or emotional disturbances (e.g. emotional lability)?
   - Is there a previous history of psychiatric problems or memory problems, or a previous history of delirium? What is the state of his current physical health and are there any other medical problems of note? Has he been prescribed any new medications (e.g. steroids or antibiotics)? Had his family expressed any concerns around previous memory and functioning?
   - What is the team's future medical plan? What have been the results of any relevant investigations?

3. Summarise findings and likely differential diagnosis to the house officer. Based on your findings, you will have to consider acute confusional state or delirium superimposed on dementia, drug-induced (steroids for COPD). You will have to advise on any further relevant investigations if necessary, such as brain imaging. The house officer may ask what delirium is and how to go about managing the patient. Be familiar with NICE delirium guidance: prevention, diagnosis and management guidance.

ADDITIONAL POINTS

1. ICD-10 defines delirium as an 'etiologically non-specific syndrome characterised by concurrent disturbances of consciousness and attention, perception, thinking, memory, psychomotor behaviour, emotion

and the sleep – wake cycle.'[1] If there is no previous psychiatric history of note and the problems are of relatively recent and rapid onset then delirium or acute confusional state should be considered. According to ICD-10 criteria, for a diagnosis of delirium, symptoms in each of the following areas should be present: (a) impairment of consciousness and attention; (b) global disturbance of cognition, with perceptual disturbances (which usually tend to be visual hallucinations); (c) psychomotor disturbances; and (d) emotional disturbances.

2. Other potential differential diagnoses might include a mood disorder, an acute psychotic episode or (pre-existing) dementia/delirium superimposed on dementia.

3. Potential causes of an acute confusional state in this case might include infection (chest infection or urinary tract infection) or medications/polypharmacy (steroids or antibiotics).

4. Risk factors for delirium include older age,[2] medical and psychiatric comorbidity,[2] underlying cognitive impairment (e.g. dementia),[2,3] psychoactive drug use,[4] polypharmacy[4] and male sex.[2] Risk factors for delirium can be characterised as predisposing versus precipitating.[2]

REFERENCES

1. WHO (1992) *The ICD-10 Classification of Mental and Behavioural Disorders: Clinical Descriptions and Diagnostic Guidelines.* Geneva: WHO Press.
2. Burns, A., Gallagley, A. & Byrne, J. (2004) Delirium. *Journal of Neurology Neurosurgery and Psychiatry*, 75, 362–7.
3. Fick, D.M., Agostini, J.V. & Inouye, S. (2002) Delirium superimposed on dementia: A systematic review. *Journal of the American Geriatrics Society*, 50(10), 1723–32.
4. Taylor, D., Paton, C. & Kerwin. R. (2007) *The Maudsley Prescribing Guidelines*, 9th edn. London: Informa Healthcare, p. 465.

The examiner's mark sheet

Domain/ percentage of marks	Essential points to pass	✓	Extra marks/comments (make notes here)
1. Rapport and communication 25% of marks	Clear communication Open and closed questions Empathy Demonstrating patience		
2. Assessment of patient 25% of marks	Explores possible aetiologies of confusion Performs brief cognitive tests		

⇧ 3. Collateral history

    25% of marks

Elicits history of premorbid functioning, change in attention and features of delirium

4. Feedback

    25% of marks

Able to summarise the positive findings and arrive at a likely diagnosis, able to address any questions from junior doctor

% SCORE _____

                  ____   **OVERALL IMPRESSION**

4   (CIRCLE ONE)

Good Pass

Pass

Borderline

Fail

Clear Fail

NOTES/Areas to improve

STATION 6: ADJUSTMENT DISORDER

INSTRUCTION TO CANDIDATE

You are asked to see 30-year-old Mr Andrew Jones, who has become increasingly anxious and depressed. He recently discovered that his partner is HIV positive. The man is accompanied by his sister; assume that he has consented to you discussing his health with her.

Assess the gentleman and finish by explaining to him what you think the problem is and how you might go about managing it.

ACTOR (ROLE-PLAYER) INSTRUCTIONS

You are Mr Andrew Jones and you are 30 years old. You have been in a relationship for the past 5 years.

Your partner revealed to you 10 days ago that she is HIV positive.

You are worried that you may have contracted HIV and you have been anxious since then.

You have been low in mood since you heard the news and have been struggling to concentrate on work.

You have difficulty sleeping, have lost appetite and energy and you spend a lot of time worrying about your own future.

You sometimes feel angry with your partner but you do not have any thoughts of harming her. You do not have any thoughts of ending your life.

SUGGESTED APPROACH

Setting the scene

Introduce yourself to the gentleman and to his sister. 'Hello, Mr_____, I am Dr_____, a psychiatrist. I gather that you are going through a tough time right now. Hopefully we can discuss your difficulties and see how we can help you.' Explain that you wanted to ask him a few questions regarding his health; it may be worth checking again if he is happy to discuss all matters in front of his sister, given the sensitive nature of the difficulties.

Completing the task

1. Take a brief history from the gentleman; his sister will be able to provide a collateral history.
   - Clarify the onset of difficulties. Has there been a discernible change in mental state, and if so, when did this occur? When did his sister notice the changes? When did the changes to mental state come on with respect to receiving the news about his partner's health?
   - What is the situation with his current partner – is it a stable and long-term relationship or more recent? How did he find out about his partner's diagnosis? When did he find this out?
   - Has he any concerns regarding his own health? Does he have any plans for HIV testing himself and pre-/post-test counselling?
   - Other relevant factors in history – previous psychiatric history of note, current medications, family history and drug and alcohol use.

2. Mental state examination.
   - Assess for psychopathology, especially for mood and anxiety symptoms.
   - Risk assessment – risk to himself (self-harm/suicide) or through neglect. Risk to others – ask about current sexual practices/other practices which could put others at risk of potential HIV infection (injecting drug use/needle sharing, etc.).
   - For the risk assessment, his sister will provide helpful collateral history, especially regarding risk to himself.

3. Summarise the main points discussed during the interview and finish with a brief differential diagnosis and management plan, explained to the patient in simple, jargon-free terms.
   - Likely differential diagnosis could include: adjustment disorder, major depression or an anxiety disorder.[1] Be familiar with the relevant diagnostic criteria.
   - Advise HIV pre-test counselling, safer practices, informing sexual partners, etc.
   - Suggest SSRI treatment if he meets clinical criteria for depression or an anxiety disorder.
   - Suggest psychological support, either CBT if depressed/anxious or supportive counselling if there are outstanding issues regarding his health and his relationships.

ADDITIONAL POINTS

Note the difference between an adjustment disorder and an acute stress reaction, as described in ICD-10.[1] To meet the criteria for an acute stress reaction (F43.0), there should be evidence of 'exposure to an exceptional mental or physical stressor,' and symptoms should come on within 1 hour of the stressor.[1] Conversely, to meet the criteria for an adjustment disorder

(F43.2), there should be evidence of 'an identifiable psycho-social stressor, not of an unusual or catastrophic type, within one month of onset of symptoms'. Symptoms may be similar to those noted within the 'neurotic, stress-related and somatoform disorders' or 'affective disorders', but should not be of a severity to indicate a separate diagnosis of these.[1]

REFERENCE

1. WHO (1992) *The ICD-10 Classification of Mental and Behavioural Disorders: Clinical Descriptions and Diagnostic Guidelines.* Geneva: WHO Press.

The examiner's mark sheet

Domain/ percentage of marks	Essential points to pass	✓	Extra marks/comments (make notes here)
1. Rapport and communication 25% of marks	Clear communication Open and closed questions Empathy Demonstrating patience		
2. Assessment 25% of marks	Able to elicit relevant history of mood disorders and adjustment disorders Identifies the role of psycho-social stressors		
3. Diagnostic formulation 25% of marks	Able to arrive at possible diagnosis Able to exclude other differentials		
4. Explanation and management 25% of marks	Explains to patient the diagnosis Briefly talks about bio-psycho-social approach to treatment		

% SCORE _____

OVERALL IMPRESSION

4 (CIRCLE ONE)

Good Pass

Pass

Borderline

Fail

Clear Fail

NOTES/Areas to improve

STATION 7: KORSAKOFF SYNDROME – EXPLANATION

INSTRUCTION TO CANDIDATE

Mr John Wright is a 66-year-old man who has been admitted with confusion to the medical ward. He had been drinking 2 L of cider every day and he required alcohol detoxification. He continues to remain confused, is confabulating and has ataxia. He has been requesting to take his own discharge. You are a specialist trainee 6 (ST6) in the liaison psychiatry service and you have assessed Mr Wright. You have made a diagnosis of Korsakoff syndrome. The nurse in charge of the ward wants to speak to you about him.

Explain your findings. Address the nurse's views, concerns and expectations.

ACTOR (ROLE-PLAYER) INSTRUCTIONS

You are the nurse in charge of the medical ward.

You are concerned that Mr Wright is very confused and wandering. He is interfering with other patients, and other patients on the ward are complaining about him.

You are of the opinion that his stay on the ward is 'inappropriate'.

You want him to be sectioned and taken to a psychiatric hospital as he is 'psychotic' and not making any sense – he is 'clearly a mental health patient'.

You are concerned that he will not cope at home if he was to take his own discharge.

SUGGESTED APPROACH

Setting the scene

Introduce yourself and offer to address any questions the nurse may have. 'Hello, I am Dr_____, the psychiatrist. Nice to meet you. I am aware that Mr Wright in your ward is quite disturbed. I hope we can discuss and think about how to go about managing him.' Be mindful that the nurse could be quite frustrated and may start asking questions or expressing her anger. Allow her to talk and listen, then address her queries.

Completing the task

This task is about explanation of a complex mental health condition to another professional, but not from a psychiatric background. Though you may use some technical terms, try and avoid a lot of psychiatric terminology. Below are some of the questions that might come up and their answers. Similar to this station, you may be asked to talk to a relative, in which you would have to adjust the language accordingly.

What is Korsakoff syndrome?

Korsakoff or Wernicke–Korsakoff syndrome is a spectrum of disease affecting memory resulting from thiamine deficiency. This usually develops in patients who misuse alcohol. Wernicke's encephalopathy is described as a triad of mental confusion, ataxia (disturbance in walking) and ophthalmoplegia (eye muscles becoming affected, causing visual disturbances). Korsakoff syndrome is a late complication of inadequately treated Wernicke's encephalopathy.

What are the features of Korsakoff syndrome?

The main symptom of Korsakoff syndrome is memory loss, particularly of events that occur after the onset of the condition. Memories of the more distant past can also be affected. Other symptoms may include:

- Problems acquiring new information or learning new skills
- Personality changes, ranging from apathy to talkative and repetitive behaviour
- Poor insight
- Confabulation, where a person invents events to fill the gaps in their memory

What causes Korsakoff syndrome?

This condition is caused by a lack of thiamine (vitamin B1), affecting the brain and the nervous system. Heavy drinkers develop thiamine deficiency because of poor diet, alcohol interfering with the conversion of thiamine to its active form and frequent vomiting (due to inflamed stomach lining) affecting the absorption of the vitamins.

Why is the patient lying/what is confabulation?

Confabulation is a cognitive problem in which the patient answers questions promptly with inaccurate answers and sometimes with bizarre answers. This happens because of falsification of the memory in clear consciousness. It is a characteristic problem in Korsakoff syndrome.

What is the treatment for this condition?

During the initial stages, intravenous thiamine infusion followed by extended treatment with oral thiamine is recommended. This, along with abstinence from alcohol, may improve the chances of recovery from the symptoms of Korsakoff syndrome.

What is the prognosis?

Mortality rates are high if Wernicke–Korsakoff syndrome is left untreated. Most deaths are the result of a lung infection, blood poisoning (septicaemia) or irreversible brain damage.

Korsakoff syndrome may continue to progress if the patient continues to drink and maintains poor dietary intake. The progression can be halted if the person abstains from alcohol and maintains adequate dietary intake with vitamin supplements. Approximately a quarter of affected people make a very good recovery. Approximately half of people make some recovery, requiring support in their lives. Recovery is slow and can take up to 2 years. There is evidence suggesting that significant recovery is possible with appropriate assessment and rehabilitation.

Why can't we take the patient to a mental health unit?

The patient is presenting with a medical complication of alcohol misuse and as such the main treatment is vitamin replacement and abstinence from alcohol. The patient does not require active psychiatric treatment warranting admission to an acute psychiatric unit. The liaison team can support the medical ward to manage the behavioural problems. We can also receive input from the drug and alcohol team.

He wants to take his own discharge. What should we do?

The Mental Capacity Act and, on occasions, the Mental Health Act may have to be considered in these patients in the early stages of the syndrome. At a later stage, it may be necessary to invoke a guardianship order. Other legal measures may be required to manage finances and debts. Until his needs are clearly established and a management plan is in place, he can be treated in his best interest. I would suggest convening a best interest meeting involving the family as soon as possible.

ADDITIONAL POINTS

- An individual with Wernicke–Korsakoff syndrome (WKS) is often mentally confused. This can make patient–doctor communication difficult. A doctor may overlook the possibility of a physical disorder when dealing with a confused patient.
- Check for signs of alcoholism and conduct a liver function test to check for liver damage, which is a common sign of alcoholism.
- The individual may also appear to be malnourished.
- Nutritional tests may include:
- Serum albumin test: a blood test that measures the levels of albumin (a protein) in the blood. Low levels may signal nutritional deficiencies, as well as kidney or liver problems.
- Serum vitamin B1 test: a blood test to check vitamin B1 levels in the blood.
- Transketolase (enzyme) activity in the red blood cells: low enzyme activity signals a vitamin B1 deficiency.
- Diagnostic imaging tests for WKS include:
- Electrocardiograph, which looks for abnormalities before and after giving vitamin B1.
- Computed tomography scan to check for brain lesions related to Wernicke's disease (WD).
- MRI scan to look for brain changes.
- Physicians may also use neuropsychological tests to judge the severity of mental deficiencies.

FURTHER READING

Alzheimer's Society (2007) *Dementia UK: A Report into the Prevalence and Cost of Dementia Prepared by the Personal Social Services Research Unit (PSSRU) at the London School of Economics and the Institute of Psychiatry at King's College London, for the Alzheimer's Society.*

Kopelman, M.D., Thomson, A.D., Guerrini, I. & Marshall, E.J. (2009) The Korsakoff syndrome: Clinical aspects, psychology and treatment. *Alcohol and Alcoholism, 44,* 148–54.

Victor, M. & Yakolev, Pl. (1955) S.S. Korsakoff's psychic disorhic disorder in conjunction with peripheral neuritis; a translation of Korsakoff's original article with comments on the author and his contribution to clinical medicine. *Neurology, 5,* 394–406.

WHO (2007) *WHO Expert Committee on Problems Related to Alcohol Consumption.* Geneva: WHO Press.

The examiner's mark sheet

Domain/ percentage of marks	Essential points to pass	✓	Extra marks/comments (make notes here)
1. Rapport and communication 25% of marks	Clear communication Open and closed questions Demonstrating patience when dealing with frustrated colleague		
2. Explanation – diagnosis 25% of marks	Demonstrates awareness of diagnostic criteria for Korsakoff syndrome and able to explain to colleague Demonstrates knowledge of symptoms and aetiology and explains to colleague		
3. Explanation – management 25% of marks	Able to formulate management plan and communicate effectively with colleague		
4. Addressing concerns 25% of marks	Able to liaise with colleague who is angry Able to address concerns in a calm manner Maintains professional behaviour under pressure		

% SCORE _____

___
4

OVERALL IMPRESSION

(CIRCLE ONE)

Good Pass

Pass

Borderline

Fail

Clear Fail

NOTES/Areas to improve

STATION 8: NEUROLEPTIC MALIGNANT SYNDROME

INSTRUCTION TO CANDIDATE

Mr John Smith is a 35-year-old patient known to services with a diagnosis of schizoaffective disorder for 10 years. He was on a prescription of lithium 1000 mg nocte and olanzapine 15 mg nocte and had been stable for 2 years. He showed symptoms of relapse and olanzapine was increased to 20 mg nocte 2 weeks ago. His mental state did not improve and he was admitted to an acute psychiatric ward 4 days ago. He had been agitated and aggressive on the ward and had been administered a few doses of haloperidol. Last evening, he developed a high temperature and became increasingly confused. He was noted to be stiff and his blood pressure was high. He was seen by the on-call senior house officer (SHO) and transferred to a medical unit.

The next day, the liaison psychiatry team has received a referral. You are a specialist trainee 5 (ST5) with the liaison team and you visit the medical ward to review John. John's father is waiting to speak to a psychiatrist about his son.

Talk to his father to clarify the situation. Address his concerns, views and expectations. You are not expected to take a history.

ACTOR (ROLE-PLAYER) INSTRUCTIONS

You are the father of John Smith and he is your only son.

You are very supportive of your son and you raised concerns with the mental health team that your son was deteriorating.

You understand that your son was very psychotic, requiring admission to psychiatric hospital, and you have been devastated that he had to go into a psychiatric hospital again.

You are angry that your son is in an intensive care unit because of complications.

You want to know why he was prescribed medication that you believe could kill your son.

You are not happy with the treatment received in the mental health hospital and want to put in a formal complaint.

SUGGESTED APPROACH

Setting the scene

Introduce yourself: 'Hello, Mr_____, I am Dr_____, the psychiatrist. I am aware of what is happening with your son's situation. Hopefully I can address your concerns.' It is important to acknowledge the concerns of the angry relative and approach the issue sensitively.

Completing the task

This task is about dealing with an angry relative and also demonstrating to the examiner your knowledge of neuroleptic malignant syndrome (NMS). The first thing to try to do is to build a rapport. It is OK to say, 'I am sorry to inform you that your son has developed a severe reaction.' It is very important not to be confrontational or defensive. It is important to explain that this is a very rare side effect and, with early treatment, the chances of recovery are very good. The following are some of the questions that may be asked and suggested answers.

Can you tell me what happened to my son?

'I am very sorry to inform you that your son has suffered from a rare reaction to the anti-psychotic medication he has been prescribed. The condition is called neuroleptic malignant syndrome.'

What is neuroleptic malignant syndrome?

'The condition is characterised by high fever, stiffness of the muscles, confusion, wide swings of blood pressure, excessive sweating and excessive secretion of saliva. NMS is a rare condition that can occur as a reaction to medication that is used to treat schizophrenia and other mental conditions.'

Why did my son develop this condition?

'NMS generally develops within the first 2 weeks of an anti-psychotic drug being initiated or after a change of dose. Abrupt stoppage of anti-psychotic medication can also result in this reaction. In the case of your son, we believe the changes to the dose and prescription of haloperidol may have resulted in this complication.'

My son is in intensive care – is this condition dangerous?

'It is a potentially life-threatening condition. However, fatality is unusual in cases where the condition is identified and treatment is initiated early.'

I was not informed that he is being transferred to the medical hospital

'I am very sorry that this did not happen. Since the situation was quite dangerous, I can only assume that the psychiatric team dealing with your son were more focussed on ensuring the safety of your son.'

You almost killed my son!

'I can assure you that the medications that have been prescribed for your son have been safely used to treat patients for decades. Your son was very disturbed due to his psychotic symptoms and I believe the ward psychiatric team had to treat him urgently to alleviate his symptoms. The team could not have necessarily foreseen this particular complication arising. However, the staff on the ward are trained to pick up early signs of this condition and it has resulted in your son being transferred quickly to a medical ward for treatment.'

Why did you use a drug that could cause this condition?

'This condition can occur with any anti-psychotic medication that we prescribe and it is unfortunate that your son had developed this rare side effect.'

What are the chances of developing this condition?

'This condition is very rare and the chances of a person developing NMS are two to three in 1000. Most of the time, the condition is mild, and the chances of developing a severe form of NMS is even more rare.'

What is the treatment for this condition?

'The treatments are mainly supportive – controlling the temperature and rigidity and preventing complications like respiratory failure and breakdown of muscle proteins leading to renal failure. The most important step is to stop all anti-psychotic medication.'

I know my son has schizoaffective disorder and you have stopped his medication – what if he gets agitated?

'We can use a class of medication called benzodiazepines such as diazepam or lorazepam to control the agitation until the condition improves.'

What is the prognosis of NMS?

'The prognosis is better when the condition is identified early and appropriate treatment is initiated. In the last two decades, the mortality rate has come down to less than 10% because of early recognition and improvement in management.'

Will you restart him on medication?

'In most cases, symptoms resolve in 1 – 2 weeks. We will reintroduce the anti-psychotic medication in a small dose and consider a medication that is chemically unrelated. We would consider a medication like quetiapine and clozapine, which have lesser propensities to cause NMS.'

I want to put in a formal complaint

'There is a trust complaints procedure and I can give you the details. I would like to reassure you that this condition is unpredictable and the ward psychiatric team could not have foreseen this happening. In my view, the ward team have been extremely vigilant and managed to get him the medical help as early as possible. If it helps, I could arrange a meeting with the ward psychiatric team and you can raise your concerns with them.'

Conclusion

Assure the relative that you are doing everything you can to ensure the safety of the patient. Assure them that you can give them details of the trust complaints procedure should they wish to complain.

ADDITIONAL POINTS

Cardinal features of neuroleptic malignant syndrome are as follows:

- Severe muscular rigidity
- Hyperthermia (temperature >38°C)
- Autonomic instability
- Changes in the level of consciousness

Clinical features of neuroleptic malignant syndrome include:

- Muscular rigidity (typically 'lead pipe' rigidity)
- Hyperthermia (temperature >38°C)
- Diaphoresis
- Pallor
- Dysphagia
- Dyspnoea
- Tremor
- Incontinence
- Shuffling gait
- Psychomotor agitation
- Delirium progressing to lethargy, stupor or coma

Risk factors

Risk factors that may predispose patients to developing NMS include male sex, learning disability, iron deficiency, high ambient temperature, depot anti-psychotic injections, alcoholism, exhaustion and dehydration. Any recent changes to anti-psychotic medication (including abrupt increases or decreases in dose) can precipitate NMS.

The examiner's mark sheet

Domain/ percentage of marks	Essential points to pass	✓	Extra marks/comments (make notes here)
1. Rapport and communication 20% of marks	Clear communication Demonstrating patience Not using medical jargon		
2. Dealing with angry relative 20% of marks	Able to remain calm under pressure Tries to build rapport Empathises with relative		
3. NMS – diagnosis and symptoms 20% of marks	Demonstrates knowledge of the symptoms and aetiology of NMS		
4. NMS – management 20% of marks	Demonstrates knowledge of the management of NMS		
5. Addressing the concerns 20% of marks	Able to address queries raised by relative		

% SCORE _____

___   **OVERALL IMPRESSION**

5   (CIRCLE ONE)

Good Pass

Pass

Borderline

Fail

Clear Fail

NOTES/Areas to improve

Chapter 9

General adult psychiatry

○ LINKED STATIONS

STATION 1(a): BIPOLAR AFFECTIVE DISORDER – TYPE II

INSTRUCTION TO CANDIDATE

A 21-year-old university student, Miss Lara Tracey, has been referred to your service with bouts of depression lasting a few weeks at a time. She takes mirtazapine and has reported no change in her depressive symptoms. You have inherited this patient from your predecessor's out-patient clinic.

Take a history of her mood and find out more about her symptoms.

DO NOT PERFORM A PHYSICAL EXAMINATION.

ACTOR (ROLE-PLAYER) INSTRUCTION

You have a 3-year history of two distinct types of symptoms:

1. Low mood: four episodes per year of periods in which you feel low throughout the day, without energy and unable to enjoy things for a few weeks.
2. Elevated mood: three to four episodes per year of periods in which you become incredibly productive with your university projects, finishing a project in a few days, as you are up most nights until very late, requiring 2–3 hours of sleep. As a result, your grades are good.

You spend most of your time when free of work at the student union and have become social secretary. You have become a little more promiscuous during this time, but do not engage in unprotected sex. You do not see this component of your presentation as a problem.

You have no suicidal thoughts or history of illicit drugs, self-harm, excessive alcohol or psychosis.

SUGGESTED APPROACH

Setting the scene

Begin by addressing the patient by name and introducing yourself. Explain your understanding of the current problem from reading the notes.

'Hello, Ms Tracey, I am Dr_____, the psychiatrist who has taken over from Dr_____. I understand that things have been difficult for you for some time, that you have had problems with low mood and that the antidepressants appear to have had little effect. Is that correct?'

'Given that we have not met before, and as part of the process of getting to know you/ understand what you have been through, would you mind if we covered some aspects of the history again?'

Completing the task

The main point of this station is that the candidate is presenting with a highly atypical presentation of depressive symptoms. This is always an indication to review the diagnosis.

This patient presents with periods of depression alternating with periods of hypomania (her symptoms are not sufficiently severe for hospital admission) suggestive of a bipolar II diagnosis. The quantification of the subtype of bipolar is not necessary to pass the station, but will highlight the candidate with a more comprehensive understanding of ICD-10.

Additionally, the frequency of mood symptoms would be consistent with a rapid cycling disorder. The antidepressant is not helping matters and may be contributing to her instability.

Depression history

The core features of depression (low mood, anergia and anhedonia) along with additional symptoms that indicate the level of severity (ICD-10 DCR) should be explored. Given that the patient has been unresponsive to therapy, it is important to explore medication history and medical history and briefly look for the presence of comorbidities. In particular, ask about anxiety disorders, alcohol, suicidal ideation and personality difficulties.

'Please tell me the problems you have been having with your mood and when it all started. What symptoms trouble you most? How have your energy levels been? What sort of things do you enjoy?'

Hypomania history

The candidate may gain marks for delineating a clear history with an exploration of potential triggers. Additionally, the shifts in mood should be explored. They should ask about physical health contributions, including thyroid disease, antidepressant-induced switching and erratic sleep patterns.

'Sometime people who suffer from low mood can also notice that they have periods where they feel the opposite, an improvement in their mood, with increased levels of energy, so they feel like they could do almost anything. Tell me more about those periods.'

Activities of daily living

'How has your life changed since your mood swings began? Are you having difficulties in carrying on with your routine because of this? What do other people think about how you are during these periods?'

Bipolar II and rapid cycling

The patient will need to meet the criteria for a present or past hypomanic episode and the criteria for a current or past major depressive episode. Rapid cycling requires four demarcated episodes of an affective disturbance in the course of a year that is sufficient to meet 'caseness' for the disorder.

FURTHER READING

American Psychiatric Association (2013) *Diagnostic and Statistical Manual of Mental Disorders*, 5th edn. Washington, DC: American Psychiatric Association.

Cooper, J.E. (1994) *Pocket Guide to the ICD-10 Classification of Mental and Behavioural Disorders: With Glossary and Diagnostic Criteria for Research: ICD-10/DCR-10.* London: Churchill Livingstone.

National Institute for Health and Clinical Excellence (2006) *Bipolar Disorder: The Management of Bipolar Disorder in Adults, Children and Adolescents, in Primary and Secondary Care. NICE Clinical Guideline 38 (Update Clinical Guideline 185, 2014).* http://www.nice.org.uk/guidance/cg185?unlid=373313324201622816295

The examiner's mark sheet

Domain/ percentage of marks	Essential points to pass	✓	Extra marks/comments (make notes here)
1. Rapport and communication 25% of marks	Clear communication Open and closed questions Empathy Demonstrating patience		
2. History taking sufficient to elicit all pertinent components of the presentation 25% of marks	There must be sufficient exploration of symptoms to demonstrate sufficient severity for 'caseness' for unipolar depression and hypomania		
3. Risk assessment 25% of marks	Exploration of risks known to be precipitants and/or consequence of both disorders		
4. Differential diagnosis exploration 25% of marks	Exploration of other conditions commonly seen as differentials, including substance misuse and personality disorders		

% SCORE _____

____ **OVERALL IMPRESSION**

4 (CIRCLE ONE)

Good Pass

Pass

Borderline

Fail

Clear Fail

NOTES/Areas to improve

STATION 1(b): BIPOLAR AFFECTIVE DISORDER – DISCUSSION WITH CONSULTANT

INSTRUCTION TO CANDIDATE

You decide from your history that the patient has bipolar II and is a rapid cycler with several cases of depression each year. She has previously unobserved episodes of hypomania and is currently hypomanic. The duration and the severity of each hypomanic phase are increasing with each relapse, but she does not yet fulfil the criteria for mania.

The patient says she would be willing to try any medications to stop the frequency of her depressive episodes.

As you are new to the job, your consultant reviews the case with you, asks what examination you did in clinic and asks how you are going to manage the condition.

ACTOR (ROLE-PLAYER) INSTRUCTIONS

You are to discuss the patient with the psychiatry trainee doctor. You ask him or her to present their history/examination and summarise the positive findings. You ask for what he or she thinks is the most likely diagnosis and why. You then ask the doctor what suggestions he or she has for managing the patient. Ask about the risk assessment if he or she does not inform you themselves.

SUGGESTED APPROACH

Setting the scene

Introduce yourself: 'Hello, Dr_____, I am Dr_____. I have assessed Ms Tracey and wonder if I can briefly discuss with you.' You should be mindful that you are discussing with a senior colleague, so you can use technical terms and psychiatric terminology to explain your findings. Be systematic in presentation and summarise at the end.

Completing the task

Present the case in a systematic way but succinctly; there is limited time, so there is no need to go into elaborate details of personal history unless there is anything significant. Focus on positive findings and conclude with a brief risk assessment. Summarise your findings and discuss likely diagnosis and management plan.

'This is a 21-year-old university student who has been to the psychiatric clinic for recurrent depressive episodes. Today she came for a review, and following a detailed history, I gathered she has been experiencing episodes of depression and hypomanic episodes. The hypomanic episodes have presented with symptoms (expand according to the patient's account), but do not meet the criteria for mania. In summary, this lady presents with frequent episodes of depression and hypomania – more than four episodes per year – affecting her activities of daily living significantly. This presentation is likely to be consistent with bipolar affective disorder type II, rapid cycling type.'

'In terms of management of this patient, I would consider investigations and treatment. Treatment would involve managing the acute phase and then consideration of prophylaxis.'

Investigations

'I would like to take some time to review the notes and perform a full history and physical examination. I also need to perform a full blood screen (including thyroid function) and urine drug screen. I would consider some form of brain imaging (computed tomography or magnetic resonance imaging) if this has not been done already. I would also seek collateral/informant history.'

'I would consider a rating scale (such as the Young Mania Rating Scale) given the variation of her symptoms, allowing for a more accurate recording of fluctuation and perhaps identifying a pattern (including any potential triggers).'

Treatment

'I would want to withdraw the antidepressant in the first instance. It may be appropriate to observe for a period as this in itself may restore the balance in mood, but I would want to see her again in out-patient or follow up by phone in 1–2 weeks to see if there was any evidence of her symptoms worsening. My preferred setting would be regular out-patient reviews, although this may change if she starts to present with any risks as a result of her mental state, alongside other factors such as home environment and any others risks brought up by the collateral.'

'If this period of watchful waiting/observation showed no improvement or a potential worsening of symptoms, I would want to initiate an anti-psychotic with proven efficacy in mania such as olanzapine or quetiapine that also have an evidence base for relapse prevention.'

'Medium and long term, I would also consider a mood stabiliser, if necessary. I would put to her the option of lithium or valproate. I would want to discuss the implications of both choices with her, especially as she is of childbearing age. I would want to emphasise the risk of relapse if she is poorly compliant with her medication.'

Psychological therapies

'Psychological work might include psycho-education, stressing the need to maintain adherence to medication (especially in rapid cycling). She warrants a referral for cognitive behavioural therapy, although NICE outlines a range of psycho-social interventions which have a range of benefits in the form of medication adherence, help with the identification of triggers, treatment of mood symptoms (in particular her depression) and help with stress and lifestyle management.'

'As part of her care agreement, I would want her characteristic symptoms of depression or hypomania documented alongside the early intervention strategies the patient and our treatment should implement when faced by these symptoms.'

'From the social point of view, I would check whether she is driving, given her mood symptoms and the likely start of further psychotropics. It would be useful to contact the university, which can often provide some psychological support and help if she has problems with exams.'

ADDITIONAL POINTS

Whilst rapid cycling has been a topic of debate over the years, there is insufficient evidence to suggest that the treatment strategy should be any different from any other form of bipolar, at least in the earlier stages.

⇧ Although not included here, examiners often attempt to differentiate the high-achieving candidates by asking about an individual's prognosis. Have a clear list of prognoses for the common psychiatric disorders that are likely to present in the examination, including depression, bipolar, schizophrenia and personality disorder.

FURTHER READING

BALANCE Investigators (2010) Lithium plus valproate combination therapy versus monotherapy for relapse prevention in bipolar I disorder (BALANCE): A randomised open-label trial. *The Lancet, 375*(9712), 385–95.

Fountoulakis, K.N. (2010) The BALANCE trial. *The Lancet, 375*(9723), 1343–4.

Macritchie, K., Geddes, J., Scott, J., Haslam, D.R. & Goodwin, G. (2001) Valproic acid, valproate and divalproex in the maintenance treatment of bipolar disorder. *The Cochrane Database of Systematic Reviews* (3), CD003196.

National Institute for Health and Clinical Excellence (2006) *Bipolar Disorder: The Management of Bipolar Disorder in Adults, Children and Adolescents, in Primary and Secondary Care. NICE Clinical Guideline 38 (Update Clinical Guideline 185, 2014).* http://www.nice.org.uk/guidance/cg185?unlid=37331332420162281629 5

Taylor, D., Paton, C. & Kapur, S. (2015) *The Maudsley Prescribing Guidelines in Psychiatry,* 12th edn, London: Wiley-Blackwell.

The examiner's mark sheet

Domain/percentage of marks	Essential points to pass	✓	Extra marks/comments (make notes here)
1. Planning and communication 25% of marks	Clear communication Structure to response Clarity of short-, medium- and long-term planning		
2. Consideration of appropriate investigations 25% of marks	Demonstration of a full bio-psycho-social approach to investigations		
3. Appropriate treatment plan 25% of marks	Demonstration of a full bio-psycho-social approach to investigations		
4. Knowledge 25% of marks	Demonstration of the additional difficulty posed by the current presentation due to ongoing antidepressant use and rapid cycling		

⇩

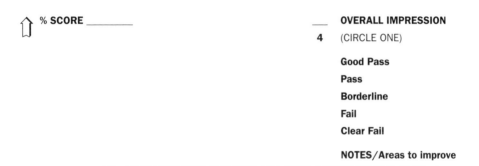

⇧ % SCORE _____

___ **OVERALL IMPRESSION**

4 (CIRCLE ONE)

Good Pass

Pass

Borderline

Fail

Clear Fail

NOTES/Areas to improve

STATION 2(a): DEPRESSION

> **INSTRUCTION TO CANDIDATE**
>
> You are asked to see a patient, Mrs Johnston, for a second opinion by a more junior colleague. She has a long-standing history of low mood and several admissions with suicidal thoughts and plans. She is currently prescribed amitriptyline.
>
> **Take a history of her mood symptoms and explore her previous psychiatric history.**

ACTOR (ROLE-PLAYER) INSTRUCTIONS

You have been low in mood for the last 2 years but have brief periods where you almost feel 'normal' again. That said, you cannot recall feeling 'happy' during this time.

You have put on a significant amount of weight (you were told by your GP that you have gone from a healthy weight to a BMI of 28 in the last 18 months).

You sleep at least 10 hours per day, as you cannot bear to face the real world. You are frequently tearful, have difficulty concentrating and are in despair about your future. On one such occasion, 2 years ago, you took all your tablets, necessitating an admission to a medical intensive care unit.

You have a partner who is not supportive, drinks heavily and has been verbally and physically abusive in the past (he has not hit the children). You left your job as you did not feel able to cope.

Your mother helped look after the children – no concerns have been raised about their recent care.

You have had further thoughts of killing yourself recently.

SUGGESTED APPROACH

Setting the scene

Begin the task by introducing yourself and explaining the purpose of the assessment.

'Hello Ms. Johnston, I am Dr_____, I am a colleague of your usual psychiatrist who asked for a review given your depressive symptoms. On some occasions when a patient is not getting better with the usual treatments, it is not uncommon to ask for a second opinion by another member of the team to see if there is more that can be done.'

Completing the task

This task is about eliciting a history of depressive disorder. One should be aware of the diagnostic criteria for depression and other differential neurotic and affective disorders.

'Tell me a little about the first episode of depression you had. What was going on at the time? What other symptoms did you experience? Tell me about further depressive episodes that you have experienced since.'

Due to limited time, it will be difficult to comprehensively cover her past psychiatric history. It is sufficient to ask about when she first became depressed, the reasons for this (the patient in the station will maintain that she has been depressed constantly since then), the number of times (approximately) she has been admitted to hospital and whether they were formal or informal admissions. As always at this stage, whether she has tried to harm herself needs to be clarified.

Finally, a medication review (still considered a part of the past psychiatric history) would include which medications she had taken for her mood and whether she felt any of them helped. One would also need to enquire about compliance, how long she took these medications for and if she had problems tolerating any of them.

'Were any of the medications that you have tried particularly helpful? What caused you to stop taking them? Did you remember to take them regularly?'

Risks

'Have you thought about harming yourself recently? Have you gone so far as to think about how you might do that? What thoughts have stopped you so far?'

Psycho-social stress factors

This will inform factors perpetuating depression. 'How bad did the difficulties with your partner get? Did it get to the stage of pushing and shoving? Did he hit you? When was the last time this happened? Why do you think he has stopped?'

'How are the children doing at school? Have any concerns been raised about them? Did they see your husband hit you previously? Where are they now?'

Finally, rule out other differentials and ask about any free-floating anxiety, psychotic experiences, obsessions/compulsions and panic attacks.

Problem solving

Some candidates may fail to identify this as a case of atypical depression. It is a somewhat controversial diagnosis with some suggesting that it is associated with increased distress, suicidal ideation and disability compared with 'typical' depression. Despite this, they should be able to highlight the psycho-social stressors that are having an impact on her mood. The differential includes dysthymia and mixed anxiety and depressive disorder. One should make an effort to exclude these as possibilities.

ADDITIONAL POINTS

A common failing in this situation is that candidates are unclear of the symptoms for differentiating moderate from major depression. For a clear understanding of this, refer to the ICD-10 diagnostic criteria. Suicidal acts are almost always associated with severe depression.

The candidate will gain extra marks for taking the history in a structured way. However, they should not be afraid to further explore the information provided by the patient, as a simple tick-list approach to symptoms will not be rewarded.

FURTHER READING

American Psychiatric Association (2013) *Diagnostic and Statistical Manual of Mental Disorders*. 5th edn. Washington, DC: American Psychiatric Association.

Brown, G.W. & Harris, T.O. (eds.) (1978) Social origins of depression. In: *A Study of Psychiatric Disorder in Women*, 5th edn. London: Routledge.

Brown, G.W., Harris, T.O. & Hepworth, C. (1995) Loss, humiliation and entrapment among women developing depression: A patient and non-patient comparison. *Psychological Medicine*, 25, 7–21.

Kendler, K.S., Hettema, J.M., Butera, F., Gardner, C.O. & Prescott, C.A. (2003) Life event dimensions of loss, humiliation, entrapment, and danger in the prediction of onsets of major depression and generalized anxiety. *Archives of General Psychiatry*, 60, 789–96.

The examiner's mark sheet

Domain/ percentage of marks	Essential points to pass	✓	Extra marks/comments (make notes here)
1. Rapport and communication 20% of marks	Clear communication Open and closed questions Empathy Demonstrating patience		
2. Exploration of the atypical presentation 20% of marks	Clarity in approach of more typical depressive features and how these differ Rules out differentials		
3. Exploration of past psychiatric history 20% of marks	Concise exploration of salient components of past psychiatric history		
4. Medication history 20% of marks	Clarity that this patient has taken previous medications for depression and adequate dose and duration		
5. Risk assessment 20% of marks	Exploration of direct and wider risks		

⇑ **% SCORE** _____

___ **OVERALL IMPRESSION**

5 (CIRCLE ONE)

Good Pass

Pass

Borderline

Fail

Clear Fail

NOTES/Areas to improve

STATION 2(b): DEPRESSION – DISCUSSION WITH COLLEAGUE

> **INSTRUCTION TO CANDIDATE**
>
> The lady you have just seen is depressed with an atypical depression. She has symptoms of variability of mood, tension, overeating, oversleeping and fatigue.
>
> She has also expressed further recent thoughts of self-harm. She lost her job as due to depression she was struggling to cope. She has a partner who is not supportive and drinks heavily. He has been both verbally and physically abusive in the past.
>
> She has had recent thoughts of self-harm, but no clear plans as to how she might do this.
>
> **You meet with your junior colleague. Give your advice on managing Mrs Johnston's condition. Try to gather more appropriate information.**

ACTOR (ROLE-PLAYER) INSTRUCTIONS

You are the junior doctor. You are grateful that the candidate has stepped in to help you with the assessment. You are talkative and inquisitive.

You want to know what the diagnosis is and how to manage it.

You are worried about her social situation and in particular the abusive relationship with her partner and that she may be at risk. You want to know what is available to the patient to support and reduce her risks.

You ask whether amitriptyline is the best choice of antidepressant and whether she should switch to an alternative and how this would be managed.

SUGGESTED APPROACH

Setting the scene

Introduce yourself; remember this can be informal as he is your colleague. 'Hello, glad we can catch up, let us discuss this patient Mrs Johnston and think about how we can go ahead.'

Completing the task

This is a management station. Give a brief summary of your findings from your previous assessment. When addressing risk, the candidate should avoid the temptation to start outlining in detail their risk history. They should mention the salient points and highlight that she has some atypical features such as overeating and excessive sleep.

'She has atypical depression that impacts on her social and occupational functioning. There are a number of social stressors, including her relationship with her husband.'

'The major issue is the management of her depressive illness and her risk of suicide. I would therefore want to perform a full risk assessment.'

'One needs to consider her treatment setting. Is her home situation currently safe? Is she living in a home situation where home treatment would be possible or desirable? Could she be treated as an out-patient? Could she go to stay with a relative? Alternatively, if the risks escalated, might a women's refuge or shelter be an option? From what I know currently of the history, I would be reluctant to admit her to a general adult ward as these can be distressing environments in their own right.'

'If we decide we can manage her as an out-patient (i.e. we can manage the risk and can contract her safety), my treatments would consist of biological and psycho-social interventions.'

Treatment

'I note this lady is on amitriptyline. I would want to know the reasons for such a choice. I would then want to explore if it had been of benefit. It does have sedative properties and may not be the treatment of choice as she is sleeping more than usual and has ideas of self-harm, which might include overdosing.'

'The social interventions in this individual will be of particular importance. I would want to contact children's social services to clarify the risk to the children and discuss the need for a safeguarded alert if this had not already been done. I would refer her to an adult social worker within our team to look into her current financial situation and ensure her basic needs are being met (e.g. is she on benefits? Does she have any money?). She may need a review of her housing. She may also need a referral to other services such as "RELATE" if she requires support for her marriage.'

ADDITIONAL POINTS

Making reference to Barbui and Hotopf's (2001) meta-analysis indicating the possibility of increased effectiveness of amitriptyline in comparison to alternative antidepressants, despite its lower level of tolerability, is impressive.

NICE suggests a selective serotonin reuptake inhibitor (SSRI) should be used for all types of depression in the first instance. That said, whilst monoamine oxidase inhibitors have largely fallen out of favour, the candidate may wish to indicate their knowledge of the literature by suggesting that they may have some efficacy in atypical depression.

The diagnosis of atypical depression, however, remains controversial. There should be a balanced approach as she has symptoms that are consistent with atypical depression and there should be awareness that understanding of this condition and treatment implications are works in progress.

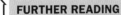

FURTHER READING

Barbui, C. & Hotopf, M. (2001) Amitriptyline vs the rest: Still the leading antidepressant after 40 years of randomised controlled trials. *British Journal of Psychiatry*, 178, 129–44.

Stewart, J.W., Tricamo, E., McGrath, P.J. & Quitkin, F.M. (1997) Prophylactic efficacy of phenelzine and imipramine in chronic atypical depression: Likelihood of recurrence on discontinuation after 6 months' remission. *American Journal of Psychiatry*, 154, 31–6.

The examiner's mark sheet

Domain/ percentage of marks	Essential points to pass	✓	Extra marks/comments (make notes here)
1. Planning and communication 25% of marks	Clear communication Structure to response Clarity of major issues		
2. Consideration of appropriate investigations 25% of marks	Demonstration of a full bio-psycho-social approach to investigations		
3. Appropriate treatment plan 25% of marks	Indications for pertinent medications Consideration of treatment setting		
4. Risk assessment 25% of marks	Adequate consideration of the social risks, risk to self and child protection		

% SCORE _____

___ 4

OVERALL IMPRESSION

(CIRCLE ONE)

Good Pass

Pass

Borderline

Fail

Clear Fail

NOTES/Areas to improve

STATION 3(a): FIRST ONSET PSYCHOSIS

INSTRUCTION TO CANDIDATE

An 18-year-old university student is referred for assessment by his GP. The patient is perplexed, frightened and expresses ideas of persecution. He is keen to be admitted to hospital. He has no previous psychiatric history.

> Your consultant catches you before you see the patient. She wants to discuss your thoughts on the differential diagnosis and how you intend to proceed over the next 48 hours.

ACTOR (ROLE-PLAYER) INSTRUCTIONS

You are the senior doctor and want to discuss this referral that has come through from the GP. You have a discussion with your junior doctor about what differential diagnoses he or she will consider for this patient and discuss treatment plans with him or her.

SUGGESTED APPROACH

Setting the scene

Introduce yourself: 'Hello, Dr_____, glad we can meet beforehand to discuss this referral. I gather from the GP letter I am about to see an 18-year-old student who is paranoid.'

Completing the tasks

This task is about demonstrating knowledge of various differential diagnoses in a young person presenting with paranoid symptoms. Be prepared to be questioned about the diagnostic criteria for those diagnoses. You will have to elaborate on a proposed management plan further. As you have not yet assessed the patient, you will have to be broad and inclusive of various presentations when considering the answers. Discuss risk assessment and risk management.

Differential diagnosis

Consultant: I just wanted to brainstorm with you what sort of differentials you have in mind for this patient.

C: In terms of Fould's hierarchy, I would consider:

- Drug-induced psychosis – he could be in a state of intoxication or withdrawal.
- Organic illness, including neurological disorders; this includes brain tumour, temporal lobe epilepsy and autoimmune conditions causing vasculitis in the brain.
- A pre-psychotic state or prodrome of psychosis, a full-blown psychotic episode or a transient psychotic experience.
- Schizoaffective state if there are affective symptoms alongside.
- Manic episode with psychotic symptoms.
- A depressive episode with psychotic features.
- An anxiety disorder due to the clear high levels of distress.
- Personality disorder (e.g. schizotypal or paranoid).

Consultant: How would you go about managing this patient?

C: I shall proceed first to obtain a full history, mental state examination and detailed physical examination. I would pay attention to biological, psychological and social vulnerabilities and possible precipitants. My management would then consist of investigations and treatment. I would want to continue monitoring his mood to pick up on any potential signs of worsening of anxiety symptoms and distress. My investigations may involve a period of watchful waiting in whichever environment we decide to treat him.

Investigations

'I would want to investigate for important comorbidities such as substance misuse. Physical investigations would include a full blood screen including glucose, liver, thyroid function and lipids. I would also want baseline physical observations. There is an increasing trend to consider screening for NMDA auto-antibodies if there is anything atypical about the presentation e.g. movement disorders, evidence of seizures etc... In line with NICE guidance, I would arrange brain imaging such as a CT head or MRI.'

Treatment

'If however, he has clear-cut first rank symptoms and these psychotic experiences have been present for some time, or he is significantly distressed, I would start an anti-psychotic immediately. I would also bear in mind (although this would not delay instigation of treatment) that both ICD-10 and DSM-IV require a 4-week history of symptoms to diagnose schizophrenia (this is important regarding what we tell him of his diagnosis). I would consider the prescription of a benzodiazepine to alleviate any significant distress or anxiety.'

Consultant: Would you consider admitting him to hospital if he wants to?

C: From the brief description outlined by the GP, there is nothing that would indicate to me a need for an admission currently, so I would want to explore the reasons for why he is asking for a hospital bed. The types of risks I would bear in mind would be:

- Those that pose a risk to self or others, including challenging or unpredictable behaviour
- Risks associated with his high level of distress
- Wider risks such as:
- Lack of engagement at this important first stage
- Damage to his social network and reputation, which may worsen with untreated psychosis
- Labelling as 'schizophrenic' at too early a stage.

ADDITIONAL POINTS

It is good to have an awareness of the National Service Framework and its suggestion of the need for early intervention and treatment to reduce levels of morbidity.

The first point of contact with mental health services is important, as it may influence engagement and counter the individual's and their relatives' prejudices and issues of stigma. This should be reflected throughout the management of this scenario.

Essentially, the candidate should deal with two main issues in the acute setting: treating the psychotic symptoms, treating factors associated with their development (including consideration of treatment setting) and wider issues relevant to their onset.

FURTHER READING

Department of Health (1999) *A National Service Framework for Mental Health: Modern Standards and Service Models*. London: Department of Health.

Foulds, G.A. & Bedford, A. (1975) Hierarchy of classes of personal illness. *Psychological Medicine*, 5(2), 181–92.

Marshall, M. & Rathbone, J. 2006. Early intervention for psychosis. *Cochrane Database of Systematic Reviews* (3), CD004718.

National Institute of Clinical Excellence (2002, updated 2010) *Schizophrenia: Core Interventions in the Treatment and Management of Schizophrenia in Primary and Secondary Care*. London: NICE.

The examiner's mark sheet

Domain/ percentage of marks	Essential points to pass	✓	Extra marks/comments (make notes here)
1. Differential diagnosis discussion 25% of marks	Clear structure and consideration of each psychiatric domain		
2. Appropriate investigations 25% of marks	Bio-psycho-social considerations		
3. Appropriate treatment 25% of marks	Bio-psycho-social considerations		
4. Risk assessment 25% of marks	Exploration of awareness of a wider variety of risk than simply direct harm		

% SCORE _____

___ **OVERALL IMPRESSION**

4 (CIRCLE ONE)

Good Pass

Pass

Borderline

Fail

Clear Fail

NOTES/Areas to improve

STATION 3(b): FIRST ONSET PSYCHOSIS – DISCUSSION WITH RELATIVE

INSTRUCTION TO CANDIDATE

You have assessed the patient and you decide that the patient has symptoms that are consistent with first onset psychosis. The patient's mother, Mrs Giles, turns up and asks what is going on. She saw a programme on bipolar disorder the other day and wonders if this is what her son has. She wants to know what the management plan is and if he will be able to go back to university (she comments that he has been struggling for the last year – he used to be top of the class but has had no evidence of a frank psychosis until now). If not, she wonders whether she should take him home. She has also heard of early-onset services, and wonders whether this is a suitable service and what other options may be available.

The patient has said he is happy for you to speak to his mother alone. Speak to her and address her concerns.

ACTOR (ROLE-PLAYER) INSTRUCTIONS

You have a limited understanding of schizophrenia, and from what you have seen on the television, you think it might be a dangerous condition (you think your son may become violent). You have therefore asked your son to stay in hospital.

You understand that schizophrenia means 'split mind' and wonder whether it's akin to a Dr Jekyll and Mr Hyde presentation. You ask the doctor to explain.

You are worried about his academic performance.

There are no risks at home, and if the candidate is sufficiently reassuring, you will agree to have your son home.

SUGGESTED APPROACH

Setting the scene

Introduce yourself and explain the purpose of the meeting. 'Hello, Mrs Giles, I am Dr_____, I have seen and spoken with your son, who has given permission to talk about what we think is going on. How can I help you?'

Try to clarify any concerns then address any negative stereotypes/fears of mental illness (and services).

Completing the tasks

This is an explanatory station; avoid medical jargon when explaining to relatives. Listen carefully to her concerns and try and address them. This station is also about psycho-education for family and alleviating the anxieties of a worried mother.

Explaining the diagnosis

Mother: You say my son is psychotic, is he a psycho? Schizophrenia means split personality, right?

C: I understand your concerns, and certainly the media has had a part to play in the misunderstanding of mental illness in today's society. Schizophrenia does not mean that one has a split personality, or is a psychopath or 'psycho' as some people put it. This reference to psychopaths is very different to what we mean when we talk about psychosis. In fact, it is an entirely different psychiatric illness. You are right that schizophrenia does mean split mind, but psychiatrists use this in relation to the split of normal links between thinking, behaviour, mood and perception or contact with reality. What you tend to see are two main types of symptoms. The first – positive symptoms – include 'delusions', which are thoughts and beliefs that no-one else knows or believes and are usually bizarre or strange in nature. They are strongly held, usually preoccupy the patient and cannot be shaken with evidence or logic. They also include 'hallucinations', in which the patient can hear, smell, feel or see something that is not there. The second set of problems, called 'negative symptoms', include loss of interest in their ability to start or persist with tasks; in other words, a lack of their previous 'get up and go'.

Explaining cause

Mother: Why has he got this illness?

C: We know one of the natural chemicals in the brain called dopamine is released in larger quantities for those who suffer from this condition. This chemical is linked with 'importance' and 'learning'. One theory behind the development of schizophrenia is that too much of this chemical leads to too great an emphasis or *meaning* in relatively normal events. The patient, like your son, starts off feeling the effects of dopamine, and starts to suspect something is wrong. They may look preoccupied (or perplexed as we call it), just like your son does. As the levels of this dopamine increase, they suddenly have a clearer idea of what was so important. For example, an entirely random event such as someone looking at them on the street may suddenly be taken to mean that the government has sent that person (or MI5) to spy on them.

Explaining impact of illness and prognosis

Mother: Is he going to get better? Can he complete his course?

C: We will need to see what happens after treatment. There are studies that indicate some patients may show a decrease in their IQ by around 4–8 points, but this does not happen in all people who suffer from the condition, and it does not necessarily mean that they will not be able to complete their course. A return to university will depend on his progress. A discussion with the university will be needed at this time as he may need some support. If he responds well to treatment, he should be able to return with support.

Explaining treatment

'Anti-psychotics reduce the action of this natural chemical in the brain, and therefore weaken the delusions and hallucination experience. It does not necessarily cure the condition, but controls symptoms in the same way a blood pressure tablet controls hypertension. They work best when taken regularly.'

'Psychological therapies can also help, including cognitive behavioural therapy to identify triggers to illness and ways of coping with them. Family therapy can also help your son and yourselves cope better with the illness.'

ADDITIONAL POINTS

- Explore their viewpoint on what might have contributed to this current state. Use predisposing, precipitating and maintaining factors rather than discussion on a purely biological basis. A blame-free approach is particularly important.
- Address practical issues such as what home life is like and whether in this situation it would be appropriate to send this patient home – provide an adequate exploration of the risks.

FURTHER READING

Kapur, S. & Mamo, D. (2003) Half a century of antipsychotics and still a central role for dopamine D2 receptors. *Progress in Neuro-Psychopharmacology and Biological Psychiatry*, 27(7), 1081–90.

Reichenberg, A., Weiser, M., Rabinowitz, J. & Caspi, A. (2002) A population-based cohort study of premorbid intellectual, language, and behavioral functioning in patients with schizophrenia, schizoaffective disorder, and nonpsychotic bipolar disorder. *The American Journal of Psychiatry*, 159(12), 2027–35.

The examiner's mark sheet

Domain/ percentage of marks	Essential points to pass	✓	Extra marks/comments (make notes here)
1. Rapport and communication 20% of marks	Clear communication Open and closed questions Empathy Demonstrating patience		
2. Explaining diagnosis 20% of marks	Clarity in discussion of hallucinations and delusions		
3. Explaining cause 20% of marks	Clarity in discussion of cause		
4. Explaining impact of illness and prognosis 20% of marks	Dealing with the current uncertainty of his concern		
5. Explaining treatment 20% of marks	Discussion of biological and psychological options		

% SCORE _____

___

5

OVERALL IMPRESSION

(CIRCLE ONE)

Good Pass

Pass

Borderline

Fail

Clear Fail

NOTES/Areas to improve

STATION 4(a): RAPID TRANQUILISATION

INSTRUCTION TO CANDIDATE

You are on your lunch break when you are called to your general adult psychiatry ward urgently. A new patient admission, Mr Clancy, has become extremely agitated and has assaulted a member of staff. He is holding a dinner fork in his hand and is shouting about the CIA coming to get him.

The patient has been escorted back to his bedroom. You enter the room with the restraint team. Perform a mental state examination.

ACTOR (ROLE-PLAYER) INSTRUCTIONS

You are a patient with new-onset paranoid schizophrenia.

You believe that the staff member you assaulted is a spy working for the Central Intelligence Agency (CIA) and that he was trying to poison you when he gave you your regular prescribed risperidone.

You will not take oral medication as you believe it is poisoned. You have a history of assault with a charge of actual bodily harm in the context of this current episode of psychosis.

You will become progressively more agitated and angry during the assessment unless the candidate is able to successfully de-escalate the situation. You are shouting and becoming extremely threatening.

You have been on the anti-psychotic risperidone for 6 weeks. You have been taking it infrequently as it makes you feel slow, tired and stiff (the stiffness is the worst of the symptoms).

SUGGESTED APPROACH

Setting the scene

Introduce yourself: 'Hello, Mr Clancy, I am Dr____, the psychiatrist.' The patient will be agitated, rude and shouting; it is important to remain calm under pressure and be professional at all times. Talk clearly and slowly and explain why you have come to see him. 'I hear that things are not going very well for you right now, can you tell me what is bothering you?'

Completing the task

This is a high-risk scenario in the ward environment. Your immediate concern is for the safety and welfare of the other patients and staff. The candidate should explore the reasons for the patient's agitation, background relevant to the ward admission and whether there were any known risks prior to the admission.

De-escalation and removal of the weapon

Despite the risk, the patient is clearly unwell. The candidate will need to engage with the patient in as positive a manner as possible, and establish some form of rapport with the patient.

The NICE guidelines on agitation and aggression are clear that staff should accept it is not realistic to expect the person exhibiting disturbed behaviour to simply calm down. In a crisis situation, staff are therefore responsible for avoiding provocation.

The interaction should involve clear statements, with one question given only at a time, a focus on questions relating to facts regarding the problem and an avoidance of minimising the patient's concerns.

'Mr Clancy, I am Dr_____, I am very sorry to see that we have upset you. I'm here to help if I can. Firstly, can you tell me what just happened now with the nurse? ... I'm sorry to hear that that happened. I think we need to come up with a plan as to how we can help you whilst you are here. However, it is very difficult for us to talk to you with you holding the fork like that. You can see that this is frightening to other people. I need you to put it on the floor over there so we can move on and focus on how to help you best ... Thank you for doing that, it really is appreciated.'

Assessment of mental state and risk

'Now, as I promised, I would like to think about how we can help you. Do you think you might get the urge to hit another nurse if they give you medication? ... I can see you are still upset – I would be inclined to suggest another tablet to help calm you down and reduce the stress that the thoughts of the CIA are giving you. I hope you are not offended by this, but it is a question I ask everyone: have you taken any illicit drugs prior to coming on the ward? A final question: the nurse you hit is actually quite hurt currently. What are your thoughts on that? Remind me, do you have any problems with your physical health? Any problems with your heart or breathing problems? Have you had a particularly bad reaction to any previous psychiatric medications?'

ADDITIONAL POINTS

In the unlikely event that the patient becomes unmanageable, the candidate should terminate the interview to allow for restraint and rapid tranquilisation.

The examiner's mark sheet

Domain/ percentage of marks	Essential points to pass	✓	Extra marks/comments (make notes here)
1. Rapport and communication 25% of marks	Clear communication Open and closed questions Empathy Demonstrating patience		
2. Verbal de-escalation and risk management 25% of marks	Negotiation of removal of the weapon Appropriate timing of decision to implement rapid tranquilisation if verbal de-escalation fails		
3. Assessment of mental state and risk 25% of marks	Discussion of risks		
4. Assessment of patient's views on assaulting the nurse 25% of marks	Checking for any level of insight or remorse into actions		

% SCORE _____

OVERALL IMPRESSION

___

4   (CIRCLE ONE)

Good Pass

Pass

Borderline

Fail

Clear Fail

NOTES/Areas to improve

STATION 4(b): RAPID TRANQUILISATION – DISCUSSION WITH NURSE

> ## INSTRUCTION TO CANDIDATE
>
> The patient has now handed the fork over and has taken a single dose of lorazepam 1 mg orally.
>
> He is still pacing the room restlessly, muttering to himself. He has punched the wall on one occasion.
>
> **Speak to the nurse in charge about further management.**

ACTOR (ROLE-PLAYER) INSTRUCTIONS

You have significant concerns about the patient staying on the ward.

You will want a clear management plan, with a clear idea of successive steps in such a plan.

You are concerned that whilst he has been taking his risperidone on the ward, there appears to have been no improvement in his symptoms.

SUGGESTED APPROACH

Setting the scene

Introduce yourself: 'Hello, Sister, I am Dr_____, the psychiatrist. I know things have been very difficult on the ward and you are concerned. Let us have a discussion on how to go about this further.' If the nurse interrupts with anger or asks questions, listen to and acknowledge her. Try to address the worry that she expresses.

Completing the task

This task tests the skill of the candidate to formulate a management plan in a difficult situation and communicate the plan effectively to a professional from a nursing background. Be mindful that a nurse on a medical ward may not have any mental health experience if this scenario is happening on a medical ward. It is important for the candidate to demonstrate that they are giving consideration to all aspects of ward management, including the welfare of the patient, other patients and staff. In particular, they should demonstrate an awareness of the impact on ward resources of the loss of a staff member, with simultaneous increased nursing care requirements of an agitated patient.

'How are the nursing staff on the ward doing? They must be a little shaken up by it all. Where is the nurse who was assaulted? Who is looking after her? Is she OK? Does she need to go to A&E? Do we have sufficient staff for the current shift now that she is off the ward? Will we need to bring in someone for additional cover at short notice?'

Medical treatment

'We need to give some time for the lorazepam to take effect. If he is still agitated after 45 minutes, I think he should have a further dose of 1–2 mg, depending on how successful the current dose has been at reducing his agitation. Ideally, we would offer this to him orally, but it should be given intramuscularly if there is no alternative. Can we check we have stocks of flumazenil on the ward? We need to be careful that he hasn't taken other illicit substances.'

'Is there a nurse who knows him well who might be able to encourage him to take something orally?'

'If he is still not settled and needs further treatment, I would prefer to use a single antipsychotic if possible. We are not sure that he has been taking his risperidone regularly in the community, and he complained of some side effects as well.'

'I would be inclined to switch it to olanzapine, which has a reasonable proven efficacy in disturbed patients. For the time being, shall we use the orodispersible Velotab to ensure he is taking it, at a dose of 10 mg if he is agitated. This can also be given intramuscularly if he refuses oral medication to a maximum dose of 20 mg in 24 hours. Remember, it cannot be given within an hour of lorazepam, as it will increase the risk of respiratory distress.'

'He will need ongoing regular monitoring of levels of alertness (GCS), blood pressure, pulse, temperature and respiratory rate if possible. If he is not cooperative, we will need the nurse to document what observations she is able to carry out.'

Psychological treatment

'I think we need to allocate a regular time for interaction with his named nurse on the ward – say hourly in the first instance to build up a rapport, if possible, and to monitor any levels or agitation or distress. If they have any concerns, they should contact me. We will discuss his care regularly during the day.'

Social treatment

'I think we should give him a period of time out in his room until he calms down, and he should currently be placed on "within eyesight" levels of observations. This needs to be done carefully so as not to increase his levels of paranoia.'

'If he has a good relationship with his family, I think we might need to enlist their help in calming him down. They certainly need to be told if we are using restraint and rapid tranquilisation measures.'

'I will go back in and tell him the current plan. Can I take two nurses with me?'

'We will also need to tell the ward consultant that this has happened. They might want to discuss the case with psychiatric intensive care, just so that they are aware that this patient might potentially need a transfer.'

'I think we need to complete an incident form or Datix as well.'

'If all else fails, we may need to consider intravenous diazepam or a dose of zuclopenthixol acetate (Acuphase) intramuscularly, or transfer to a psychiatric intensive care unit, but let's see how he responds to the current treatment plan. I will discuss these with my consultant if he is not improving.'

'The nurse who was assaulted should not return to the ward for the time being whilst the patient remains an in-patient and a risk. I would speak to the ward manager about ensuring that she goes to see occupational health. Additionally, we will need to think about arranging a suitable time for a ward debrief with any of the nurses who wish to attend.'

'Finally, each of the patients should have some time with their key worker to see if they were upset by the situation.'

ADDITIONAL POINTS

There is some conflation in the literature of the studies of rapid tranquilisation and how they relate to clinical practice. Most used a single psychotropic and most patients were given their medications orally. Most relevant to the day-to-day clinical scenario were the Tranquilização Rápida-Ensaio Clínico (TREC – Rapid Tranquillisation-Clinical Trial) studies performed in Brazil and India, which tested the effectiveness of parenteral treatments.

FURTHER READING

Alexander, J., Tharyan, P., Adams, C., John, T., Mol, C. & Philip, J. (2004) Rapid tranquillisation of violent or agitated patients in a psychiatric emergency setting. Pragmatic randomised trial of intramuscular lorazepam v. haloperidol plus promethazine. *The British Journal of Psychiatry*, 185(1), 63–9.

Huf, G., Coutinho, E.S. & Adams, C.E. (2002) TREC-Rio trial: A randomised controlled trial for rapid tranquillisation for agitated patients in emergency psychiatric rooms. *BMC Psychiatry*, 2(1), 11.

National Institute for Health and Care Excellence (NICE) (2015) *NG10: Violence and Aggression: Short Term Management in Mental Health, Health and Community Setting*. https://www.nice.org.uk/guidance/NG10

Taylor, D., Paton, C. & Kapur, S. (2015) *The Maudsley Prescribing Guidelines in Psychiatry*, 12th edn. London: Wiley-Blackwell.

TREC Collaborative Group (2003) Rapid tranquillisation for agitated patients in emergency psychiatric rooms: A randomised trial of midazolam versus haloperidol plus promethazine. *BMJ*, 327(7417), 708–13.

The examiner's mark sheet

Domain/ percentage of marks	Essential points to pass	✓	Extra marks/comments (make notes here)
1. Rapport and communication 25% of marks	Appropriate enquiry into welfare of assaulted nurse Empathy Demonstrating patience		
2. Medical treatment 25% of marks	Clarity with medication planning and potential risk of co-prescribing		
3. Psychological treatment 20% of marks	Appropriate reference to psychological input		
4. Social management 30% of marks	Demonstration of the wider impact that such an event might have on the staff and patients		

⬆ **% SCORE** _____

___ **OVERALL IMPRESSION**

4 (CIRCLE ONE)

Good Pass

Pass

Borderline

Fail

Clear Fail

NOTES/Areas to improve

O SINGLE STATIONS

STATION 5: SSRI DISCONTINUATION SYNDROME

INSTRUCTION TO CANDIDATE

You are seeing in your out-patient clinic a 50-year-old lady, Ms Gibson, who called you 3 days after stopping her paroxetine. She thinks she is relapsing as she is feeling increasingly anxious and nauseous. She wants to know if this is normal.

Assess her symptoms and explain how you are going to manage them.

ACTOR (ROLE-PLAYER) INSTRUCTIONS

You have a discontinuation syndrome precipitated by stopping your medication abruptly. Your symptoms include your old anxiety symptoms (shortness of breath, nausea, palpitations, diaphoresis and a feeling of loss of control), but on direct enquiry, you will reveal you also have diarrhoea, electric shock-like sensations, vivid dreams and brief twitching (myoclonic jerks) the previous night.

You previously suffered from panic disorder with agoraphobia, but have been well for 3 months. You stopped your medication without consulting a health professional, as you felt well.

You are annoyed that no one told you that you could not stop your medications when you wanted.

You wonder if you were misinformed about their 'addictive' potential.

Your symptoms have been so bad that you have at times thought of killing yourself, but know you will not do this as you have so much to live for.

You are insistent you want to stop your medications.

SUGGESTED APPROACH

Setting the scene

Introduce yourself and explain the purpose of the meeting: 'Hello, Ms_____, I am Dr_____, the psychiatrist. I understand you are feeling unwell after you stopped your psychiatric medication. I hope we will be able to discuss this and find a solution to your problems.'

Completing the task

The key aim is to differentiate the patient's panic symptoms from the new phenomenon of discontinuation syndrome. As such, dizziness, palpitations, shortness of breath, diaphoresis and paraesthesia may carry less weight, as they are commonly found in panic, whilst diarrhoea, vivid dreams and electric shock-like sensations should be viewed with concern.

'Can you tell me what anxiety symptoms you used to suffer from 6 months ago? What was the worst of these symptoms for you?'

'Are any of the symptoms different from then; for instance, the ones we worry most about when antidepressants are stopped quickly are muscle jerks, electric shock-like sensations, diarrhoea and vivid dreams. Have you experienced any of these?'

One should enquire about suicidal ideation: 'Has things been so difficult lately that any thoughts of ending your life may have crossed your mind?'

Management

Management should start with psycho-education, including a collaborative discussion on a time frame for discontinuing a medication. It is worthwhile normalising the process to an extent, indicating that paroxetine is one of the most well-known medications for this condition and that, whilst these symptoms can happen while on any antidepressant to some extent, her symptoms are significant enough that we would want to act on them.

There should be brief discussion about alternative therapies, such as cognitive behavioural therapy, if she relapses and no longer wants tablets.

There should be some exploration of the differentials, including neuroleptic malignant syndrome.

'We normally recommend that you only stop your medication after discussion with our team or your GP, ordinarily over a 4-week period.'

'I am not sure what you were told previously, as it is true that antidepressants are not addictive; for instance, they are not like the benzodiazepine tablets that used to be used so readily several years ago, and needed increased doses over time in order to have the same effect. Paroxetine is generally maintained on the same dose.'

'Like all medications (even physical health medications like blood pressure tablets), one should never stop them suddenly, as this can cause problems.'

'If you are happy with this, in order to manage these symptoms, I would be inclined to restart you back onto your full dose, let you settle for about a week, then slowly taper off the dose by 5 mg per week until completely discontinued.'

'It is important to watch to see if thoughts of self-harm start to increase, and to let us know immediately if this is the case.'

The examiner's mark sheet

Domain/ percentage of marks	Essential points to pass	✓	Extra marks/comments (make notes here)
1. Rapport and communication 20% of marks	Clear communication		
	Open and closed questions		
	Empathy		
	Demonstrating patience		

⇧ 2. Exploration of symptoms

20% of marks

Systematic approach to symptoms, including exploration of current symptoms in comparison to previous history

3. Consideration of differential diagnoses

20% of marks

Brief consideration of alternative diagnoses that impact on current management

4. Patient explanation

20% of marks

Clarity of diagnosis and symptoms

5. Treatment plan

20% of marks

Clarity of treatment plan

% SCORE _____

___ **OVERALL IMPRESSION**

5 (CIRCLE ONE)

Good Pass

Pass

Borderline

Fail

Clear Fail

NOTES/Areas to improve

STATION 6: TREATMENT-RESISTANT SCHIZOPHRENIA

INSTRUCTION TO CANDIDATE

Mr Chan is a 30-year-old male with an established diagnosis of paranoid schizophrenia who has tried two anti-psychotics for 6 months each. He is still troubled by distressing persecutory delusions and auditory hallucinations.

Discuss ongoing management with him.

ACTOR (ROLE-PLAYER) INSTRUCTIONS

You are very distressed by these ongoing symptoms and have tried risperidone 6 mg, which you had to discontinue due to side effects. You are currently taking olanzapine 20 mg, which had very little effect on your symptoms. Both medications have been prescribed for approximately 4 months.

You might forget to take medications on the odd day, but were otherwise fully compliant.

You are interested in learning more about clozapine.

SUGGESTED APPROACH

Setting the scene

As always, begin the task by introducing yourself: 'Hello, Mr Chan, I am Dr_____, the psychiatrist.' Acknowledge your understanding of his current problem: 'I gather you are troubled by hearing voices and are feeling unwell. Let us talk about this.'

Completing the task

This task is about demonstrating knowledge of the management of treatment-resistant schizophrenia. You will have to establish other factors that may be perpetuating the psychosis, such as non-compliance with medication, substance misuse, coexisting affective disorder and psycho-social stressors. Clarify what treatment he has received so far.

'I am sorry to hear you are still troubled by these distressing thoughts and unpleasant experiences. It looks like we need to make a decision about your next treatment. Can I ask what anti-psychotics you have tried? Did you take them regularly?'

'Essentially, we have three choices: we can try another anti-psychotic that you have not yet tried; for instance, a tablet like amisulpride. We can add in another tablet to your current treatment plan or we can follow the recommended National Institutes of Clinical Excellence (NICE) guidance and switch you to clozapine.'

'If you are willing to try, I would suggest the last of the three options: a switch to clozapine. It has by far the largest evidence base for what we call treatment-resistant schizophrenia (defined as lack of response to two anti-psychotics given at a treatment dose for a sufficient period of time for them to able to take effect).'

Information on starting clozapine

'There are a number of important things to know when starting clozapine. It is the most effective of the anti-psychotics, with improvement in around 60% of patients who take it. The first thing to say is that, on the whole, it is tolerated well, certainly just as well as any of the other anti-psychotics you have tried. That said, there are some important side effects to be aware of. The common ones are tiredness, problems with too much saliva (causing some people to slur their words) and constipation. Some also experience an increase in heart rate and a drop (or rise) in blood pressure. These are mostly seen in the first month and tend to wear off over time.'

'In the longer term, like most of the anti-psychotics, a lot of people put on quite a lot of weight (up to 4 kg). As such, exercise and healthy diet are very important.'

'Then there are rarer problems, such as a decrease in production of the white blood cells in the body, which are used to fight off infection. For every 100 people who take the medication, an average of three people (or 3%) will experience this, but we can decrease this risk to around half a percent if we monitor your blood closely with weekly blood tests. Again rarely, there is an increased risk of seizures and there can be a problem with inflammation of the heart muscle.'

'I must stress that these complications are all rare. The risks I have mentioned are increased in *relative* terms; however, *total* numbers of people who suffer these complications are very low. It is important to tell you about them so that you can make a fully informed decision about your treatment and also so that you know what to look for should any of these symptoms start to occur.'

Patient requirements

'There are a number of things we would need to do before starting treatment. The first thing would be a blood test, including measurement of the cells that fight infection – your white blood cells – and those that measure your blood sugar (glucose) and natural fat (or lipid) levels. We would need to weigh you and also measure the function of your heart using a heart trace machine called an electrocardiogram or ECG.'

'On the day that you start, you will need to come to the clinic in the morning and take a tablet. We will observe you for a period to see if you tolerate it. On the second day, we would repeat this, but give you a tablet to take home. We can then arrange for people to come and visit you at home in order to monitor you physically as we increase the dose. They will see you daily for the first 2 weeks.'

'We will wean you off the olanzapine that you are taking now. After 2 weeks, we would start to decrease your olanzapine and would decrease this by 5 mg every 2 weeks until you were off it.'

'The one thing I would say is that if you are not confident that you will be able to take these tablets regularly, we would need to think of another way to manage your illness. Stopping the tablets suddenly puts you at high risk of a relapse.'

FURTHER READING

Royal Pharmaceutical Society of Great Britain (2015) *British National Formulary 70*. London: Royal Pharmaceutical Society.

Taylor, D., Paton, C. & Kapur, S. (2015) *The Maudsley Prescribing Guidelines in Psychiatry*, 12th edn. London: Wiley-Blackwell.

The examiner's mark sheet

Domain/ percentage of marks	Essential points to pass	✓	Extra marks/comments (make notes here)
1. Rapport and communication 25% of marks	Clear communication		
	Open and closed questions		
	Empathy		
	Demonstrating patience		
2. Explanation of treatment options 25% of marks	Evidence of a collaborative approach		
	Explores any other perpetuating factors for ongoing psychosis		
3. Information on clozapine 25% of marks	Balanced discussion of benefits and risks		
4. Patient requirement 25% of marks	Clarity in discussion of necessary investigations and need for compliance		

⇧ **% SCORE** _____

___ **OVERALL IMPRESSION**

4 (CIRCLE ONE)

Good Pass

Pass

Borderline

Fail

Clear Fail

NOTES/Areas to improve

STATION 7: POST-TRAUMATIC STRESS DISORDER

INSTRUCTIONS TO CANDIDATE

You are seeing Mark, a 32-year-old man who has been referred by his GP for anxiety and lack of sleep. He has stopped working recently and is worried about his future.

Speak to Mark and elicit the history of his symptoms with a diagnostic approach.

ACTOR (ROLE-PLAYER) INSTRUCTIONS

You have been suffering from anxiety for approximately 8 months; it all began after the car accident that you experienced on your way to work. You suffered some injury to your shoulder, which is now being treated well. Since then, you have been waking up from sleep with vivid nightmares of the accident. Every time you drive past the place of accident, you feel panicky and you feel your heart is racing and as if you are going to faint. Therefore, you decided that you would change your route, but recently you have become terrified of driving itself. This has limited your activities, as without driving you cannot go anywhere; you have started to stay at home. This has caused problems at work and you are at risk of losing your job. You are anxious about your future and would appreciate any help from the health services.

SUGGESTED APPROACH

Setting the scene

Begin the task by addressing the patient by name and introduce yourself. Acknowledge that they may be anxious to see the psychiatrist and explain the purpose of your assessment: 'Hello, Mark, I am Dr_____, a trainee psychiatrist. I understand you have been going through a tough time. I am here to understand your difficulties and see if we can help you manage them.'

Allow the patient to tell you what their understanding of this appointment is. As he is experiencing anxiety already, he may be reluctant to freely explain the symptoms and will need some encouragement.

Completing the task

After introduction, allow the patient to tell you what his problems are and how they began. Take a history of post-traumatic stress disorder (PTSD), including the presenting complaints and duration of illness. Begin with open-ended questions and then ask about specific symptoms. The differential diagnosis would include panic disorder, generalised anxiety disorder and comorbid condition such as depression. Therefore, ask briefly about low mood, anhedonia and biological symptoms of depression. A brief risk assessment is required in order to assess any suicidal tendencies.

Elaborate on history

Begin the interview using the information given by the GP: 'I see you have been experiencing anxiety/nervousness. Can you tell how this started?' Ask about the chronology of events: 'How long has this been affecting you? When did this begin? Have there been any changes in your condition over these few months? How has this affected your life?'

The most characteristic symptoms of PTSD are re-experiencing symptoms. PTSD sufferers involuntarily re-experience aspects of the traumatic event in a very vivid and distressing way. This includes flashbacks in which the person acts or feels as if the event were recurring, nightmares and repetitive and distressing intrusive images or other sensory impressions from the event. Reminders of the traumatic event arouse intense distress and/or physiological reactions. Ask about such symptoms in a sensitive manner, as talking about them can make the person uncomfortable. 'Have there been any instances where you felt as if you were reliving that terrible moment again? When do you experience this? How often does this happen? Can you describe how you feel during those times?'

Avoidance of reminders of the trauma is another core symptom of PTSD. This includes people, situations or circumstances resembling or associated with the event. PTSD sufferers often try to push memories of the event out of their mind and avoid thinking or talking about it in detail, particularly about its worst moments. On the other hand, many ruminate excessively about questions that prevent them from coming to terms with the event; for example, about why the event happened to them, how it could have been prevented or how they could take revenge. Explore these symptoms in a gentle manner by asking, for example, 'You have been through such traumatic events lately, I can imagine how difficult it must have been for you. How do you cope in situations when you are reminded of that accident? How has your life changed following this event?'

People with PTSD experience symptoms of hyperarousal, including hypervigilance for threat, exaggerated startle responses, irritability, difficulty concentrating and sleep problems. On the other hand, PTSD sufferers also describe symptoms of emotional numbing. These include an inability to have any feelings, feeling detached from other people, giving up previously significant activities and amnesia for significant parts of the event. You can explore such symptoms by asking questions like, 'Do you find yourself to be excessively sensitive to what goes on around you? Are you getting startled by things that normally wouldn't surprise you that much? Have your feelings/emotions towards others changed? Do you think your personality has changed in the recent months? If so, how have they changed?'

Many PTSD sufferers experience other associated symptoms, including depression, generalised anxiety, shame, guilt and reduced libido, which contribute to their distress and impact on their functioning, all of which need to be briefly explored. Ask about any relationship difficulties or financial difficulties that may have ensued from his anxiety.

At the end, briefly rule out other anxiety disorders such as generalised anxiety disorder (free-floating anxiety), panic disorder (frequent and regular panic attacks with no obvious triggers) and depression. Do a risk assessment, mainly to consider any suicidal tendencies and use of alcohol as a coping mechanism.

Conclusion

Here you can summarise what you have assessed, any information you may need and what the next steps will be:

'Mark, from what we talked about today, I gather you have been feeling increasingly anxious since you met with an accident 8 months ago. You have been experiencing periods where you are almost reliving the incident again and again. You therefore have been avoiding the route, now you started to avoid driving and it looks like this has been significantly affecting your activities of living and your emotions. I think you may be experiencing post-traumatic stress disorder. Most people when faced with severe trauma get over such experiences in time. In some people, though, traumatic experiences set off a reaction that can last for many months or years. This is called post-traumatic stress disorder, or PTSD for short. We shall meet again to discuss the possible options to manage your condition. This will include talking therapies and medications. In the meantime, can I recommend to you some self-help books for you to consider?'

FURTHER READING

American Psychiatric Association Steering Committee (2010) Practice guideline for the treatment of patients with acute stress disorder and posttraumatic stress disorder. www. psychiatryonline.org/pb/assets/raw/sitewide/practice_guidelines/guidelines/acutes tressdisorderptsd.pdf

http://www.rcpsych.ac.uk/healthadvice/problemsdisorders/posttraumaticstressdisorder. aspx

Post-Traumatic Stress Disorder: Management. NICE Guidelines (CG26). Published date: March 2005. https://www.nice.org.uk/guidance/cg26?unlid=38893879820164179 4355

The examiner's mark sheet

Domain Percentage of marks	Essential points to pass	✓	Extra marks/comments (make notes here)
1. Rapport and communication 20% of marks	Introduces self appropriately Uses clear communication Makes appropriate use of open and closed questions Demonstrates an empathic and caring approach		
2. History taking – core symptoms 20% of marks	Core symptoms – flashbacks, nightmares, avoidance and hypervigilance		
3. Exploring symptoms 20% of marks	Explores the impact on life activities and general wellbeing Psycho-social adversities – lack of job and any financial or relationship difficulties that have arisen out of this situation		

4. Exploring differentials and risk assessment

20% of marks

Explores differentials, mood disorders, panic disorder and generalised anxiety disorder (GAD)

5. Ascertaining diagnosis and conclusion

20% of marks

Diagnosing PTSD

Advises patient on the rationale for diagnosis and offers further help

% SCORE _____

___

5

OVERALL IMPRESSION

(CIRCLE ONE)

Good Pass

Pass

Borderline

Fail

Clear Fail

NOTES/Areas to improve

Chapter 10

Neuropsychiatry
Derek Tracy

○ LINKED STATIONS

STATION 1(a): ASSESSMENT OF A HEAD INJURY

INSTRUCTION TO CANDIDATE

An orthopaedic specialty trainee, Dr Arun, wants to discuss one of his in-patients who was admitted 10 days ago following a serious road traffic accident. The patient underwent external fixation of fractures in both femurs and required suturing for multiple superficial injuries.

Over the past few days, this 40-year-old man has been behaving 'strangely' on the ward; for example, trying to climb out of his bed and walk despite his leg injuries and nursing requests to remain in bed. Your colleague advises you that all blood tests have been within normal limits for several days, though a magnetic resonance imaging (MRI) scan of the patient's head taken yesterday shows frontal lobe contusions.

Dr Arun would like your opinion on what might, from a neuropsychiatric point of view, be causing this behaviour, and advice on management.

Discuss the differential diagnoses you are considering and how you might confirm or refute these. In general terms, discuss the treatment options available.

ACTOR (ROLE-PLAYER) INSTRUCTIONS

The details of the accident are somewhat sketchy, but witnesses told the ambulance service that a lorry broke a red light and hit the man as he crossed the road.

As far as you are aware, he has otherwise been fit and well physically and mentally, but you have not been able to trace any medical records or family.

The patient accepts that he has probably 'annoyed' the nursing and medical staff, but he does not think his behaviour has been unreasonable.

Your patient is persistently distractible during interviews and finds it hard to stick to the questions asked; his manner with staff is overly familiar and personal.

SUGGESTED APPROACH

Setting the scene

'Thank you for referring this very interesting patient, Dr Arun; I'm Dr_____, the neuro-psychiatry specialty doctor. I'd like to clarify some issues you previously mentioned.'

Clarifying the recent background history

The differential diagnoses are numerous, so it is important to be as structured as possible when discussing this. Organic causes include a traumatic brain injury (TBI) and delirium with multiple potential causes. There might be withdrawal from alcohol or drugs, medication-induced confusion and mental illness including depression and psychosis. The history, examinations and investigations to date will help shed light on the likelihood of each of these differentials.

It will be necessary to clarify the circumstances surrounding the RTA: is there any evidence of the crash being intentional or of the patient having consumed drugs or alcohol prior to the accident? Although not expected to be an expert in orthopaedics, the neuropsychiatric specialty trainee should obtain a brief description of the nature of the initial injuries and subsequent surgery – the time frame and how complicated the procedure(s) was/were. Was there initial loss of consciousness, and if so, how long did this last – comas lasting more than a few days have a poor prognosis. Is there any evidence of post-traumatic amnesia? Did the patient have any seizures? Peri-operative confusion might well be expected, particularly in a traumatic emergency case. The candidate will need to be satisfied that physical examination and investigations are both thorough and recent. Is there evidence that the patient's behaviour is related to physical changes in their health? Were there any abnormalities on examination, especially neurologically? How is the patient being physically managed at present?

Clarifying potential psychopathology

'Strange behaviour' is quite vague: it is necessary to expand on this. Check the time frame – are the symptoms changeable? Is there confusion or disorientation? Is the patient agitated? Could it be related to anaesthesia or analgesia? Is there evidence of withdrawal from any substances? The candidate is looking for evidence of delirium, which would be suggested by a fluctuating pattern of abnormal behaviour in the context of disorientation. This might be caused by post-operative haematological abnormalities, withdrawal from drugs or alcohol or medication-induced or concussion injury. Neuroimaging suggests frontal lobe damage: enquire about symptoms of disinhibition and apathy.

As well as physical causes of apparently unusual behaviour, it is vital to ask about the mental state: could the patient be suicidal and trying to harm himself intentionally? Is there any evidence of psychotic symptoms? Is there any past psychiatric history? Psychiatric symptoms could either precede the injury or be caused (or exacerbated) by them. TBI psychosis is not particularly common, but depression occurs in about a quarter of these cases.

Considering management

Management will depend upon identifying the cause of the behaviour; for example, rectifying electrolyte imbalances, treating alcohol withdrawal and reducing (where practicable) opiate analgesia.

Environmental management of a distressed or confused patient should not be underestimated and simple measures such as ensuring adequate lighting and provision of location and time cues (e.g. a board with the ward name, day and date) can be invaluable.

Sedation could be considered, taking into account the fact that additional medications may in fact worsen confusion. Options might include a benzodiazepine such as lorazepam. Of course, should a mental illness be identified, this would need to be treated appropriately.

ADDITIONAL POINTS

1. An understanding of the potential for drugs (whether illicit, legal but potentially harmful, such as alcohol, or prescribed) to cause confusion is essential. It would look professional and structured to delineate drugs into the categories above and to display awareness of how both initiation and withdrawal from many substances can alter the mental state. Drugs to specifically enquire about include alcohol, opiates and benzodiazepines.

2. Management of confused hospital in-patients is a common neuropsychiatric problem. Medication is frequently less helpful than clear communication with the patient and staff. The introduction of simple procedures, such as ensuring staff always identify themselves to the patient and environmental cues such as good lighting, can be hugely helpful.

FURTHER READING

David, A.S., Fleminger, S., Kopelman, M.D., Lovestone, S. & Mellers, J.D.C. (2012) *Lishman's Organic Psychiatry: A Textbook of Neuropsychiatry*. 4th edn. Hoboken, NJ: Wiley-Blackwell.

Fleminger, S., Greenwood, R.R.J. & Oliver, D.L. (2006) Prescription drug use for managing agitation and aggression in people with acquired brain injury. *Cochrane Database of Systematic Reviews*. http://www.cochrane.org/CD003299/INJ_prescription-drug-use-for-managing-agitation-and-aggression-in-people-with-acquired-brain-injury

Levin, H.S. & Diaz-Arrastia, R.R. (2015) Diagnosis, prognosis, and clinical management of mild traumatic brain injury. *Lancet Neurology, 14*(5), 506–17.

Reis, C., Wang, Y., Akyol, O. et al. (2015) What's new in traumatic brain injury: Update on tracking, monitoring and treatment. *International Journal of Molecular Sciences, 16*, 11903–65.

The examiner's mark sheet

Domain/ percentage of marks	Essential points to pass	✓	Extra marks/comments (make notes here)
1. Clarifying recent history	Clear communication		
	Open and closed questions		
40% of marks	Clarifying circumstances of accident		
	Clarifying post-accident treatments		
2. Clarifying any psychopathology	Asking about symptom variability		
	Considering insight		
40% of marks	Establishing current risks		
3. Considering management	Considering environmental strategies		
20% of marks	Recognising medication also carries risks		

⇧ **% SCORE** _____

___ **OVERALL IMPRESSION**
3 (CIRCLE ONE)

Good Pass

Pass

Borderline

Fail

Clear Fail

NOTES/Areas to improve

STATION 1(b): TESTING OF A HEAD INJURY

INSTRUCTION TO CANDIDATE

The orthopaedic specialty trainee is grateful for your advice, although he admits that he is not confident he has given an adequate history and requests a review of this 40-year-old man. You are given the most recent set of blood tests, which include FBC, U&Es and LFTs – all of which are normal – and a copy of the radiologist's report, noting frontal lobe contusions on his MRI scan.

The patient says that he cannot recall much about the accident but believes his memory since his operations has been fine, which is corroborated by the nursing staff. He felt well in himself in the preceding weeks: he denies ever suffering from any mental health problems, describing himself as a 'chirpy, happy sort of guy'. He denies illicit drug use and says he rarely drinks alcohol.

He admits that his mother has said he has been acting 'a bit weird' since the accident – she complained that he cursed frequently and told sexually explicit jokes in her presence, something she says he would never normally do. The only change he has noticed is that he cannot operate his mobile phone properly because 'there are too many buttons and controls to work out'.

In light of the neuroimaging results and the patient's comments, assess the relevant cognitive domains. Explain your findings to the patient, Keith.

ACTOR (ROLE-PLAYER) INSTRUCTIONS

You will engage with the tests, although you are bemused by them.

Your answers will show some errors in all domains.

SUGGESTED APPROACH

Setting the scene

'Thank you for seeing me, Keith. I'm sorry to hear about the accident. It seems as if you may be having some difficulties that you didn't have before; I'd like to do a few tests with you to check this in more detail if I may – they're not too difficult, and I'll explain each one before we do it, but don't worry if you make mistakes.'

Undertaking frontal lobe testing

The history and investigations suggest frontal lobe impairment. The frontal lobes are involved in higher cognitive and executive functioning, although fully assessing and quantifying a so-called dysexecutive syndrome is clinically difficult without extensive neuropsychological batteries. However, 'bedside testing' can explore established subdomains of frontal lobe function such as abstract reasoning, mental flexibility, executive motor programming, interference resistance, inhibitory control and autonomy.

The order of the following tests is not especially important once all domains are covered.

Abstract reasoning

Neuropsychologists employ complex tests such as card-sorting tasks to assess abstract reasoning, but at the bedside, either proverb interpretation or categorisation/conceptualisation tasks can be utilised. Proverb interpretation involves getting the subject to explain the metaphorical meaning of a well-known proverb such as 'people in glasshouses shouldn't throw stones'. Categorisation/conceptualisation tasks involve asking subjects to state how two objects are similar to each other and how they differ from one another; for example:

'I know this might sound like an unusual thing to do, but I'd like you to tell me, as best you can, how you think a "car" is similar to a "train".' After allowing the patient time to give their response, follow up with, 'Thank you, and now can you tell me how a "car" is different to a "train".'

Frontal lobe dysfunction may lead to impaired abstract reasoning, with resulting concrete interpretations of proverbs and categories; for example, 'Throwing stones will break the glass', or 'Trains and cars are both red'.

Mental flexibility

The subject is challenged to list as many words (barring the names of people and places) beginning with a given letter (traditionally 'f', 'a' or 's') or by a given category (e.g. 'animals') in 1 minute. This tests the subject's ability to design a cognitive strategy: 'normal' functioning depends on the scale utilised, but a healthy individual should be able to name more than 20 words or animals.

'Now I'm going to time you doing this next task. In 1 minute, I'd like you to tell me as many words as you can that begin with the letter "f" for "Freddy." They can be any words except the names of people or places. Is that clear? OK, we'll start the minute *now*.'

Motor sequencing

This involves copying and continuing a complex multistage motor sequence, such as the Luria series of 'fist, palm, and edge'. Frontal lobe impairment can lead to difficulty learning or executing the demonstrated sequence.

Interference resistance

The Stroop test involves subjects naming the colours of printed words whilst ignoring what the word actually says. At the bedside, a finger tap test can be employed. When the examiner taps their finger once, the subject should tap theirs twice; when the examiner taps twice, the subject should tap once. This test explores the subject's ability to override competing stimuli.

'We're going to do a "tapping" test next. When I tap my finger *once*, like this, I'd like you to tap your finger *twice*: let's try that. OK, and when I tap my finger *twice*, like this, I'd like you to tap your finger *once*: let's try that. Is that clear?'

Inhibitory control

This is a 'go-no-go' variation of the finger tap test above. In this version, the subject taps twice when the examiner taps once, but does nothing when the examiner taps twice. Impairment can lead to loss of inhibitory control, with subjects continuing to tap even when they should not.

'The next test is another "tapping" test, but the rules are slightly different. When I tap my finger *once*, you tap your finger *twice*, like the last time: let's try that. Now when I tap my finger *twice*, you *do nothing* – don't tap at all: let's try that. Is that clear?'

Autonomy

This is the subject's independence from environmental cues. It can be assessed by telling the subject to do exactly what you command, then placing your hands on the subject's palms telling them 'do not grab my hands'. Lack of environmental independence will result in the subject grabbing the examiner's hands.

'In this last test, I'd like you to listen very carefully to what I say, and do what I tell you. Could you place your hands on your lap with your palms facing upwards like I'm doing? Great, now *do not grab my hands*.'

Explaining the results

Explaining the results of all investigations requires tact and delicacy, especially when results are suboptimal. The reason for getting candidates to explain these results include assessing this communication skills, as well as checking their knowledge of what the test assesses and their ability to record performance.

In this example, the candidate can remind the subject that the brain scan showed some 'bruising' on the front parts of the brain after the accident, and that this might explain some of the difficulties the patient and his mother had noted. The tests were a good way of looking at this further and measuring any difficulties so that any necessary help can be given and future improvements noted.

ADDITIONAL POINTS

1. Although test ordering is not important, once the major subdomains are reviewed, candidates should have their own structured examination method: this will allow them to appear more professional in testing, as well as reducing the chance of omitting a test.

2. In the abstract reasoning task, categorisation/conceptualisation is usually a preferable test to proverb interpretation. This is because proverb interpretation is culturally, linguistically and educationally biased: many subjects will not have heard a given proverb before. If this task is utilised, one should ask the subject, 'Have you heard the phrase _____ before?' and only ask for its interpretation if the subject says yes.

3. Time is obviously short and precious in examinations: a single trial of each test will probably suffice, although ambiguous performance on any given test may warrant a second example. In a similar vein, it should prove

possible to abort a verbal fluency task after less than 30 seconds: in an examination, the point is to demonstrate familiarity and competence with the test, with the caveat that if the candidate does end the task early, they should identify that they are doing so for reasons of time, and explain how ordinarily one should continue for the full minute.

4. It is usually easy to discern candidates who have only theoretical knowledge of frontal lobe tests from those who have actually clinically administered them. The tests are beguilingly simple, but can be difficult to explain to others (and indeed difficult to perform – try explaining what 'A rolling stone gathers no moss' means to someone!). Practise these tests, especially on 'non-medical' friends – it is all too easy to think one knows them and can therefore explain them.

5. Whilst not essential, use of a recognised scale such as the Frontal Assessment Battery demonstrates structure (and aids recollection), as well as enabling scored measurement using a validated tool and affording the opportunity to retest and monitor change.

FURTHER READING

Dubois, B., Slachevsky, A., Litvan, I. & Pillon, B. (2000) The FAB: A frontal assessment battery at bedside. *Neurology, 55,* 1621–6.

Hodges, J. (2007) *Cognitive Assessment for Clinicians.* Oxford, UK: Oxford University Press.

Tracy, D.K. (2014) Evaluating malingering in cognitive and memory examinations: A guide for clinicians. *Advances in Psychiatric Treatment, 20,* 405–12.

The examiner's mark sheet

Domain/ percentage of marks	Essential points to pass	✓	Extra marks/comments (make notes here)
1. Undertaking frontal lobe testing	Covers an appropriate range of frontal lobe domains		
60% of marks	Clear explanation of tests		
2. Explaining the results	Uses appropriate language		
40% of marks	Checks the patient understood		

% SCORE _____

___
2

OVERALL IMPRESSION

(CIRCLE ONE)

Good Pass

Pass

Borderline

Fail

Clear Fail

NOTES/Areas to improve

STATION 2(a): ASSESSMENT OF NON-EPILEPTIC SEIZURES

INSTRUCTION TO CANDIDATE

You are asked to see a 19-year-old college student, Karen, who has been admitted by the neurologists for further assessment of seizures. She has been having fits for over 2 years, and recalls having her first episode in school prior to an examination. Anticonvulsants over the past 2 years have not been helpful and video-telemetry during this admission has failed to show any epileptiform activity on electroencephalography (EEG) during bouts of fitting.

In light of the telemetry findings, take a neuropsychiatric history from the patient.

ACTOR (ROLE-PLAYER) INSTRUCTIONS

You are somewhat defensive initially at seeing a psychiatrist, and fearful he/she thinks you are 'making it up'.

You accept that the neurologist's tests were 'normal', but are persistent on the point that you are having fits.

The seizures get worse if you are distressed; for example, during college examinations.

You are open to other explanations of causes of your difficulties, if they are sensitively addressed.

SUGGESTED APPROACH

Setting the scene

'Hello, Karen, I'm Dr_____, one of the psychiatrists in this hospital. My colleague has asked me to have a chat with you about the seizures you've had to see if we can find what's causing them and ways we might help.'

Establishing a positive, constructive rapport

Good initial engagement is critical. Patients with non-epileptic seizures can be understandably resistant and guarded about seeing psychiatrists, especially if the rationale has not been sensitively explained to them. It can make people fear they are being accused of being 'mad' or of feigning illness. It is important to start gently with the facts and to remember – unless malingering is suspected – that they *are* having seizures, just not epileptic ones. Careful consideration needs to be given to the precise phraseology used: it can be helpful to follow the patient's lead in how they describe their seizures (e.g. 'fits', 'episodes', 'turns' or 'shaking'), being careful, however, not to use the word 'epilepsy'. It is often useful to educate the individual that there are different types of seizures, but that not all are due to epileptic activity in the brain; furthermore, it is 'good news' not to have epilepsy, although this means that the actual cause needs to be sought.

Ask about the patient's understanding of the results

It is important to assess the patient's understanding of the results; unfortunately, it has occurred on many occasions that patients have rather brusquely been told, 'You don't have epilepsy', with no further explanation.

Clarifying the history and pattern of the seizures

Although video-telemetry failed to show epileptic activity during filmed seizures, it is important to remember that dissociative seizures are more common in those who also have and who have had epilepsy. Check for possible organic causes such as head injuries, and ask about alcohol and illicit drug use. Was there any history in the past of epilepsy or seizures? Were there any positive findings such as an abnormal EEG?

A good history of the seizures is required, even if the information has already been relayed to you by the neurologists – they will be looking for and giving salience to different aspects of the history to neuropsychiatrists. How long have the fits been occurring, how frequently do they occur, are there any obvious precipitating factors and how do they resolve? Have others described the nature of the seizures; for example, the pattern of movement and any variation? Is the pattern changing over time?

Looking for potential non-epileptic features

There are no pathognomonic features of dissociative seizures. However, factors that might make one more suspicious of dissociative seizures include retained consciousness, violent or thrashing movements, shutting of eyes (including resistance to opening), lack of tongue biting and urinary incontinence and a general lack of physical injuries due to 'controlled' falling. Dissociative seizures are more likely to have a gradual onset and fluctuating course. It is also extremely pertinent to explore psychological factors, such as exacerbation of seizure frequency in the face of increased distress and, conversely, a noted decrease when more relaxed. Whilst the patient may be unaware of this or deny it, a general sense of the pressure they are under and their overall mood is important. Seizures may also occur more frequently in emotionally salient environments; for example, only in front of friends but not at home. Family history is similarly important: there is an increased risk of dissociative seizures where there is someone to, albeit subconsciously, model on. This also extends to friends with epilepsy.

ADDITIONAL POINTS

1. Candidates may find patient engagement and building a rapport a difficult component of this station. This can be due both to potential patient hostility to a psychiatric review and the doctor's concern about offending the patient or choosing the 'wrong' term to explain what's happening. Openness and honesty is essential. It has been the author's experience that it can be very helpful to talk about how common seizures are and to note that some are caused by abnormal firing of brain cells (epilepsy) but that some are not, without giving weight or primacy to either.

2. Whilst the station is leading towards a diagnosis of dissociative seizures, the possibility of an alternative undiagnosed psychiatric illness, whether aetiological (panic attacks, in particular, may mimic the 'aura' of a seizure) or comorbid, must be considered.

3. Non-epileptic seizures, pseudo-seizures, non-epileptic attack disorder and dissociative seizures are mistakenly used as interchangeable synonyms, although they are in fact not identical. The different terminology is confusing both for patients and doctors: pick a term and stick with it. Many people find terms such as hysterical or pseudo-seizures to be pejorative, with the implicit meaning that the seizures are 'fake'. Furthermore, non-epileptic seizures include provoked seizures caused by various conditions such as arteriovenous malformations, cerebrovascular accidents, drug intoxication and withdrawal and head injury. ICD-10 uses the diagnosis of dissociative seizures, and from a neuropsychiatric viewpoint, this is probably the most sensible term to use. Up to a fifth of individuals in epilepsy clinics may have dissociative seizures; determining the actual diagnosis often takes considerable time, and prognosis can be poor, with limited data on psychological treatment despite its remaining the treatment of choice.

FURTHER READING

Goldstein, L.H., Mellers, J.D., Landau, S. et al. (2015) Cognitive behavioural therapy vs standardised medical care for adults with Dissociative Epileptic Seizures (CODES): A multicentre randomised controlled trial protocol. *BMC Neurology, 15,* 98.

Sahaya, K., Dholakia, S.A. & Sahota, P.K. (2011) Psychogenic non-epileptic seizures: A challenging entity. *Journal of Clinical Neuroscience, 18*(12), 1602–7.

Schmutz, M. (2013) Dissociative seizures – A critical review and perspective. *Epilepsy & Behavior, 29*(3), 449–56.

The examiner's mark sheet

Domain/ percentage of marks	Essential points to pass	✓	Extra marks/comments (make notes here)
1. Establishing a positive, constructive rapport 30% of marks	Clear communication Active listening Open and closed questions Demonstrating patience A non-judgemental attitude		
2. Asking about the patient's understanding of the results 30% of marks	Clear communication Not avoiding explaining or downplaying negative neurology findings		
3. Clarifying the history and pattern of the seizures 20% of marks	Checking for possible organic aetiology Good history of seizure time frame Establishing the nature of the seizures		

⇧ 4. Looking for potential non-epileptic features

20% of marks

Considering psycho-social triggers

Looking for atypicalities, such as no seizure injuries or confusion

% SCORE _____

___
4

OVERALL IMPRESSION
(CIRCLE ONE)

Good Pass

Pass

Borderline

Fail

Clear Fail

NOTES/Areas to improve

STATION 2(b): DISCUSSING NON-EPILEPTIC SEIZURES WITH A RELATIVE

The investigations and history are strongly suggestive of dissociative seizures. The patient is quite upset, both by being referred to psychiatry and by the facts that her brain scan and blood tests were normal and no epileptiform activity has been found on video-telemetry. Since your last review, she has repeatedly been telling her sister that staff thinks she is 'making it up'. She has asked for you to talk to her sister about dissociative seizures.

Discuss with Karen's sister, Robyn, what the findings mean, what treatment(s) are available and what the prognosis is for non-epileptic seizures.

ACTOR (ROLE-PLAYER) INSTRUCTIONS

You are upset and concerned about your sister's wellbeing.

You are angry about how the neurologists have looked after her and incredulous that you are talking to a psychiatrist.

You will challenge psychological models, as you have witnessed the seizures yourself.

SUGGESTED APPROACH

Setting the scene

'Hello, Robyn, I'm Dr_____, one of the psychiatrists in the hospital. As you know, I met with your sister Karen recently and she'd like me to explain to you what we've discussed and where we might proceed from here. Of course, please feel free to interrupt me if I use any terminology or phrases of which you're not sure. Before I start, are there any questions you'd like answered?'

Establishing a good rapport

A sensitive approach to a potentially upset and confused relative is required. Affording time at the start for the sister to voice the major areas of concern may help build a relationship, show you are interested in her particular worries and point out areas that must be covered.

Explaining the nature of non-epileptic seizures

Adequate explanation of any terminology that is used is essential. A suggested approach to the relative is as follows:

- A seizure or fit is caused by abnormal brain functioning and can result in unusual movements, behaviour and changes in consciousness. Different things can cause fits, and it is important to identify the cause so that the correct treatment can be started.
- A common cause of fits, and one that many people are aware of, is epilepsy. Epilepsy is caused by abnormal excessive firing of brain cells, and is treated with anticonvulsant medications that work by reducing this increased activity. Epilepsy can be measured by an electroencephalogram, or EEG. This is a simple, painless and relatively quick test where electrodes are placed on the head and the underlying activity is monitored.
- A problem with EEGs is that they are frequently normal or inconclusive between fits, and it can be difficult to demonstrate that epileptic changes are occurring. In some cases, as occurred with your sister, the doctors set up an EEG to run over 24 or 48 hours whilst simultaneously videoing the patient. In that way, they can see on the video footage when the fit occurred and look for the relevant part of the EEG. With this information, they can decide whether or not it is epilepsy that is causing the fits.
- In this instance, no epileptic activity was detected, and so epilepsy is not the cause of her problem. In addition, the blood tests and brain scan she had were normal, all of which is good news, ruling out some other serious potential causes of seizures, such as infections, multiple sclerosis (MS) and problems with the brain's blood supply.
- A common cause of non-epileptic seizures are what are known as dissociative seizures. Whilst this is not yet fully understood, it seems that some individuals are prone to 'break off' or 'dissociate' subconsciously from everyday life in light of distress, although they may not be able to identify this distress clearly. This can manifest in different ways, including, as appears to be the case with your sister, having seizures or fits.
- Dissociative seizures are involuntary and outside of the patient's control: they are not 'faking' or 'making up' symptoms.

Discussing therapeutic options

Identifying that the *cause* is psychological enables appropriate psychological *treatment*. The current treatment of choice is known as cognitive behavioural therapy (CBT). Explain how this explores the thoughts and feelings an individual experiences in various settings and how they can interplay to affect behaviour. An aim is to look at what might be happening around the time of her fits and how altering this might lessen the number and severity of her fits.

The facts that epileptic activity has not been detected and that antiepileptic drugs (AEDs) are not required should be portrayed as positive outcomes.

ADDITIONAL POINTS

1. Dissociative seizures are more common in those who have had epilepsy in the past, and approximately a fifth of those with dissociative seizures will have current comorbid epilepsy. Given these facts and the frequent desire for a 'medical' cause, patients and relatives may challenge the diagnosis, citing, for example, ambiguous EEGs (and remember that non-specific EEG abnormalities are seen in approximately a sixth of healthy individuals) or the concept that the EEG might have 'missed' some fits. Such arguments are impossible to refute, and usually best avoided. If directly challenged, the clinician should not become defensive, accepting the raised points, but trying to move the discussion past this. For example, in such a situation, it would be correct to note that the seizures filmed were non-epileptic, and therefore the treatments offered should reflect this. Symptoms and investigations can always, and should be, revisited.

2. The issue of whether or not symptoms could be feigned for psychological gain (a factitious disorder) or fraudulent gain (malingering) may be at the back of the clinician's mind. Clearly, this is an extremely sensitive area to explore, and guidelines on this topic cannot be prescriptive. Dissociative seizures are, by definition, considered unconscious, and it is worth bearing in mind that dissociative seizures are frequently quite dissimilar to epileptic seizures, and most patients admitted for video-telemetry have a fit in an environment where they know they are being closely scrutinised – factors that militate against intentional deception.

FURTHER READING

http://www.epilepsy.org.uk/info/nonep.html

http://www.patient.co.uk/showdoc/40026034/

The examiner's mark sheet

Domain/ percentage of marks	Essential points to pass	✓	Extra marks/comments (make notes here)
1. Establishing a good rapport 30% of marks	Clear communication Open and closed questions Demonstrating patience		
2. Explaining the nature of non-epileptic seizures 50% of marks	Being clear that there is no epileptiform activity Being clear that the seizure is 'real' Being clear that her sister is not 'faking'		
3. Discussing management options 20% of marks	Describing a psychological model Explaining that medication is not appropriate or useful		

⇩

⇑ **% SCORE** _____

___
3

OVERALL IMPRESSION
(CIRCLE ONE)

Good Pass

Pass

Borderline

Fail

Clear Fail

NOTES/Areas to improve

STATION 3(a): UNUSUAL BEHAVIOUR IN PARKINSON'S DISEASE

INSTRUCTION TO CANDIDATE

You have been referred to a 68-year-old woman, Katherine, with Parkinson's disease who, during an admission for management of worsening tremor, has been difficult to manage on the ward. She has appeared agitated at times and has been frequently noted to lie naked and fully exposed on her bed.

Take a relevant history from the patient, with a particular focus on exploring the behavioural change and possible causes of this.

ACTOR (ROLE-PLAYER) INSTRUCTIONS

You are aware that you have Parkinson's disease, and believe you were admitted to hospital as your tremor has been getting worse. However, you are not insightful into behavioural disturbances. You slept naked as that is how you always sleep at home; it is inconvenient to put on pyjamas just to go to the bathroom at night.

If asked about your general health, you had a chest infection last week, and are still coughing up green phlegm.

You admit that you do sometimes feel a bit 'muddled' and confused about things, and your recollection of events to the doctor can be erratic and contradictory.

You have seen what appears to be a 'ghost', whom you've named 'Tommy'; he is not frightening but distracts and annoys you, and you cannot explain why he appears at night.

During the interview, you believe you are at home, and occasionally call for your husband Neil to 'stick the kettle on, dear'.

SUGGESTED APPROACH

Setting the scene

'Hello, Katherine, I'm Dr_____, one of the psychiatrists in this hospital. I've been asked by my colleagues to have a chat with you about how you've been getting on in hospital.

Some of what I'm going to ask you may seem a little personal, but it's important information for me to obtain, so I hope you'll bear with me.'

Sensitively approaching unusual behaviour

There is a lot of ground to cover in this station, so it is essential to be as focussed and structured as possible. A leading introductory question is likely to be required in order to quickly open the area for discussion.

'I understand from some of the staff on the ward that at times you haven't seemed yourself recently. For example, there was some concern that perhaps you've been feeling a bit irritated or fed up recently, and sometimes you haven't been taking care of your personal dress as well as you might. Does this ring a bell with you?'

This rapidly establishes what you want to talk about with the patient. An immediate observation should be the patient's level of insight: is she aware that there is a problem?

Considering symptoms and their causes

The differentials are numerous, so the candidate must remain structured to keep a grip on the station. From even this most brief of introductory vignettes, one should be thinking of the following:

- Part of the pathology of Parkinson's, for example:
- Cognitive impairment (dementia)
- Delirium
- Psychosis
- Depression
- Anxiety
- Personality changes including apathy and emotional lability
- Medication caused
- Drug (dopamine)-induced delirium
- Drug-induced psychosis
- Drug-induced personality changes such as disinhibition and hypersexuality
- A comorbid psychiatric illness, such as depression

Whilst this is a reasonably large list for a timed exam (and it is not exhaustive; e.g. it presumes the behaviour is truly pathological), it allows for suitable probes to be asked: what is the time frame of such behaviour? Is it related to any medication changes? What have the patient's mood and anxiety levels been like? Is the memory as good as it has been? Has the patient seen or heard things that no one else does, or seem to have any new and unusual ideas? Have friends and family noticed any differences or thought the individual was not quite the same person as before?

ADDITIONAL POINTS

1. It is important not to be seduced by 'finding' the diagnosis. Even if early questioning heavily points to, for example, a depressive disorder, it is essential to continue to screen for other causes and comorbidities; for example, coexisting cognitive decline.

2. Time will likely militate against a full cognitive examination, so the candidate needs to show awareness of the importance of this task and highlight that it is an area to return to:

'You feel your memory isn't what it once was. When I've more time, I'd like to examine this in some depth. For the moment, would you mind if I asked you a few quick memory questions? Could you tell me:

- What date it is today?
- What your date of birth is?
- Our whereabouts at the moment?'

3. In practice, it is seldom possible to confidently state that low mood is 'comorbid' or 'psychologically reactive' as opposed to a neuropsychiatric complication of a Parkinsonian picture. However, the candidate should look for a past psychiatric history, including prior to diagnosis with Parkinson's disease, and get a sense from the patient regarding beliefs surrounding any low mood. Even if the patient does not attribute any salience to the Parkinsonian medication, it is helpful to establish what the patient is taking, and in clinical practice, it is important to ask specific questions around disinhibitory hypersexuality and gambling.

4. Parkinson's disease, like multiple sclerosis, has a higher-than-expected rate of affective disorders when the overall disability of the disease is taken into account, with typical figures showing an approximately 50% prevalence for depression of at least mild severity. However, it is often difficult to clearly determine whether a mood or anxiety disorder is directly 'caused' by Parkinson's pathology or is psychologically secondary or independent of it, although some authors have argued that thoughts of self-harm are less frequent when part of the neurological disease. A diagnostic difficulty is the fact that several overlapping symptoms with different causes may coexist. For example, apparent psychomotor retardation may be part of a depressive disorder or simply part of the Parkinson's disease. Similarly, apathy and mild cognitive impairment might falsely suggest depression.

FURTHER READING

Averbeck, B.B., O'Sullivan, S.S. & Djamshidian, A. (2014) Impulsive and compulsive behaviours in Parkinson's disease. *Annual Review of Clinical Psychology, 10*, 553–80.

Weintraub, D., Simuni, T., Caspell-Garcia, C. et al. (2015) Cognitive performance and neuropsychiatric symptoms in early, untreated Parkinson's disease. *Movement Disorders, 30*(7), 919–27.

The examiner's mark sheet

Domain/ percentage of marks	Essential points to pass	✓	Extra marks/comments (make notes here)
1. Sensitively approaching unusual behaviour 40% of marks	Clear communication Open and closed questions Able to address unusual behaviour		

⇧ 2. Considering symptoms and their causes	Good awareness of the numerous differentials	
60% of marks	A structured approach to symptoms	
	Consideration of psychological ill-health	
	Consideration of the role of medication	

% SCORE _____

___
2

OVERALL IMPRESSION

(CIRCLE ONE)

Good Pass

Pass

Borderline

Fail

Clear Fail

NOTES/Areas to improve

STATION 3(b): DISCUSSING UNUSUAL BEHAVIOUR IN PARKINSON'S DISEASE WITH A RELATIVE

INSTRUCTION TO CANDIDATE

Your assessment of Katherine shows that she has been suffering from fleeting visual hallucinations of a 'ghost' that distracts and irritates her, and these hallucinations have led to much of her agitation on the ward. She was somewhat disorientated, thinking she was at home with her husband Neil, but besides intermittent agitation, her affect seemed generally euthymic. The symptoms have been there for some time, although her husband feels they have worsened since starting her new medication with this admission.

Her husband, Neil, wants to know what you can do to help his wife. Discuss with him in lay terms what might be happening and how you might be able to help.

ACTOR (ROLE-PLAYER) INSTRUCTIONS

You are concerned about your wife's health and distressed by her hallucinations.

You are afraid that she is 'going mad' or that she has dementia.

You feel her new medications have worsened her condition, and are therefore concerned about the introduction of any new drugs.

You also want to know what you can do to help.

SUGGESTED APPROACH

Setting the scene

'Hello, Neil, my name is Dr_____, and I'm a psychiatrist. I understand you wanted to talk about what we can do to help your wife. I think it's important to state at this point that we're not completely certain about the exact cause of her symptoms, as there are a number of possibilities, and treatment options will depend on the cause.'

Explaining differential diagnoses in lay terms

The potential differentials must now be explicitly stated, with the added requirements of tact and avoidance of unduly technical medical terminology. A major mood or anxiety disorder has largely been excluded, but there is evidence of disorientation and hallucinations that have been exacerbated by recent medication changes. At this stage, there is insufficient information to state a diagnosis – and thus a definitive management plan – with confidence. However, the station design allows the candidate to demonstrate their logical thought processes to the examiner. A further benefit (to the candidate) of this particular station is that by asking for explanations in lay terms, it avoids the need to mention some specifics such as medication doses and so forth.

Differentiating delirium from dementia

The disorientation may be a delirium or a dementia, and both may manifest with hallucinations and other psychotic phenomena. Of course, a delirium may also be an acute problem over a chronic dementia. To further complicate things, the psychotic symptom(s) may be independent of the cognitive impairment. Clarifying questions are required, and aetiology and management options will follow from the answers.

'When I asked your wife some memory questions recently, she got some answers wrong. I wonder is this something that has been happening for a while. Does this change from day to day or has it been stable? Have the medications made this part worse?'

'Has she been having other memory problems before she came in – perhaps problems with names or faces, or getting lost when out?'

'I want to ask some questions about the "ghost" she's been seeing. Has "Tommy" only been there since she came into hospital? Has she had any other problems seeing or hearing things that no one else seems able to see or hear? I know these questions may seem unusual, but have you noted that she's been having unusual ideas recently, and or any concerns about anyone trying to harm her or to control her or her thoughts in any way?'

The suggestion is of a delirium, whether or not on top of pre-existing dementia, and apparently caused or exacerbated by medication.

'Some of the problems Katherine seems to be having with her memory look like they might be what we call a "delirium." That's to say, it's a sudden change in the ability to focus attention or remember or think clearly. It can vary, sometimes dramatically, from hour to hour and day to day, and it can have many causes. We'll have to arrange some further tests to see if, for example, there are any underlying infective or metabolic problems that might be causing this. Treatment will depend on what we find.'

Discussing various effects of medication

Medication as a *cause* of the delirium needs to be addressed, given the fact that the vignette mentions this directly. However, reducing medication can bring about its own problems by exacerbating the Parkinson's disease. The candidate needs to exercise tact by accepting that the problem could be iatrogenic without attributing blame, and by discussing possible medication changes without promising something they cannot necessarily deliver.

'It is possible that the new medication, or indeed interactions with other medications, could be causing some of these symptoms. However, the medications are obviously very important, and we'll have to think carefully and perhaps consult expert colleagues in the pharmacy department and the neurologists before making any changes, and any changes will probably be done quite gradually.'

Discussing therapeutic options

Simple, but crucial, environmental factors must be addressed:

'Often, simple things such as keeping lights on, and reminding staff and visitors to keep things simple and repeat themselves frequently can be very useful.'

Treating psychotic symptoms in Parkinson's disease is difficult and the point of such a station is to allow the candidate to demonstrate their knowledge of these problems and suggest possible treatment options with reference to them. A stepwise rationale is required with awareness and active seeking of any side effects of treatment:

- If thought likely to be secondary to a delirium, no active treatment for the hallucinations, besides management of the underlying delirium, may be required.
- Similarly, in cases where hallucinations are not unduly troublesome, watchful waiting may be sufficient.
- Medications with anticholinergic side effects should be reduced or stopped *where possible*.
- The dose of any dopaminergic drugs may need to be reduced. This should be done gradually to watch for evidence that it is effective at reducing symptoms as well as worsening of Parkinson's disease.
- An anti-psychotic may be added. Typical anti-psychotics should be avoided due to the high propensity to cause EPSE and worsen Parkinson's disease symptoms. Choose an atypical anti-psychotic: there is some evidence for quetiapine having fewer motor side effects than other atypical anti-psychotics.
- In severe cases, other options such as electro-convulsive therapy and clozapine can be considered.

ADDITIONAL POINTS

1. A temptation in a station such as this is to get caught up in pharmacological management, whether by adding or removing medications; however, good environmental management is just as important in delirium and dementing processes. Simple examples in a hospital environment include adequate lighting, cues such as clocks, calendars and photos from home and assigning regular members of staff to look after the patient who can repeat information in non-technical terms as required. Finally, do not forget that psychotic symptoms are not necessarily caused by dopaminergic treatments – dyskinesias are more common as side effects of such drugs – and psychotic symptoms may be part of a progressive neurodegenerative disease. Dementia and psychosis frequently coexist and the presence of one increases the risk of developing the other. ⇩

2. Ten of the 25 most commonly prescribed medications in the elderly are associated with delirium. Polypharmacy and poor physical health are general risk factors, and watch in particular for medications with anticholinergic properties.

FURTHER READING

Bastide, M.F., Meissner, W.G., Picconi, B. et al. (2015) Pathophysiology of L-dopa-induced motor and non-motor complications in Parkinson's disease. *Progress in Neurobiology, 132,* 96–168.

Taylor, D., Paton, C. & Kapur, S. (2015) *The Maudsley Prescribing Guidelines,* 12th edn. London: Informa Healthcare.

Wong, C.I., Holroyd-Leduc, J., Simel, D.L. & Straus, S.E. (2010) Does this patient have delirium? Value of bedside instruments. *JAMA, 304*(7), 779–86.

The examiner's mark sheet

Domain/ percentage of marks	Essential points to pass	✓	Extra marks/comments (make notes here)
1. Explaining differential diagnoses in lay terms 30% of marks	Clear communication Open and closed questions Demonstrating patience		
2. Differentiating delirium from dementia 30% of marks	Clear explanations Checking they have been understood		
3. Discussing various effects of medication 20% of marks	Awareness that medications can cause symptomatology Clear lay explanation of how this occurs		
4. Discussing therapeutic options 20% of marks	Addresses environmental options A logical, structured approach to treatments Clear lay explanations of these		

% SCORE _____

___
4

OVERALL IMPRESSION

(CIRCLE ONE)

Good Pass

Pass

Borderline

Fail

Clear Fail

NOTES/Areas to improve

O SINGLE STATIONS

STATION 4: ASSESSMENT OF TEMPORAL LOBE EPILEPSY

INSTRUCTION TO CANDIDATE

On the advice of her neurologist, Dr Sean, a local GP refers to you a young woman with established temporal lobe epilepsy (TLE). The neurologist noted an increase in inter-ictal hallucinations following a recent increase in her fluoxetine; the antidepressant had been commenced by her GP in the management of a comorbid mild depressive episode.

Take a history of seizures from this patient, Sunita, focussing on the TLE and key areas of mental state and discuss management options with her.

ACTOR (ROLE-PLAYER) INSTRUCTIONS

You can predict a seizure is pending as you get a strange sensation that your legs are lengthening. You are not usually aware of the seizures once they commence and, as far as you are aware, you have never had 'convulsions' or 'fitting'.

If asked, during fits, which last a couple of minutes and have been occurring at least weekly since the medication increase, you have been told that you look 'blank' and move your lips as if talking to yourself. You typically suffer an irritating sense of déjà vu and derealisation (not feeling 'real') for a day or so afterwards.

You feel that the depression is primarily related to stress at work and not, to your mind, related to the epilepsy, although a lack of sleep can make the latter worse.

Your memory has been adversely affected, hindering your job and social life, but this is only discussed if directly asked by the candidate.

Your neurologist has discussed a referral to a neurosurgeon for an opinion on brain surgery, but you are very much against this line of action.

SUGGESTED APPROACH

Setting the scene

'Thank you for coming to see me today. Can I call you Sunita? I'm Dr_____, a specialty doctor in psychiatry. I understand that you've been seeing your neurologist about your epilepsy, but they thought it might be helpful to have a psychiatric review of your medication and difficulties.'

It is important, as ever, to remain structured. There are several obvious lines of enquiry opened through the vignette, and they will each need to be tackled: epilepsy, the novel psychopathology, the depression and the therapeutic and/or side-effect aspects of medication.

Clarifying the nature of the seizures

A clear history of TLE is necessary, including first onset and any putative aetiological factors, as well as seizure precipitation, auras, frequency, duration and typical manifestation. Individuals are often unaware of the aspects of these, and the actor may thus be primed to be a vague historian: direct probing will be important.

Temporal lobe epilepsy can manifest with a range of neuropsychiatric symptoms, and candidates might feel uncertain about these and potential treatment options. It is easy to confuse the concepts of partial and complex seizures, or to mistakenly only consider the perhaps more widely conceptualised complex type. Some individuals will have *both*, and TLE spreads to become a secondary generalised tonic–clonic seizure for many; all of these factors will need to be enquired into. Alcohol and illicit drug use are essential areas for exploration in all psychiatric histories, and they have obvious potential as exacerbants of epilepsy.

Partial seizures have preserved consciousness but altered autonomic, sensory, affective and cognitive symptoms; complex seizures manifest with impaired consciousness and usually a blank stare and idiosyncratic automatisms. A wide range of potential symptoms is possible, which can be divided by time frame (before, during or after the seizure) and symptom domain:

- Autonomic: palpitations and nausea/abnormal gastric sensations.
- Sensory: illusory disturbances or frank hallucinations. The modality may be atypical to that usually seen in psychiatry (e.g. olfactory or gustatory).
- Affective: sudden changes in mental state, including agitation, aggression, elation or depression.
- Cognitive: memory impairment is a signature feature of TLE, but can also affect other cognitive processes, including IQ, executive functioning and language skills. Individuals can suffer déjà and jamais vu, derealisation and depersonalisation and oneiroid states.
- Automatisms: repetitive movements of the face or hands; may be dystonias.

Seizures usually last for a few minutes, and are commonly followed by fatigue, headache and confusion.

Explore the current mental state

Depression and epilepsy have well-established links both neurobiologically and psychologically, but the association in this vignette might well be coincidental; the candidate will need to explore for any links. Similarly, there are complex pharmacological possibilities, so a clear history of medication instigations is critical: some AEDs are mood stabilisers, but some are pro-depressive; most psychotropics (barring benzodiazepines) lower the seizure threshold.

Cognitive problems can have several causes, including peri-ictal confusion, medication (both AEDs and benzodiazepines) and cortical scarring/lesions. Premorbid intellectual functioning, such as educational attainment and employment type, may be of assistance in establishing any changes.

Asking about treatments to date

Current and previous management of TLE should be determined. AEDs are the mainstay of treatment, but neurosurgery is a treatment for refractory TLE. Clearly, surgical interventions have the potential to produce psychiatric and behavioural sequelae. The patient should be asked about any such procedures, and if they were undertaken, whether there were any obvious complications.

The efficacy of antidepressants and anti-psychotics in epilepsy has not been well studied in robust double-blind randomised controlled trials. In general, selective serotonin reuptake inhibitors (SSRIs) and SNRIs have reasonable safety profiles regarding inducing seizures, although there can be considerable variation between individuals, and any given agent (or dose) might need altering, being mindful of the risks of such actions. Fluoxetine and paroxetine are cytochrome P450 interacting, and might necessitate alteration of AED dosage. The psychopharmacology of AEDs is complex. Phenobarbital, vigabatrin, tiagabine and clobazam can cause depression. Topiramate can cause word-finding difficulties, and levetiracetam has had reports of agitation, aggression, depression and psychosis. Carbamazepine, valproate, lamotrigine and pregabalin are established mood stabilisers.

ADDITIONAL POINTS

1. TLE is the most common focal epilepsy, with seizures originating in one or both temporal lobes. However, its epidemiology is not well established, in part due to its complex presentation, and also due to the fact that it can spread to become a generalised seizure. It has been estimated that approximately a quarter of those with a partial epilepsy have TLE; it is twice as common on the medial aspect of the lobe as the lateral. Early-life febrile seizures, central nervous system infections and traumatic brain injuries are risk factors, as is a positive family history, although there can be a considerable 'latent period' of some years after any insult before seizures become apparent. The illness burden can be quite considerable, heavily impacting many sufferers in terms of their psycho-social functioning. Inter-ictally, approximately a third will suffer depressive symptoms and one in ten will suffer psychotic symptoms. Overall, the lifetime prevalence rates of depression and generalised anxiety disorders are approximately double those of the general population, with a fivefold increase in suicide. Seizures can occur in sleep, some might not be witnessed and it can be difficult to get an accurate sense of their frequency. Patients might downplay or deny seizure frequency, particularly if there are concerns over their fitness to drive. A collateral history is very helpful where possible, including to check on the individual's responsiveness during a seizure.

2. Approximately half of patients are successfully treated on single-dose AEDs, and approximately a third are refractory to pharmacological intervention. The illness can be both progressive in symptomatology and cause structural brain damage. Pathologically, there are hallmark temporal lobe lesions, sclerosis or gliosis, particularly on the hippocampi, with permanent cognitive impairment. However, damage can include areas well outside of the temporal lobes. Neurosurgery is a therapeutic option where pharmacotherapy has failed; it is a reasonably effective intervention, particularly if any lesions have been demonstrated on neuroimaging. Understandably, many are hesitant to undergo this, although decisions must be balanced against the fact that the longer a refractory illness is untreated, the greater the potential for permanent cognitive damage. Research has shown that patients are typically referred for surgery after 20 years of seizures, lessening the chance of positive outcomes. A randomised trial has shown that amongst those with *newly intractable* TLE, surgery plus medication had a better outcome over a 2-year follow-up than AEDs alone. Actual rates of surgery-induced serious injuries, including verbal memory impairment, are 1–5/100. Anterior temporal lobectomy was the classical surgical approach, with removal of the mesial and lateral structures, although there are more specific, area-sparing techniques such as selective amygdalohippocampectomy and dominant mesial temporal lobe resection.

⇧ 3. Geschwind (or Gastaut–Geschwind) syndrome is a (debated) eponymous inter-ictal TLE phenomenon seen in some individuals, manifesting with behavioural changes of deepening emotions, circumstantiality, altered sexual or religious thinking and hypergraphia: it has been purported to have been suffered by, and contributed to the output of, numerous historical geniuses, including van Gogh and Dostoyevsky.

FURTHER READING

Bell, B., Lin, J.J., Seidenberg, M. & Hermann, B. (2011) The neurobiology of cognitive disorders in temporal lobe epilepsy. *Nature Reviews Neurology, 7,* 154–65.

Brodie, M.J. & Kwan, P. (2012) Newer drugs for focal epilepsy in adults. *British Medical Journal, 344,* e345.

Engel, J. Jr, McDermott, M.P., Wiebe, S. et al.; Early Randomized Surgical Epilepsy Trial (ERSET) Study Group (2012) Early surgical therapy for drug-resistant temporal lobe epilepsy. A randomized trial. *JAMA, 307(9),* 922–31.

The examiner's mark sheet

Domain/ percentage of marks	Essential points to pass	✓	Extra marks/comments (make notes here)
1. Clarifies the nature of the seizures 50% of marks	Clear communication Open and closed questions Delineating partial from complex seizures Explores autonomic, cognitive, affective, sensory and automatism symptoms		
2. Explores the current mental state 30% of marks	Actively looking for psychopathology Attempts to see how this might be linked to the TLE		
3. Review of treatments to date and further management 20% of marks	Consideration of how medication might impact Awareness of neurosurgery as a possibility		

% SCORE _____

$$\frac{}{3}$$

OVERALL IMPRESSION

(CIRCLE ONE)

Good Pass

Pass

Borderline

Fail

Clear Fail

NOTES/Areas to improve

STATION 5: EXPLANATION OF THE NEUROPSYCHIATRY OF A GLIOMA

INSTRUCTION TO CANDIDATE

A core trainee in psychiatry, Dr Morgan, asks for advice about one of his out-patients. The patient, Shri, is a 46-year-old man recently diagnosed with a malignant glioma, with purported subsequent personality change. He is undergoing radiotherapy combined with the oral chemotherapeutic agent temozolomide, and is currently rather angry, wanting to know why he is seeing a psychiatrist. The junior doctor admits to feeling out of his depth, and asks that you speak with the patient.

Discuss the rationale for seeing a psychiatrist, elicit any relevant psychopathology and discuss potential multidisciplinary care options.

ACTOR (ROLE-PLAYER) INSTRUCTIONS

You were diagnosed 'out of the blue' with a brain tumour 2 months ago, following a period of ongoing nausea and headaches that would wake you from your sleep and an acute episode of a collapse and urinary incontinence.

You have had a course of external radiotherapy, which involved powerful x-rays to your brain and chemotherapy medication; these have left you feeling very tired and often nauseous. If asked directly, you had a brief course of steroids a month ago, but have not been on any for some time; you have not had any seizures.

You are very scared about the future – your neurosurgeon has not given you a firm prognosis – and wonder how you and your wife will cope.

You admit you have been 'flying off the handle' a lot, but think this is reasonable given your situation. If pushed on the issue, you admit that others have said you seem different to your normal self; you are ruder, have made out-of-character sexually explicit comments to strangers and you have felt paranoid that NHS staff are performing an experiment on you.

You are sceptical of psychiatry having a role, but are persuadable that pharmacological and/or psychological interventions might be of benefit.

SUGGESTED APPROACH

Setting the scene

'Hello, Shri, I'm Dr_____, one of the psychiatrists. I know you just saw Dr Morgan, and he has requested, given the complexity and difficulty of all you have been through, that a more senior doctor assists with some of your queries – I hope that's alright. I appreciate this must have been a hugely trying time for you and your family; would you like to start by asking me any questions or identifying important issues you would like us to cover?'

Although the neuropsychiatry is complex, many of the principles of this vignette should be second nature to a good candidate, irrespective of their knowledge of the gliomas. Active listening to an upset individual, providing thoughtful and appropriate (but not false) reassurance and considering the range of supports are core psychiatry skills.

Similarly, even if caught on a technical point of factual knowledge, holding a situation, accepting some limitations and seeking senior support are always perfectly acceptable practice; one will not fail this station due to a lack of knowledge of tumour grading stages, but may for a lack of suitable empathy and awareness of the need for multidisciplinary interventions.

Several things are asked for in this station: engaging with an upset and potentially hostile patient; an awareness of primary brain tumours and their potential for neuropsychiatric sequelae; consideration of the various effects of anti-tumour and psychotropic medications; and the need for a broad package of care. The station is not asking for neuropsychometric testing or complex analysis of personality change, but there needs to be an awareness of the areas that might be affected, and that such formal testing would be appropriate.

Engaging the patient

This station will need time at the beginning for the patient to unburden their worries, hopes and frustrations, and for the candidate to take a lead from this.

Clarifying the neurological/neurosurgical history

Even if the histology is not clear, it will be important to obtain a history of the onset of the tumour, the types and time frames of the interventions – including if there was any neurosurgery, and possible complications thereof – and future neurological/neurosurgical plans.

Assessing the mental state

From a mental state viewpoint, given the patient's putative anxiety or scepticism towards psychiatry, it might be best to first establish this in terms of a reaction to having a serious illness before dealing with personality change. One should sensitively approach issues regarding depression and thoughts of not wanting to be alive, as well as life supports; mania can also accompany gliomas, and pathological mood highs should be looked for. General levels of activity and functioning, and how the tumour impacts this, should be sought.

Assessing personality change

Having hopefully established a constructive rapport, one can try to elicit any direct neuropsychiatric problems. 'Personality change' is broad, but several obvious large domains should be explored: social interactions and disinhibition and impulsive or risky behaviour (broadly orbitofrontal); planning and executive functioning (dorsolateral); and apathy and abulia/amotivation (medial frontal). These should be tested with real-world examples, such as changes in relationships or conversations with friends and strangers, taking undue or unusual risks and so forth. Cognitive functioning and memory should also be enquired after. It is worth 'thinking aloud' for the examiner's benefit that a more thorough scored neuropsychological battery might be required in due course. Paranoia can be approached as one ordinarily would in psychosis, with gentle probing for the degree (overvalued versus delusional) and other psychotic symptoms.

Evaluating potential therapeutic needs

The interventions that are necessary will depend on the information provided by the patient, but the scenario is pointing towards joint mental health and neurosurgery working, with a likely need for a care coordinator. Obvious areas to explore will be psychological support for the patient (directly for a depression or health psychology, with the latter potentially provided by the physical health team) and/or family members, as well as possible psychotropic medication.

A glioma is not a contraindication to an antidepressant or anti-psychotic, but of course it might lower the seizure threshold, and this will need to be discussed with the individual. There are no well-powered randomised controlled trials on the use of psychotropic medications in this population group; prescribing is typically pragmatic, based on usual best psychiatric practice while being mindful of the additional vulnerabilities of the patient. Side effects, including seizures, sedation and (further) hampering cognition, should be explicitly noted.

The station does not need to establish whether each one of these intervention types is definitively necessary, but should start the exploration of each, and conclude with an agreement for ongoing work and collaboration.

ADDITIONAL POINTS

1. The incidence of primary brain tumours is a little over 6/100,000 per annum; unfortunately, early diagnosis and treatment do not improve outcomes, and the prognosis is generally very poor. Their classification can be confusing, and they are histologically quite disparate. Gliomas – tumours arising from the brain's stromal or support glial cells (as opposed to neurons, which are – fascinatingly – non-oncogenic despite their proliferation through even adult life) – can be classified by grade, by glial cell type and by cortical location.

2. The World Health Organisation divides them into four categories (I–IV) of increasing aggressiveness, anaplasia (lack of morphological characteristics of mature cells) and pleomorphism (increased variation in cellular appearance). The most common type, accounting for over three-quarters of all cases, are *de novo* grade III and IV anaplastic malignant gliomas that did not arise from preceding lower-grade tumours.

3. Neurological/neurosurgical treatments include relief of pressure symptoms arising from oedematous swelling via corticosteroids and antiepileptic drugs if there are seizures, although there is no evidence to support their prophylactic use. Surgical excision will debulk and allow histological identification, although the tumour site may preclude this. Combination radiotherapy and chemotherapy are usual, although the protocols vary according to tumour factors such as type and location. Median 5-year survival rates vary according to these factors and the individual's health, from 85% for some well-differentiated low-grade tumours to less than 5% for grade IV glioblastomas.

4. Whilst personality change, impairments of cognition and psychiatric symptomatology are well recognised in the literature on gliomas, there are no good data on their prevalence.

FURTHER READING

Boele, F.W., Rooney, A.G., Grant, R. & Klein, M. (2015) Psychiatric symptoms in glioma patients: From diagnosis to management. *Neuropsychiatric Disease and Treatment, 11,* 1413–20.

Omuro, A. & DeAngelis, L.M. (2013) Glioblastoma and other malignant gliomas. A clinical review. *JAMA, 310*(17), 1842–50.

Westphal, M. & Lamszus, K. (2011) The neurobiology of gliomas: From cell biology to the development of therapeutic approaches. *Nature Reviews Neuroscience, 12,* 495–509.

The examiner's mark sheet

Domain/ percentage of marks	Essential points to pass	✓	Extra marks/comments (make notes here)
1. Engaging the patient 25% of marks	Clear communication Open and closed questions Demonstrating patience		
2. Clarifying the neurological/ neurosurgical history 15% of marks	Establishes a good neurological history and time frame		
3. Assessing the mental state 20% of marks	Consideration of a psychological reaction to a serious illness Consideration of risk		
4. Assessing personality change 20% of marks	Sensitive approach Addresses a range of domains in a structured fashion		
5. Evaluating potential therapeutic needs 20% of marks	Considers family needs Considers multidisciplinary working Considers varying psychological approaches Considers medication, including risks		

% SCORE _____

___
5

OVERALL IMPRESSION
(CIRCLE ONE)

Good Pass

Pass

Borderline

Fail

Clear Fail

NOTES/Areas to improve

STATION 6: MEDICALLY UNEXPLAINED SYMPTOMS

INSTRUCTION TO CANDIDATE

The neurology team has admitted Radha, a 35-year-old woman, for a full workup and investigations on the background of 15 years of full body pain and generalised weakness, which have never been successfully managed. This admission has included an MRI of the patient's head, an EEG, an auto-antibody screen including rheumatoid markers and routine bloods and physical examination – all of which have been unremarkable, in keeping with past findings. Prescribed analgesia and a trial with a TENS machine have been unsuccessful at treating her pain. The neurology SpR, Dr Sean, requests a neuropsychiatric review, advising you that their team feel 'it is all in her head'. They have advised her of the negative findings, the fact that they have no further investigations planned and that they aim to discharge her shortly.

Take a *brief* symptom history from this patient, who admits that she is surprised at being referred to a psychiatrist as she has never had to see one before.

Focus on possible psychiatric diagnoses and feed back a suitable model of her symptoms.

ACTOR (ROLE-PLAYER) INSTRUCTIONS

You are quite irate at seeing a psychiatrist, and remain petulant throughout the assessment.

You accuse the psychiatrist (and other doctors) of treating you as if you were mad, and of not believing you.

You are adamant that further testing (perhaps by 'better doctors') might elicit the real cause of your problems.

SUGGESTED APPROACH

Setting the scene

'Hello, Radha, my name is Dr_____, a psychiatrist. I'd like to have a chat with you about some of the problems you've been having. Would that be okay?'

Sensitivity and tact are needed. In this station, the idea of somatoform or hypochondriacal illnesses can be raised, but the patient need not be directly challenged – something that is unlikely to occur on a first assessment in clinical practice. Ultimately, a time may occur in treatment at which the patient will need to be confronted and told that further investigations should not occur and that the diagnosis is a psychological one, but this could be catastrophic at a first appointment. Rather, the candidate's role is to introduce the idea of body–mind interactions in order to explain the symptoms and how psychological theory can offer avenues for treatment.

Establishing a positive, constructive rapport

The patient may be sceptical or even hostile to seeing a psychiatrist, and a positive start is essential. Adding to the pressure of this, however, is that good time management will also be critical – the past history is undoubtedly long and complex, and it will be impossible to obtain as full a history as one would like. Rather, the aim is to obtain a brief overview of the main symptoms whilst keeping possible psychiatric diagnoses in mind.

Considering depression and anxiety as causes

A useful way to begin would be to ask the patient's opinion of what might be causing the symptoms and why investigations have been negative and treatments ineffective. Precipitants, exacerbants and relieving factors, especially psychological ones, should be looked for.

One conceptual model of medically unexplained symptoms is:

- Possible organic illness, but not fully understood, and with evidence of psychological component. Examples include fibromyalgia, IBS, chronic fatigue and neurasthenia. An important point is that whilst the pathology might be poorly understood and at times controversial, there is good evidence that psychological interventions help *regardless* of the aetiology.
- A primary psychiatric illness, in particular depression, anxiety and obsessive compulsive disorder (OCD). Patients might be alexithymic, have poor insight into their mental state or have cultural difficulties talking about feelings.
- Somatoform disorders, including somatisation disorder and hypochondriacal disorder, and dissociative disorders.
- Factitious and malingering disorders, whereby the patient is consciously feigning symptoms for psychological or external gain, respectively.

It is important to explore any obvious psychopathology of depression, anxiety and OCD (and if suggested, albeit rarely, psychosis), both as possible primary diagnoses but also as secondary exacerbating phenomena. Patients may be reluctant to talk about such feelings for fear of being labelled 'psychiatric', so sensitivity is required. One might normalise the situation; for example, noting how 'things frequently appear worse when we feel a bit down; for example, we might find that pain felt worse when we were more tired. Have you ever noticed this?' Or, 'Given the amount you've been through, it wouldn't be surprising to get a bit fed up or blue about things – has this happened?' A few quick questions on mood, anxiety and obsessional and compulsive symptoms can follow, although be careful with biological symptoms of depression – these could be manifestations of either a depressive or somatoform disorder.

Delineating somatisation, hypochondriacal and dissociative symptoms

Although less common, dissociative disorders (with the exception of dissociative seizures) are usually obvious by their physiological improbability, combined with a psychogenic aetiology and frequent lack of concern (*la belle indifference*). Candidates can have difficulty differentiating somatoform disorders – perhaps the most likely diagnosis in this case from the brief information given – which is exacerbated by ICD-10's multiple sub-categories, eponymous syndromes and nebulous terms such as 'Briquet's', 'Da Costa's syndrome', 'psychasthenia' and 'neurocirculatory asthenia'! The most important categories, and those that are diagnostically sufficient for membership candidates, are somatisation disorder and hypochondriacal disorder. In broad terms, whilst both have medically unexplained symptoms, individuals with somatisation disorder will have long-standing multi-system *complaints*, which frequently cannot be physiologically reconciled, for which they seek *treatment*. Conversely, again in crude terms, individuals with hypochondriasis tend to seek *investigations* to rule out *illnesses* (classically tumours), with an undue focus and misinterpretation of normal body signals. Therefore, it is essential to quickly explore the patient's understanding and concerns about their symptoms: have they been reassured by negative investigations, or do they need 'one more scan'?

Addressing a psychological illness model

This broaching of the psychological leads on to the final part of the station: discussing possible psychological causes and, through this, psychological management. This is a sensitive area and one needs to be careful to avoid the patient assuming that the implication is that the symptoms are not real. A general, non-judgemental opening statement could consist of the following:

'We talked about how the psychological can affect the physical – for example, how one can feel "butterflies in your stomach" when nervous, or how a stubbed toe feels worse in cold weather – and how common this is to all of us. Given all of the negative findings to date, I wonder if it's possible that there could be a psychological component to some of your symptoms? Could, for example, stress have made you pay more attention to your body's signals? I know these symptoms are real and uncomfortable when you feel them.'

A follow-up to this, considering treatment, avoids the need for direct confrontation at this early stage of engagement:

'Your doctors have mentioned how treatments to date have unfortunately been unsuccessful. We commonly find that psychological help can be really valuable, regardless of the cause of the illness; for example, managing pain in arthritis or helping people manage illnesses we poorly understand, like IBS. I think this might be something that would be really useful in helping you, and one of the great things about psychological treatment is that it doesn't have side effects like medications can. How would you feel about this?'

ADDITIONAL POINTS

The term 'psychosomatic' has become common parlance and should be avoided lest it be misinterpreted as 'making it up'. If asked for a diagnosis directly, an honest and direct approach must be adhered to, no matter how uncomfortable this may feel. 'Somatoform disorder' is an overarching diagnostic umbrella that might help explain how the mind and body can interact in the first instance. Assessment of medically unexplained symptoms is a common scenario in both liaison and neuropsychiatry.

FURTHER READING

Creed, F. & Barsky, A. (2004) A systematic review of the epidemiology of somatisation disorder and hypochondriasis. *Journal of Psychosomatic Research, 56*, 391–408.

Hatcher, S. & Arroll, B. (2008) Assessment and management of medically unexplained symptoms. *BMJ, 336*, 1124–8.

Röhricht, F. & Elanjithara, T. (2014) Management of medically unexplained symptoms: Outcomes of a specialist liaison clinic. *Psychiatric Bulletin, 38*(3), 102–7.

van Dessel, N., den Boeft, M., van der Wouden, J.C. et al. (2014) Non-pharmacological interventions for somatoform disorders and medically unexplained physical symptoms (MUPS) in adults. *Cochrane Database of Systematic Reviews, 11*, CD011142.

The examiner's mark sheet

Domain/ percentage of marks	Essential points to pass	✓	Extra marks/comments (make notes here)
1. Establishing a positive, constructive rapport 25% of marks	Clear communication Open and closed questions Demonstrating patience Not being defensive		

2. Considering depression and anxiety as causes

15% of marks

Awareness that depression and anxiety might be causes

Consideration of cultural or personal issues regarding expression of distress

3. Delineating somatisation, hypochondriacal and dissociative disorders

30% of marks

Clear understanding, as demonstrated through questioning, of the differences between these conditions

4. Addressing a psychological illness model

30% of marks

Sensitivity, but an ability to be appropriately direct

Not agreeing to any requests for further investigations or physical treatments

% SCORE _____

___

4

OVERALL IMPRESSION

(CIRCLE ONE)

Good Pass

Pass

Borderline

Fail

Clear Fail

NOTES/Areas to improve

STATION 7: LOW MOOD IN MULTIPLE SCLEROSIS

INSTRUCTION TO CANDIDATE

A consultant neurologist, Dr Byron, requests a ward review of Ms Kay, a 48-year-old woman with a 10-year history of MS. Whilst an in-patient for assessment and management of a relapse of her MS, she has become quite tearful and low in mood, saying that she does not wish to 'carry on' anymore.

Assess her mental state and past psychiatric history and discuss treatment options with her.

ACTOR (ROLE-PLAYER) INSTRUCTIONS

You are very upset about your MS, which has been getting worse.

You are fearful of the future; if directly asked, you have considered taking your own life if things got too bad.

SUGGESTED APPROACH

Setting the scene

'Hello, Ms Kay, I'm Dr_____, a psychiatrist in this hospital. Dr Byron has asked me to have a chat with you about how you've been feeling recently, is that okay?'

Assessing current mental state

Depressive criteria will need to be assessed, including a risk history. The past psychiatric history needs to be explored, looking at previous episodes of depression, if any, and the effectiveness of any treatment given. It is important to check for evidence of previous periods of euphoria, anxiety or psychosis, all of which may be neuropsychiatric complications of MS.

Consideration of MS as an organic cause

The fact that the patient is currently in hospital infers a MS relapse, although this needs to be confirmed – what has happened, and what is the degree of disability at this time? Is the patient's low mood clearly based on this relapse or fear of her ability to cope in the future? What support – from family and friends, professionals and charitable organisations – is in place after discharge? Does this need to be re-evaluated during this admission (e.g. with a home OT or physiotherapy visit)? Have there been any recent changes or additions to the patient's medications, particularly steroids or β-interferon?

Cognitive impairment occurs in up to half of all MS sufferers, and it can both cause and exacerbate other psychological symptoms: ask about problems with memory, apathy, paying attention and ability to carry out day-to-day activities (not due to physical impairment, but rather motivational and higher executive dysfunction).

Consideration of treatment options

Treatment options will depend on the history taken. Concern about iatrogenic low mood secondary to steroids or β-interferon use must be tackled cautiously – one might be wrong and also create damage in the patient's relationship with the treating neurologist. However, if the patient has noted recent changes, then it is important to recognise (and be seen to recognise) this fact:

'All medications can have side effects, and some people have become lower in mood due to steroids/β-interferon. However, we must consider the possible benefits you're getting from these medications, the risks of stopping them and the fact that the low mood may not be due to them. I know this is quite a complex business, so perhaps we can have a joint discussion with your neurologist present in which we can weigh up the pros and cons of changing these drugs.'

Should depression be diagnosed, then it is perfectly reasonable to discuss antidepressant medication – just make sure that there is no current or past history of elation. Check to see if the patient is already on an antidepressant – this may be prescribed for other reasons, such as TCAs for pain or bladder control. Previous response, if any, to antidepressants will guide prescribing, but in general, SSRIs are considered the first-line treatment, as TCAs can be poorly tolerated in MS.

Psychological support should be considered, especially CBT. Other psycho-social routes might include local support groups, the Multiple Sclerosis Society, appropriate home help and OT. This will be guided by the patient's concerns.

Mood stabilisers can be used during periods of elation, although lithium should be prescribed with care due to its propensity to cause polyuria, which can be enormously problematic if there is a concomitant problem with continence. The literature on the treatment of psychotic symptoms in MS is small, although there is evidence to support the use of atypical anti-psychotics. Remember that cognitive impairment may be due to low mood or a side effect of medication.

ADDITIONAL POINTS

1. Remember to ask about current and past symptoms of elation. Pathological laughter and crying is a syndrome that occurs in approximately one in ten MS sufferers, particularly in late-stage disease. Psychotic symptoms seldom if ever progress to a full schizophrenia-like picture: just because the patient does not present as 'obviously psychotic', do not fail to ask about hallucinations, which occur in approximately 20% of patients.

2. It is unlikely that there will be time to do a formal cognitive assessment; the usual 'trick' of asking about poor memory and concentration and mentioning how one would like to revisit this domain for 'more formal and thorough testing' at a later time should suffice to demonstrate that the candidate is aware of and understands the significance of these symptoms.

3. All chronic illnesses are associated with higher-than-average rates of depression. Multiple sclerosis has a higher rate than expected for degree of disability, suggesting at least a partial organic basis. Whilst there is evidence for β-interferon causing low mood, the significance of this may have been overstated.

FURTHER READING

Feinstein, A., Magalhaes, S., Richard, J.F., Audet, B. & Moore, C. (2014) The link between multiple sclerosis and depression. *Nature Reviews Neurology, 10*(9), 507–17.

Fernie, B.A., Kollmann, J. & Brown, R.G. (2015) Cognitive behavioural interventions for depression in chronic neurological conditions: A systematic review *Journal of Psychosomatic Research, 78*(5), 411–9.

Koch, M.W., Glazenborg, A., Uyttenboogaart, M., Mostert, J. & De Keyser, J. (2011) Pharmacologic treatment of depression in multiple sclerosis. *Cochrane Database of Systematic Reviews, 16*(2), CD007295.

Reder, A.T., Oger, J.F., Kappos, L., O'Connor, P. & Rametta, M. (2014) Short-term and long-term safety and tolerability of interferon β-1b in multiple sclerosis. *Multiple Sclerosis and Related Disorders, 3*(3), 294–302.

www.mssociety.org.uk

The examiner's mark sheet

Domain/ percentage of marks	Essential points to pass	✓	Extra marks/comments (make notes here)
1. Clarifying recent history and past psychiatric history 35% of marks	Clear communication Open and closed questions Demonstrating patience Clarifies recent and past history		

⇧ 2. Mental state
   examination: clarifying
   any psychopathology

   35% of marks

3. Management

   30% of marks

Looks for symptom variability

Tests insight

Establishes current risks

Considers environmental
strategies

Recognises medication also
carries risks

% SCORE _____

___
3

OVERALL IMPRESSION

(CIRCLE ONE)

Good Pass

Pass

Borderline

Fail

Clear Fail

NOTES/Areas to improve

Personality disorder

○ LINKED STATIONS

STATION 1(a): BORDERLINE PERSONALITY DISORDER – ASSESSMENT

INSTRUCTION TO CANDIDATE

You receive a referral asking that you review a 24-year-old woman who initially presented to accident and emergency (A&E) having taken an overdose of ibuprofen and paracetamol. She is now physically fit and the charge nurse has informed you that she is 'a right nuisance', taking up an acute bed when it could have been used more appropriately. You are told of several presentations to the same unit over the last 6 months.

You are also told that she has been known to mental health services for a number of years since moving to this area. In that time, she has had a number of different care coordinators and believes her team to be 'useless'.

Gather relevant information that will help you in considering a diagnosis.

She has been told in the past that she has a personality disorder and wants to know what this means.

ACTOR (ROLE-PLAYER) INSTRUCTIONS

You took an overdose due to being distressed and angry after an argument with your partner. You do not feel suicidal right now.

You are fed up with mental health services because you have never had any help from them despite them having seen you many times.

You feel you are depressed or bipolar because your mood is up and down all the time, but you have been told you have a personality disorder.

You want to know what this means and whether there are any tablets that can help you feel better.

SUGGESTED APPROACH

Setting the scene

Address the patient by name, introduce yourself and explain what you are there for: 'Hello, my name is Dr_____, I'm one of the psychiatrists. I've been asked by the medical team to see you. Would it be OK if we spoke about what led you to come into hospital?' Or, 'Could you tell me what happened?'

Allow time for the patient to respond and explain what their concerns are.

Completing the tasks

We have been told that she has been diagnosed with a personality disorder in the past. From the history, an emotionally unstable personality disorder appears likely, and the interview should focus on this, but it is important to screen for other psychopathologies and evaluate the patient's needs at this point in time, as rates of comorbid mental disorder and social problems are high in this patient group.

Gather relevant information that will help you in considering a diagnosis

An empathic response is needed, as are firm boundaries. Explore the events leading up to the overdose and her intentions at the time of taking the overdose. 'I know you have been through a tough time. Can you take me through the events that led you to the decision of taking an overdose? What were your intentions at that time?'

Enquire about the previous attendances at A&E due to self-harm or suicidal feelings and the context of these presentations. 'I gather you have been to A&E on previous occasions due to similar difficulties. Could you tell me a bit more about that?'

Ask what diagnosis she was given when she first came into contact with mental health services, the treatments she received and whether they helped her. What happened in the relationships with her care coordinators and why did they break down? 'You told me that you are seeing mental health professionals. What are your views on their role? What do you understand by the diagnosis that you have been given?'

Screen for affective disorder, anxiety disorders, psychotic illness and other personality disorders. 'How have you been feeling lately? How would you describe your mood? Have you ever experienced feeling tense or worried all the time? Have you had any unusual experiences such as seeing people who are not there or hearing voices that you don't understand where they are coming from?'

You must attempt to elicit the following features for an emotionally unstable personality (although all are not necessary).

Emotionally unstable personality disorder (PD)

There are two subtypes of emotionally unstable PD: impulsive and borderline. Both subtypes show impulsive behaviour, affective instability and a lack of self-control.

Unstable mood – 'Do you find your mood varies a lot from day to day or from week to week?'

Impulsivity – 'Do you tend to make quick decisions without thinking too much about what the outcome might be?'

Emotionally unstable PD (impulsive type)

Desultoriness – 'Do you often find your goals changing depending on how you feel?'

Explosiveness – 'We all get upset from time to time. Do certain people upset you from time to time? What usually happens when you become upset?'

Quarrelsomeness – 'We all have arguments and often these are important in relationships. Do you have many arguments in your everyday life?'

Lack of control – 'Do you find yourself losing control in certain situations and perhaps becoming upset, even aggressive?' Outbursts of violence or threatening behaviour are common, especially when subject to criticism.

Emotionally unstable PD (borderline type)

Relationship difficulties/crises – 'Have you had any relationship difficulties recently?' Such difficulties are often involved in intense and unstable relationships, with frequent emotional crises and excessive effort at avoiding feelings of abandonment in the form of self-harm and suicide threats.

Recurrent self-harm – 'Sometimes people's unwanted thoughts and feelings become so much that they feel like harming themselves. Has anything like that happened to you? Have you harmed yourself in the past?'

Emptiness – chronic feelings of emptiness or boredom. 'Is it difficult to find things that you're interested in? Do you often feel low or empty?'

Unstable self-image – 'How do you feel about yourself most of the time?' Their self-image, aims and sexual preferences are often unclear or disturbed.

Pt: The psychiatrist told me that I have a personality disorder. What does that mean? Am I a bad person?

C: By the time we are young adults, we have usually developed our individual personalities so that we think, feel and behave in our own ways. Most people's personality remains fairly constant throughout their lives, allowing them to get on fairly well with people most of the time. For some of us, this doesn't happen and we develop personalities that are less comfortable with others and sometimes ourselves. Often these differences in personality have been present for a long time, usually from childhood. We're not exactly sure why this happens. Some of it may be due to things like heredity and genes, and some of it can be due to our experiences while growing up. This can mean that some people have difficulties with personal relationships and friendships, dealing with feelings or emotions and difficulty controlling their temper.

Risk

Self-harm and suicidal threats might lead to admission and this process can often be counter-therapeutic for such people. However, a diagnosis of borderline personality disorder (BPD) should not compromise a thorough risk assessment and each presentation should be considered in its own rights. A drug overdose as described could have been a serious suicide attempt and requires an appropriate approach, especially in an acute A&E setting. Although in this station you have not been asked to make such decisions, you should always consider risk, and a few screening questions, including asking about illicit substance misuse and alcohol, will let the examiner know that you are a sensible psychiatrist.

Problem solving

Bear in mind that the patient is likely to be angry and dissatisfied with the help they have received so far. While you might be the focus of their distress, it is important to remain calm and in control.

Pharmacological treatment

Only indicated if specific target symptoms are present, such as antidepressants if depressed, hypnotics for insomnia, anti-psychotics for psychotic symptoms, mood stabilisers, and so forth. Be mindful of the potential for dependence and tolerance to hypnotics and benzodiazepines, as well as the potential for overdoses, so there is a need to restrict the supply of medications.

Psychological treatment

Various types of psychological treatment are available, usually longer term and community based, with varying degrees of evidence.

Mentalisation-based therapy is a combination of group and individual therapy. It aims to help you better understand yourself and others by being more aware of what is going on in your own head and in the minds of others. It is helpful in borderline personality disorder.

Dialectical behaviour therapy uses a combination of cognitive and behavioural therapies in individual and group settings and is helpful in borderline personality disorder.

Cognitive behavioural therapy is a way of changing unhelpful patterns of thinking.

Schema-focussed therapy is a cognitive therapy that explores and changes collections of deep, unhelpful beliefs. Again, it seems to be effective in borderline personality disorder.

Transference-focussed therapy is a structured treatment in which the therapist explores and changes unconscious processes. It seems to be effective in borderline personality disorder.

Dynamic psychotherapy looks at how past experiences affect present behaviour. It is similar to transference-focussed therapy, but less structured.

Cognitive analytical therapy is a way to recognise and change unhelpful patterns in relationships and behaviour.

Treatment in a therapeutic community involves treatment in a place where people with long-standing emotional problems can go (or sometimes stay) for several weeks or months. Most of the work is done in groups. People learn from getting along – or not getting along – with other people in the treatment group. It differs from 'real life' in that any disagreements or upsets happen in a safe place. People in treatment often have a lot of say over how the community is run. In the United Kingdom, it is more common now for this intensive treatment to be offered as a day programme, 5 days a week.

Rapport and communication

Display a calm and consistent approach to the patient's anger and distress. Be empathetic, but maintain appropriate boundaries.

Conclusion

Suggest the appropriate support and follow-up (crisis team/referral to CMHT/admission/referral to personality disorder service) based on your assessment of the current mental state and risk.

The examiner's mark sheet

Domain/percentage of marks	Essential points to pass	✓	Extra marks/comments (make notes here)
1. Rapport and communication 20% of marks	Clear communication Open and closed questions Empathy Demonstrating patience		
2. History taking 20% of marks	Elicits history suggestive of personality disorder		
3. Differentials 20% of marks	Rules out comorbid mental disorder (e.g. depression, anxiety disorder or psychosis)		

⇧ 4. Risk assessment   Risk assessment of further
     20% of marks   self-harm, suicide or harm to
                       others

5. Explanation   Explains diagnosis and
     20% of marks   management options to patient

% SCORE _____

___   **OVERALL IMPRESSION**

5   (CIRCLE ONE)

             Good Pass

             Pass

             Borderline

             Fail

             Clear Fail

             NOTES/Areas to improve

STATION 1(b): BORDERLINE PERSONALITY DISORDER – MANAGEMENT

> **INSTRUCTION TO CANDIDATE**
>
> The A&E consultant wants to speak to you after you have finished assessing the patient. They are not happy with the repeated presentations of the patient, which they feel take time away from caring for more deserving patients. They ask why psychiatry services are not doing anything to prevent this patient attending often in crises.
>
> **Talk to the A&E consultant about the management of patients with borderline personality disorder.**

ACTOR (ROLE-PLAYER) INSTRUCTIONS

You are the A&E consultant; your team is under pressure to clear patients within a stipulated time to meet the hospital targets.

You come across frustrated at the repeated attendances of the patient, and want to ask why the mental health services have not done anything to cure her. Why can she not have some tablets to make her better?

You think that the patient is very manipulative and does not actually require hospital treatment. You know that BPD means such individuals seek attention and have trouble getting along with people.

SUGGESTED APPROACH

Setting the scene

Introduce yourself: 'Hello, Dr_____, I am Dr_____, the psychiatrist. Can we have a discussion about patient_____?' Be mindful that although you are talking to someone from the same professional background, this person is from a different specialty. He or she may come across impatient, but allow them to speak and listen to their frustrations.

Completing the tasks

Explaining the symptoms of BPD

Highlight that you understand that staff in A&E might view the patient as manipulative and not deserving of care due to the repeated presentations. You could also acknowledge that the patient might induce strong feelings (counter-transference experiences) in some staff members, as we know that she has fallen out with health professionals and believes them to be unhelpful. It would be useful to explain to the consultant about the chaotic and unstable lifestyle a person with BPD tends to have. 'People with BPD may do things on the spur of the moment, act without thinking through the consequences and generally tend to have poor coping mechanisms.' While the patient may appear manipulative, they are not to be dismissed as less deserving of care, as they tend to have poor coping skills and problem-solving skills. Discuss why you believe she needs a thorough assessment on the occasions that she presents to emergency services – the risk of completed suicide in BPD is as high as with other major mental illnesses. 'Patients with BPD may come across as manipulative and cause strong feelings against them; however, they can act without planning, which puts them at high risk of self-harm. Therefore, they should be assessed thoroughly during a crisis.'

You could then set about discussing how psychiatry and acute hospital services together could manage the patient. It is important to explain that the hospital, as a place of safety, will provide her with some temporary stability at a time when everything else in her life is extremely chaotic. 'The psychiatry services will aim to provide consistent support to her; she will have a named nurse who will primarily oversee her care with a mutually agreed care plan. The services also provide support during crisis situations; the hospital will be a safe place to contain her anxiety right now.'

Discuss your management plan with the A&E consultant

Explain that you will complete a full history and physical examination of the patient, as well as obtaining the results of the investigations she has had at the hospital. You will be looking to obtain as much information from collateral sources, including the general practitioner (GP), community mental health team (CMHT) and family members/partner (with her consent). Gabbard's (2000) principles in managing patients with BPD would be a sensible approach:

Maintain flexibility: Take into account the patient's ego strength, psychological mindedness, intellect and emotional state when considering supportive or interpretive psychological treatment.

Establish conditions that keep the patient safe: Set boundaries regarding repeated hospitalization, suicidal behaviour, use of drug and alcohol and inappropriate crossing of professional boundaries.

Tolerate anger, aggression and hate: Defensive countermeasures, trying to prove staff are in fact good, angry responses and rejections are likely to lead to disengagement.

Promote reflection: 'What do you think are the consequences of the overdose?' 'How do you think I felt when you said that to me?'

Set necessary limits: Particularly when behaviour threatens staff or the therapeutic relationship.

Establish and maintain the therapeutic alliance: Regularly revisit the aims and goals of therapeutic contract.

Avoid splitting between psychotherapy and medication: Responses to prescribed medication must form part of the therapeutic interactions and be openly discussed if medication is resisted, sabotaged or abused. They may need reminding that medication effects are modest.

Avoid or understand splitting between members of staff: Recognize they may show opposing attitudes within short periods, which can be confusing for staff.

Monitor counter-transference feelings: Allow staff to share embarrassing or difficult feelings induced by the patient.

General
Good communication with all parties involved is essential.

Problem solving

You should offer to discuss concerns that the staff have and consider ways you might deal with these. Suggesting a session with staff in which you could discuss the case and personality disorders in more detail would be useful. It is important to have a consistent approach to the patient.

ADDITIONAL READING

http://www.rcpsych.ac.uk/healthadvice/problemsdisorders/personalitydisorder.aspx

NICE guidelines for treatment and management of borderline personality disorder. https://www.nice.org.uk/guidance/cg78

The ICD-10 Classification of Mental and Behavioural Disorders (1992) *Clinical Descriptions and Diagnostic Guidelines*. Geneva: WHO Press.

Gabbard, G.O. (2000) *Psychodynamic Psychiatry in Clinical Practice*. Washington, DC: American Psychiatric Press.

The examiner's mark sheet

Domain/ percentage of marks	Essential points to pass	✓	Extra marks/comments (make notes here)
1. Rapport and communication 20% of marks	Clear communication		
	Empathy		
	Demonstrating patience and acknowledging the anger of other professionals		
	Remains calm under pressure		
2. Addressing the concerns 20% of marks	Allows the A&E doctor to talk about their frustrations		
	Demonstrates empathy and listening skills		
	Able to respond to their concerns in appropriate manner		
3. Symptoms 20% of marks	Explains the symptoms of BPD and the underlying feelings behind the behaviour		

⇑ 4. Risk assessment   Highlights the risks involved

    20% of marks   Discusses management in order
to contain the risks

5. Treatment   Explains what treatment options
    strategies   can be offered and in what
    20% of marks   settings these can be helpful

Aware of the limitations of
medications in BPD

% SCORE _____   ___ **OVERALL IMPRESSION**

    5 (CIRCLE ONE)

Good Pass

Pass

Borderline

Fail

Clear Fail

NOTES/Areas to improve

○ SINGLE STATIONS

STATION 2: PARANOID PERSONALITY DISORDER

INSTRUCTION TO CANDIDATE

You have been asked to assess this patient who has attended the clinic. He
has a diagnosis of paranoid personality disorder (PPD). He did not turn up for
his previous two appointments.

**As part of your consultation, elicit the main features of PPD and discuss
management options with him.**

ACTOR (ROLE-PLAYER) INSTRUCTIONS

You have come to see the psychiatrist as your GP has told you to do so. You are reluctant
to talk to him or her as generally you do not trust anyone. You are annoyed because you
think this is another tactic of the NHS to get patients into their clinics and feel cheated.
You look a bit suspicious and come across as guarded when talking. You did not attend
the previous appointments because you thought they were ploys to keep you within the
mental health system so that they can make money.

SUGGESTED APPROACH

Setting the scene

Introduce yourself: 'Hello, my name is Dr_____, I'm one of the psychiatrists. Thank you
for coming to see me in the clinic today. We have not met before this time, how have you
been?' The patient may seem guarded – reassure them about confidentiality. Explain that

this appointment is to look at how he is coping with life generally and to identify whether he may need any help. Inform him that this consultation is confidential and his consent will be obtained before sharing information with other professionals.

You could also mention that he had missed several appointments: 'I notice that we haven't seen you for a while. Sometimes when people have a lot going on in their lives or they're stressed, they don't want to attend appointments. Has anything like that been happening to you?'

Completing the tasks

Elicit the main features of PPD
According to the ICD-10 diagnostic guidelines, PPD is characterised by:

- Excessive sensitiveness to setbacks and rebuffs: 'How do you cope when things don't turn out well or go the way you expect them to?'
- Bearing persistent grudges: 'How do you react when people do not treat you well? Do you find you are able to forgive them?'
- Suspiciousness and misconstruing neutral or friendly actions of others as hostile or contemptuous: 'What would you say about your ability to place trust in others? How do you think you are being treated by others generally? Have you felt that you are being looked at in an unusual way?'
- Combative and tenacious sense of personal rights: 'Would you consider yourself to have a strong sense of entitlement? How do you go about protecting your rights?'
- Recurrent suspicions, without justification, regarding sexual fidelity of partner: 'Have you experienced any betrayal? Have there been times in which you have felt more suspicious than normal? Can you tell me a bit more about that?'
- Excessive self-importance: 'How do you see yourself in the general day-to-day world? What role do you play in the lives of others around you?'
- Preoccupation with unsubstantiated 'conspiratorial' explanations of events both personal and in the world at large: 'Have you felt victimised? Have you experienced that something is going on around you that make you a bit suspicious? What happened?'

Often others become frustrated with such persistent suspiciousness and accusations. These individuals tend to distort reality, but their thoughts are not actually delusional. They continuously look to seek confirmation of their suspicions and conspiratorial explanations of events. You would want to take a full history and mental state examination. A collateral history would also be informative.

Discuss management options with him
'It seems like there are a few things in life that may be difficult for you to deal with; for example, forming trusting relationships, getting along with people who may have offended you and so forth. Sometimes, our personality traits that are formed during developmental stages can remain maladaptive, causing these effects in later life. I wonder if you may have considered this in this light before. If it is OK with you, we can discuss some therapies to help you overcome this.'

Psychotherapy
Psychological approaches are difficult, as building a trusting and intimate relationship with a therapist is often unworkable, but they are the treatment of choice so long as the patient demonstrates insight and is prepared to engage. Psychodynamic psychotherapy may be too demanding, but if successfully initiated, the therapist should be aware that ambitious interpretations may be met with resistance and breaking off of treatment. Group psychotherapy can help reduce suspiciousness and improve socialisation, but frequently such sessions are not tolerated.

Medication

The evidence base for effective pharmacotherapy is weak. Anti-psychotics can help with agitation and hypervigilance. Antidepressants can help with affective and anxiety symptoms. Short periods of benzodiazepines have also been used for marked anxiety and agitation, although there is the risk of dependence and they are generally out of favour.

Risk

Occasionally, the thoughts of these individuals can lead to violence against those they suspect. If during the course of the interview they express anger towards others, explore this further.

You can limit the likelihood of aggression towards yourself by not invading their space (i.e. not getting too close), not embarrassing them and not using an accusational interview style.

Problem solving

You need to be aware of his likely sensitivity and suspiciousness. The use of normalisation can be helpful here. Typically, these individuals do not do well with authority figures, such as doctors. This is often an obstacle to engaging with services. Such individuals feel that others are trying to get the better of them or to deceive or fool them. It is likely that during the interview you will be subject to accusations and insults, and you need to remain polite but not defensive. It is possible that any suggestions you make will be rejected or criticised.

ADDITIONAL POINTS

PDD patients are hypersensitive to potential slights, are suspicious and have a hypervigilant view of the world. They persistently scan for signs of potential danger and rarely relax their suspicions. These features make it difficult to form enjoyable relationships and others often drift away. Acquaintances will view them as secretive, prickly and devious. Unlike paranoid syndromes, in PPD, ideas or themes are not of a delusional nature and there are no hallucinatory experiences.

FURTHER READING

Bateman, A.W. & Tyrer, P. (2004) Psychological treatment for personality disorder. *Advances in Psychiatric Treatment*, 10, 378–88.

Carroll, A. (2009) Are you looking at me? Understanding and managing paranoid personality disorder. *Advances in Psychiatric Treatment*, 15(1), 40–8.

The ICD-10 Classification of Mental and Behavioural Disorders (1992) *Clinical Descriptions and Diagnostic Guidelines*. Geneva: WHO Press.

The examiner's mark sheet

Domain/ percentage of marks	Essential points to pass	✓	Extra marks/comments (make notes here)
1. Rapport and communication 20% of marks	Clear communication Empathy Demonstrating patience and acknowledging the mistrust from the patient		

⇧ 2. History taking
      20% of marks

Able to elicit information from paranoid patient

Dealing with hostility and suspiciousness

Explores relevant areas in relation to PPD

3. Diagnosis and differentials

      20% of marks

Demonstrates knowledge of the diagnostic criteria of PPD

Excludes differentials: psychotic disorder

4. Risk assessment

      20% of marks

Explores risk to self

Risk to others – any incidents of violence/aggression

5. Treatment strategies

      20% of marks

Explains what treatment options can be offered and what will be the benefits

% SCORE _____

___ **OVERALL IMPRESSION**

5   (CIRCLE ONE)

Good Pass

Pass

Borderline

Fail

Clear Fail

NOTES/Areas to improve

STATION 3: PERSONALITY ASSESSMENT

> **INSTRUCTION TO CANDIDATE**
>
> You are seeing this 24–year-old gentleman in your clinic. The GP has written to you as he believes that this gentleman has an unusual personality. He gives you little useful information as he is really not sure what to do. There is no significant past psychiatric or medical history and no regular medication. He hopes you are able to shed some light on what is going on.
>
> **Assess this patient's personality.**

ACTOR (ROLE-PLAYER) INSTRUCTIONS

You are here to see the psychiatrist, as your GP has referred you. You have been consulting your GP as you are having difficulties in forming sustained relationships and long-term friendships. You feel that there is a long-standing emptiness in the way you feel; you would like to make friends but do not know how. You answer the doctor's questions, hoping you will get to the bottom of your problems.

SUGGESTED APPROACH

Setting the scene

Introduce yourself: 'Hello, my name is Dr_____, I'm one of the psychiatrists.' Explain that you have received a letter from his doctor and ask if he knows why the GP has referred him. If he is unsure, then you could describe how his doctor felt that things did not seem to be going so well for him in his personal life and relationships, which is why he had asked that you see him. Did this seem correct to him? Ask if you could talk to him in order to find out how things have been recently.

Completing the tasks

Assess this patient's personality

In an attempt to avoid this scenario ending up as a list of questions (examiners do not like lists), useful information can be gleaned from identifying how the individual has behaved in certain situations. You should have questions in mind from each personality disorder that will allow you to tease out which is most likely (some examples are given below). Try to obtain an overall impression and scan for personality traits.

Ask about:

Character

'Can you tell me what kind of person you are?'

'How would you describe your own personality?'

'If you were with other people, say at a party or at work, how do you behave?'

Reserved/timid (anankastic)

Shy/self-conscious/anxious (avoidant)

Fussy/difficult/meticulous/punctual (anankastic)

Selfish/self-centred (paranoid)

Centre of attention (histrionic)

Sensitive/suspicious (paranoid)

Resentful/jealous (paranoid)

Attitudes of others – 'How would people that know you describe your personality?'

Attitudes to others – 'What do you think of other people; for example, your friends or people at work?'

Habits

Risk-taking behaviour (with or without criminal behaviour) (dissocial) – 'Would you consider yourself as a risk taker? Can you give some examples of risky things you have done? Have they got you into any trouble?'

Food, smoking, alcohol and drugs – 'Tell me about your dietary habits. What about alcohol? Do you smoke or take any street drugs?'

Reactions to stress

'How would you cope in an extremely stressful situation; for example, you lose your job or have broken up with your partner?'

Temperament

'What are you like if you get angry? What is the worst thing you have done out of anger?'

'Has your temper ever got you into trouble?' (Dissocial)

'Do you ever think you are irresponsible?' (Dissocial)

'Do you get into lots of arguments?' (Impulsive)

'How do you respond to criticism?' (Anxious/paranoid)

'Are you ever very emotional?' (Histrionic/borderline)

Friendships and relationships

'How do you get on with other people?' (Paranoid)

'Do you have many friends?' (Schizoid)

'Do you feel close to your friends?' (Schizoid/dissocial)

'Do your friendships last?' (Dissocial)

'Do you trust other people?' (Impulsive/paranoid)

'Have you ever had serious arguments with a partner? How did you handle this?' (Borderline)

'Do you think you depend on other people to get by?' (Dependent)

Fantasy thinking

'What do you dream of or wish for?'

'Do you ever daydream about things? Tell me more about this.' (Schizoid)

Prevailing mood

'What is your mood like for most of the time?'

'Are you predominantly cheery or gloomy?'

It is important to exclude an affective disorder by screening for depressive/manic psychopathology. If confirmed, establish a time course.

Leisure

Asking about their free time and what they enjoy can provide information on whether they prefer social or more solitary activities, as well as sedate or energetic activities.

Risk

When asking about mood and dissocial traits, this is an opportunity to screen for suicidal and homicidal ideation.

Problem solving

It can be a tense moment in a scenario if the actor turns to you and asks, 'Do I have a personality disorder?' It would be prudent to say that it is difficult to make this diagnosis after one meeting and without the benefit of more collateral information. However, do mention if they have traits of a particular personality disorder (ICD-10).

It is challenging to form an accurate opinion on personality in such a short time and also based entirely on the individual's opinion of himself. However, such is the nature of the exam that one at least needs to attempt this.

It could be quite depressing to focus on entirely negative personality traits, and the person might feel somewhat persecuted. Also enquire about their positive qualities. At the end of the interview, conclude by saying that you would ideally like to speak to his parents, partner and close friends for collateral information. If it turns out that he has features of PD, inform him that based on the information gathered, there is a likelihood he may have the features of a certain type of PD and give your rationale for this.

ADDITIONAL POINTS

A useful mnemonic for personality assessment is 'CHART FAME':

Character

HAbits

Reaction to stress

Temperament

FAntasy thinking

Mood (prevailing)

Enduring relationships

FURTHER READING

Leff, J.P. (1992) *Psychiatric Examination in Clinical Practice*. 3rd edn. Oxford: Wiley Blackwell.

The ICD-10 Classification of Mental and Behavioural Disorders (1992) *Clinical Descriptions and Diagnostic Guidelines*. Geneva: WHO Press.

The examiner's mark sheet

Domain/ percentage of marks	Essential points to pass	✓	Extra marks/comments (make notes here)
1. Rapport and communication 20% of marks	Clear communication Empathy Demonstrating patience and acknowledging that patient may feel uncomfortable with personal questions		
2. Addressing concerns 20% of marks	Listens to patient and tries to answer the questions Keeps the interview in a conversational style rather than an interrogational style		

⬆ 3. Symptoms

    20% of marks

Explores the main themes of personality

Asks relevant questions, demonstrating knowledge of the various types of personality

4. Risk assessment

    20% of marks

Asks about risks to self and others when indicated

5. Conclusion

    20% of marks

Able to conclude whether the person has any type of personality disorder

Able to give feedback to patient as to why this is the case and to explain rationale

% SCORE _____

___   **OVERALL IMPRESSION**

5   (CIRCLE ONE)

Good Pass

Pass

Borderline

Fail

Clear Fail

NOTES/Areas to improve

Chapter 12
Perinatal psychiatry   Ruaidhri McCormack

O LINKED STATIONS

STATION 1(a): POSTNATAL DEPRESSION

INSTRUCTION TO CANDIDATE

Ms Rachel Carmichael has been referred to you by her general practitioner (GP). She is a 27-year-old lady who has given birth to a baby boy 2 months ago. Over the last 5 weeks, she has been feeling low. Her partner works in a very busy city job and comes back late in the evenings. She has no other children. Her parents live in Spain and she sees them perhaps once a year. Several of her close friends do have children and live in the area, but she has preferred not to socialise with them for several weeks now.

Elicit a psychiatric history from this woman.

ACTOR (ROLE-PLAYER) INSTRUCTIONS

You are downcast with initial poor eye contact, but are keen to be helped and know you are not coping; say early that you think you need antidepressants and ask the doctor's opinion.

You have been consistently low with no energy and terrible sleep for 4 weeks; you have had suicidal thoughts and considered an overdose, but do not think you could go through with it because of the impact it would have on your partner and new baby.

You had depression after an abortion at age 16 and took an overdose resulting in intensive care unit (ITU) admission, but have been well since.

You were sexually abused by a woman as a child, but absolutely will not discuss this in more detail except to say (if specifically asked) that you have not seen this woman in 20 years; become angry and upset if the doctor belligerently and repeatedly asks about this.

You feel like a terrible mother and are very guilty and ashamed about this, but are managing to adequately care for the baby simply because of the live-in assistance of your sister; your partner works a lot because of heavy financial debts and you do not feel like inviting friends.

You love the baby (your first child) and would never do anything to harm him.

SUGGESTED APPROACH

Setting the scene

Begin the task by addressing the patient by name and introducing yourself. Acknowledge her current circumstances and begin with an open question: 'Hello, Ms Carmichael, I am Dr_____, a psychiatrist. I have a letter from your GP who is concerned about you. Can you tell me a bit about what has been happening?' Allow the patient to respond to your introduction and maintain a flow in your conversation. Supportive statements will demonstrate your understanding of her situation and encourage good rapport; for example, 'The weeks after delivery can be extremely stressful', and 'It's very common to feel this way after the baby is born'. Then proceed to hone in by using more closed questions where appropriate.

Stick to the task. The question about antidepressants is designed to distract you. Acknowledge the question but immediately come back to the task: 'Antidepressants might well have a role, but it's important at this stage that I ask a few questions so I can best understand how to help you.'

The targeted history

When taking a psychiatric history in this situation, it is important to consider the differential diagnoses; in particular, baby blues, postnatal depression (PND) and puerperal psychosis. The ICD criteria for postnatal depression are the same as for any other depressive episode. Symptoms (particularly feelings of guilt and shame) are often linked to the new role as mother. Postnatal depression occurs in 10%–15% of women post-delivery, usually within 4–6 weeks. It is not uncommon for the onset to be *before* delivery.

You should pursue the structure of a normal history, moving naturally through history of presenting complaint, psychiatric and medical histories (including medications), family history, social circumstances, alcohol and substances consumption and personal history. The network of relationships is very relevant in postnatal depression, including the effects and impacts on, and the response from, partner, baby, other children, friends and other family.

The history should make reference to the risk factors for postnatal depression:

- Anxiety or depression during pregnancy
- Stressful life events (including problems with the delivery or health of the baby)
- Poor social supports (especially from partner or parents)
- Psychiatric or family history of depression
- Baseline low self-esteem
- History of miscarriage or termination of pregnancy
- Being the victim of abuse in earlier life
- Lower socioeconomic class and lower educational level
- Personality factors (e.g. perfectionism, introversion and neuroticism)

History of presenting complaint

Ask about the duration and nature of symptoms: 'How long have you been feeling like this?' Enquire about the core criteria for an ICD-defined depressive episode – pervasive low mood, anergia and anhedonia. The minor criteria should also be sought as part of a natural dialogue – guilt and shame (particularly feelings of inadequacy as a mother), poor concentration, sleep disturbance, pessimism, low self-esteem and suicidality.

In addition to asking about symptoms, one should also ask about their impacts and associated functional impairments. The dynamic between the mother and baby is key. Ask about any concerns the mother may have regarding the baby and its health and how she and the baby are coping with new routines. Is she breast feeding, and if so, has this been problematic? Does she feel she is an adequate mother?

Psychiatric history

Ask about past episodes of depression and other mental disorders. You need to know when any episode occurred, how severe it was, what risks were associated (with their nature and severity), what and how diagnoses were made and how episodes were treated (which treatments did/did not work).

Social circumstances

Ask about prevailing stressors and the network of social supports. Screen for relationship, financial and employment-related pressures, and ask an open question about other stressors.

Risk assessment

The best risk assessments always include the history of risk as well as current risk and best impressions regarding future risk.

- Intentional self-harm – thoughts/plans/intent and history of self-harm.
- Harm to baby – where the baby is now, any fears/wishes to harm the baby and evidence she has been unable to adequately care due to mental health symptoms or other reasons.
- Harm to others – contact with other children and any wish to harm others.
- Harm from others – any ongoing contact between alleged sexual abuser and patient/baby is relevant.

Other risks can be considered as appropriate – risks of vulnerability, self-neglect or non-engagement with treatment.

If there are concerns about the safety of the child or the mother, you will need to discuss the case with her partner and social services.

Brief mental state examination to elicit psychopathology

While the station does not explicitly ask for a mental state examination, neither does it exclude it. A brief mental state examination (MSE) is absolutely essential to screen for psychosis in particular. It is also particularly pertinent to ask about anxiety symptoms (worry, apprehension, panic attacks, autonomic features, motor tension and obsessionality). Many questions normally covered in 'mood' will have already been asked in your history.

Rapport and communication

Be sensitive when inquiring about issues to do with her role and perceived ability as a mother; insensitively approaching questions to do with risk can be catastrophic to rapport. When a patient closes up about past traumas, you have to think about what relevance that incident has *now* in this encounter. Any ongoing contact between abusers and the patient and baby is relevant, but further detail may not be. 'I completely understand that you don't want to talk about this, but it is important for me to know that this person is no longer in a position to harm you or the baby.'

Conclusion

If unclear about parts of the history, summarise back to the patient to confirm or clarify.

FURTHER READING

Milgrom, J., Gemmill, A.W., Bilszta, J.L. et al. (2008) Antenatal risk factors for postnatal depression: A large prospective study. *Journal of Affective Disorders, 108*, 147–57.

Musters, C., McDonald, E. & Jones, I. (2008) Management of postnatal depression. *BMJ, 337*, a736.

> National Institute for Health and Clinical Excellence (2014) Antenatal and postnatal mental health: Clinical management and service guidance. http://www.nice.org.uk/guidance/cg192
>
> World Health Organisation (1993) *International Classification of Diseases (ICD)*. 10th edn. www.who.int/classifications/icd/en/

The examiner's mark sheet

Domain/ percentage of marks	Essential points to pass	✓	Extra marks/comments (make notes here)
1. Rapport and communication 25% of marks	Clear communication Open and closed questions Empathy Sensitivity		
2. History of presenting complaint 20% of marks	Symptoms (duration and nature) Impact (on function, role as mother and relationships)		
3. Other history 20% of marks	Medical and psychiatric Social circumstances Family and personal		
4. Risk assessment 25% of marks	Relevant risks		
5. Brief MSE 10% of marks	Psychotic symptoms		

% SCORE _____

___ **OVERALL IMPRESSION**

5 (CIRCLE ONE)

Good Pass

Pass

Borderline

Fail

Clear Fail

NOTES/Areas to improve

STATION 1(b): DISCUSSION WITH PARTNER

INSTRUCTION TO CANDIDATE

You meet with her partner (David), who has taken time off work to see you. He explains that he is trying to be as supportive as he can, but that his job is extremely demanding. He wants to know what is wrong with his girlfriend and what he should do to help.

Answer his questions and address his concerns.

ACTOR (ROLE-PLAYER) INSTRUCTIONS

You initially appear stressed, disorganised and very concerned about your partner Rachel; despite help from her sister, who is staying with you, Rachel has been crying all the time for the last 4 weeks, isolating herself and saying life is hopeless and pointless.

You love Rachel but fear she no longer feels the same way and that the relationship is over; she looks through you, ignores you and is completely disinterested in sex.

You ask the following questions: 'What is wrong with my girlfriend? What can I do to help? What is the treatment? Will she need admission?'

You eagerly answer any questions the doctor may have at any stage; you have no concerns about Rachel's interaction with the baby.

You have an extremely demanding job and need to pay off household debts; if the doctor allows you to think through your job and its demands, you realise there might be some flexibility with hours/time off if you talk to your boss.

You say at one point: 'When Rachel gets really bad, I never know who to contact', and leave a pause; do not pursue this unless the doctor takes the cue.

SUGGESTED APPROACH

Setting the scene

Begin the task by introducing yourself, confirming David's relationship to Rachel and making reference to consent: 'Hello, David? My name is Dr_____, a psychiatrist, and I've just seen Rachel, who has given me consent to speak with you. I understand you are her partner?' Allow him to respond. He may simply confirm his identity, make some opening statements or immediately start asking questions – if questions are asked, say something like, 'I certainly want to answer your questions, but in order to do that effectively, I need a bit more information first'. If you defer a question, make sure you return to it – the actor may not ask again.

The collateral history

In order to effectively answer David's questions and concerns, it is relevant to ask for his impression of Rachel's symptoms and his perspective on key risk issues.

In terms of symptoms, you can initially ask open questions: 'How do you think Rachel has been coping? How has she been feeling/behaving?' Ask more specific questions as appropriate. For example, you can ask about:

- Feeling low, unhappy or miserable.
- Being irritable with family, other children or the baby.
- Showing disproportionate tiredness (bearing in mind a new baby) or sleeplessness with early morning wakening and low energy levels.
- Showing reduced enjoyment in things previously enjoyed, including sex; does he feel rejected?
- Showing feelings of guilt.

It is also important to get a sense of what supports they have as a family unit.

You can revisit the risk issues relevant to the previous station. In particular, you could ask the following questions:

- Has Rachel ever expressed thoughts that she or the baby would be better off dead?
- What are his thoughts on the interaction between mother and baby?
- Does he have concerns about Rachel's ability to care for the baby?
- Has *he* ever felt at the end of his tether with Rachel or the baby? How has he coped and behaved?

Answering questions and addressing concerns

What is wrong with my girlfriend?

Explain that you believe she has postnatal depression. Ask what he already knows about this. Explain that depression is not just 'feeling sad'. When depressed, one's mood is pervasively low most of the time, most days, over weeks; it is not possible to just 'snap out of it', and Rachel needs help to prevent a prolonged episode. Approximately one in ten women will have postnatal depression after giving birth. There is not always a clear precipitant for PND. It can occur without any obvious stressors.

A skilful interviewer might find it effective to merge parts of the collateral history and information giving. One can explain postnatal depression and its constituent symptoms by asking David if he has recognised these symptoms in Rachel. You can then say something like: 'These symptoms that you have recognised Rachel to experience are the symptoms of postnatal depression.' It is important to say that postnatal depression is a treatable illness, and similarly, any PND-related malfunctioning in their relationship is remediable.

What is the treatment?

Consider place of care – if severely depressed or risk factors preclude community treatment, ask his opinion on admission (e.g. to a Mother and Baby Unit).

- From a medical perspective, conduct a physical examination and blood tests to rule out reversible organic causes of depression. Antidepressants are often useful (sertraline or tricyclic antidepressants [TCAs]), but can take 1–4 weeks to take effect. Discuss follow-up with a specialist perinatal mental health service or community team as applicable. Electro-convulsive therapy [ECT] is not contraindicated, but would only be considered if the mother is severely unwell and if other options have failed.
- From a psychological perspective, self-help groups, counselling or formal psychotherapy (cognitive behavioural therapy [CBT] or interpersonal therapy) can help. Many general practices have a counsellor, and health visitors can help treat PND. There may be a waiting list for CBT.
- From a social perspective, explore how supports can be augmented. Can he negotiate more hours away from work or take time off? Who else in the network of family and friends can help? Suggest charities that could help. What is his opinion on social services? Based on the risk profile, you may have to explain that a social services referral is essential.

If the partner is severely distressed or you suspect the partner has mental illness, you should suggest that they see a GP or other service as appropriate.

Other support

- Association for Postnatal Illness – provides support to mothers suffering from postnatal illness.
- PANDAS – a support service for patients and families affected by antenatal or postnatal illnesses.
- CRY-SIS – provides self-help and support for families with excessively crying and sleepless babies, 365 days a year.
- National Childbirth Trust – advice, support and counselling on all aspects of childbirth and early parenthood.
- The Samaritans – provide confidential emotional support to any person who is suicidal or despairing.

Risk management

Take time to confirm that your management plan as discussed has addressed the risks identified in Station 1(a).

Rapport and communication

It is important to correctly gauge a relative's knowledge of postnatal depression; David may have no experience or some prior experience. The interaction needs to be correctly pitched so as not to be patronising yet starting with the very basics of what depression is depending on David's experience. It is important to be reassuring yet pragmatic about the situation and any associated risks.

Conclusion

It is sensible to summarise what you have discussed and where you go from here. Offer written information about postnatal depression and charitable support. Offer a crisis leaflet for his reference and ensure he knows who to contact or where to go if Rachel is in crisis.

FURTHER READING

British Association for Psychopharmacology (2008) Evidence based guidelines for treating depressive disorders with antidepressants (revision). http://www.bap.org.uk/pdfs/antidepressants.pdf

Taylor, D., Paton, C. & Kapur, S. (2015) *The Maudsley Prescribing Guidelines in Psychiatry*, 12th edn, London: Wiley-Blackwell.

Musters, C., McDonald, E. & Jones, I. (2008) Management of postnatal depression. *BMJ*, *337*, a736.

National Institute for Health and Clinical Excellence (2009) Depression in adults: The treatment and management of depression in adults. https://www.nice.org.uk/guidance/cg90

National Institute for Health and Clinical Excellence (2014) Antenatal and postnatal mental health: Clinical management and service guidance. http://www.nice.org.uk/guidance/cg192

The examiner's mark sheet

Domain/ percentage of marks	Essential points to pass	✓	Extra marks/comments (make notes here)
1. Rapport and communication 20% of marks	Clear communication Open and closed questions Empathy		
2. The collateral history 20% of marks	His report on symptom profile Social supports Risk assessment		
3. Answering questions and addressing concerns 25% of marks	Explains PND Discussion on treatment of PND in bio-psycho-social model with reference to place of care		
4. Management plan 25% of marks	Reaches decisions on treatment in bio-psycho-social model with reference to place of care		

⇧ 5. Risk   Effective risk management
   10% of marks

% **SCORE** _____   ___   **OVERALL IMPRESSION**

                                        5   (CIRCLE ONE)

                                                Good Pass

                                                Pass

                                                Borderline

                                                Fail

                                                Clear Fail

                                                NOTES/Areas to improve

STATION 2(a): PUERPERAL PSYCHOSIS

INSTRUCTION TO CANDIDATE

Melanie Leighton is a 25-year-old lady with a 2-week-old baby girl. Her sister has reported that Melanie is behaving quite strangely. You have been asked to see her as a home visit.

Elicit the relevant features from the mental state examination and assess the risks.

ACTOR (ROLE-PLAYER) INSTRUCTIONS

You have dishevelled hair and sit sideways on your chair; you are occasionally distracted by something in an empty corner of the room and occasionally exclaim 'leave me alone'.

You are suspicious of the doctor and do not elaborate when questioned, but none-theless open up gradually if the doctor is patient and reassuring.

You occasionally completely forget what you are saying mid-sentence and lapse into silence.

You admit (only if asked specifically) that you occasionally hear an unknown man's voice coming from the corner of the room saying, 'You are a useless mother.'

You absolutely believe that baby snatchers are on a mission to steal your baby; you say (only if asked) that you know this having received 'messages' in the newspapers and say you might lock the baby in a cupboard to protect her as you love her so much.

You do not believe you have any mental illness and think everybody is conspiring to lock you up with the baby snatchers and sedate you with drugs.

SUGGESTED APPROACH

Setting the scene

Begin the task by addressing the patient by name and introducing yourself: 'Hi, Melanie. My name is Dr_____, and I've been asked to come and see how you are. I often see people who might have concerns or worries after the birth of their babies.' Identifying yourself immediately as a psychiatrist could be threatening for this patient who has not elected to see you, although you must always be honest if directly asked. See how the patient responds and try to develop a rapport by asking open questions: 'How have you been since the baby was born? How is the baby?'

The mental state examination

Solely being asked to do an MSE in isolation is not a real-life scenario; nonetheless, this is the task and it is a common request in CASC stations. For the purposes of the CASC, unless it is clearly specified that you should not conduct one, a risk assessment should be included with any MSE. Furthermore, in order to perform an effective risk assessment, you need to ask some traditional 'psychiatric history' questions (e.g. history of self-harm and harm to others, including forensic history, and alcohol/substances). Demonstrating you are not going off task is best done in the way that you structure your interview – start with the MSE and then ask relevant questions in each section of your risk assessment.

Proceed through the normal sections of an MSE – appearance and behaviour, mood and affect (anxiety symptoms), speech and thought, perception, cognition and insight.

You will not always have an opportunity in CASC to 'present' your MSE, so you may need to openly make observations in order to demonstrate an understanding of the MSE structure. For example, regarding appearance and behaviour, you can make comments like: 'I can see you are very restless. I can see you are anxious, are you worried about something?' Another section is speech and thought: 'I've noticed that you can suddenly forget what you were saying sometimes, have you noticed that? ... I haven't heard that word before, what does it mean?' This shows the examiner that you have registered the mental state phenomenon and know that it is relevant.

In the event of a linked station, however, you should anticipate having to present the MSE. In such a situation, one needs to be familiar with speech and thought phenomena, for example. There are a myriad of terms in the literature regarding subcategories of thought form disorders (see 'Further Reading' for a helpful paper). In particular, look for a loosening of associations (including related concepts of derailment, knight's move thinking and tangentiality), flight of ideas, circumstantiality and thought block. With regards to speech, look out for pressured speech, alogia, neologisms and clanging. Consider taking notes, although be careful not to inhibit the doctor–patient relationship.

Other sections of the mental state examination can be explored by more direct questioning.

Mood

Screen for the major and minor ICD criteria for depression (see Station 1[a]) and features of (hypo)mania and suicidality. You can make an observational comment about affect: 'You seem a bit flat.'

Perception

You can start with open questions: 'Does your mind ever play tricks on you? Have you had any experiences which you've found difficult to explain?'

When asking about *hallucinations*, always screen for the five sensory modalities:

- Do you ever hear voices or noises when nobody else is around? If voices, ask about their nature and content – where they come from, what they say and any commands.
- Do you ever have any funny tastes or smells?
- Do you ever feel things, like somebody touching you, when nobody else is around?
- Do you ever see things, like visions, that cannot be explained or other people cannot see?

It is easiest to remember to screen for *thought echo* when asking about auditory hallucinations: 'Do you ever hear your thoughts spoken out loud?'

When asking about delusions, you can ask the following:

- 'Do you ever feel under the control or influence of somebody or something?' (*Delusions of control and influence*)
- 'Do you ever get messages from the environment especially for you, perhaps from the TV, radio or newspapers?' (*Delusions of reference*)
- 'Do you feel safe? Is anybody or anything out to hurt or harm you or the baby in any way?' (*Persecutory delusions*)
- 'Has anything of great significance to you happened recently, something very meaningful to you?' (*Delusional perception*; e.g. 'The traffic light turned red and I just *knew* then that I was chosen to lead my people')

Other delusions to consider include *delusions of misidentification* (including Capgras and Fregoli delusions), *grandiose delusions and delusions of guilt*. You should test (although not 'argue' about) any delusion, asking what evidence they have of such a belief. You can say something like: 'That seems very unlikely to me, I don't understand what grounds MI5 would have for chasing you. Are you absolutely sure this is happening?' If the patient gets angry that you do not believe them, use a statement like, 'Of course I believe this is your experience, I'm just trying to really get a sense of what is happening.'

Thought possession

Start with an open question: 'Are you able to think clearly? Is anything interfering with your thoughts?' Then ask about *thought broadcasting* ('Do you ever feel that people can read your mind?'), *thought insertion* ('Are thoughts ever put in your head that are not your own?') and *thought withdrawal* ('Are thoughts ever taken out of your mind by someone or something?').

Cognition and insight

Test orientation in time and place and do a basic test of concentration (e.g. spelling the word 'world' backwards). Expand the cognitive assessment if relevant, although an mini-mental state examination (MMSE) would not be routinely expected. Insight will be tested to some extent when you 'test' any delusional ideas. Propose the idea that her experiences are 'tricks of (her) mind' or possibly related to mental illness; see what she says and what her opinion of treatment is.

Risk assessment

This will be similar to the risk assessment performed in Station 1(a) covering harm to self and others, including the baby and any other children. Do not forget alcohol and drugs, stressors and supports and history of self-harm. The risk of non-engagement is very relevant in this case; discern whether she has engaged with services during any prior episodes and what her views on treatment are.

Rapport and communication

Developing a rapport will often be more difficult when the patient has not elected to see you. This will be aggravated by paranoia. Do not rush the start of the interview; it is OK to dedicate some time simply to rapport. Pay attention to (body) language and cues. Be calm, reassuring and patient. When screening as part of a mental state examination, normalising lines of questioning is key: 'These are routine questions we ask everybody. Lots of people we see experience these things, so I'm just checking to see if you do.'

Conclusion

This station does not ask you to give the patient a diagnosis or discuss a management plan. It may, however, be relevant as part of insight to evaluate views on treatment – does she think it is required and would she comply? You can summarise back to the patient if you require clarification or more detail on a section of the mental state examination. It may be appropriate to thank the patient at the end for talking to you and for being honest about her experience.

FURTHER READING

National Institute for Health and Clinical Excellence (2014) Antenatal and postnatal mental health: Clinical management and service guidance. http://www.nice.org.uk/guidance/cg192

Rule, A. (2005) Ordered thoughts on thought disorder. *Psychiatric Bulletin*, 29, 462–4.

The examiner's mark sheet

Domain/ percentage of marks	Essential points to pass	✓	Extra marks/comments (make notes here)
1. Rapport and communication 25% of marks	Clear communication Open and closed questions Empathy Demonstrating patience		
2. MSE 1 25% of marks	Observational comments Mood Speech and thought		
3. MSE 2 25% of marks	Perception Cognition Insight		
4. Risk assessment 25% of marks	Self-harm Harm to others Other		

% **SCORE** _____

___

4 OVERALL IMPRESSION

(CIRCLE ONE)

Good Pass

Pass

Borderline

Fail

Clear Fail

NOTES/Areas to improve

STATION 2(b): DISCUSSING THE MANAGEMENT PLAN WITH A PROFESSIONAL COLLEAGUE

INSTRUCTION TO CANDIDATE

You return to the community team base where you meet the team manager Linda. She had been concerned about Ms Leighton following the referral. She wants to know what your care plan is following assessment.

Tell her about your assessment and plans.

ACTOR (ROLE-PLAYER) INSTRUCTIONS

You are the team manager of a community team which *is not* a specialist perinatal mental health team; you know a lot about depression but are considerably anxious about the baby in the picture.

Your team is busy; your duty team cannot see patients more frequently than every 3–4 days.

You are professional in approach and normally work well with the doctor, although require clear and unambiguous plans from members of your team; you do not tolerate 'maybes.'

You ask the following questions as appropriate: 'How is she?', 'So what are you thinking in terms of diagnosis?', 'What are the risks here?', 'What's your plan?', 'Does the patient need admission?', 'Can admission be avoided?' and 'Who is going to follow this patient up in the community?'

You are willing to discuss treatment options and give an opinion of the facts of the case, but ultimately you have not met the patient and require that the doctor finalises the plan.

SUGGESTED APPROACH

Setting the scene

You know the team manager; a simple greeting is appropriate with a clear identification of the patient to be discussed: 'Hi, Linda, how are you? I've just been to see Melanie Leighton. Do you have some time to discuss the case?'

The assessment

Give a clear and succinct case summary. Present the main findings in terms of psychopathology and the risk issues. Remember that this is also a management station. You can refer to any notes you have taken in the first station. Pause at the end of this section to see if the team manager has any comments, thoughts or questions at this stage. Do not forget to present your diagnostic formulation or differential diagnosis.

Discussion of management plan

Do not assume that your team manager is completely familiar with postnatal mental disorders and their management. Better candidates will not 'list' a plan; rather, they will develop a structured narrative using broad headings and draw on supporting information from the symptom profile and history, as well as risk concerns. They might start by outlining priorities or key concerns.

Place of care and multidisciplinary team (MDT) working

It helps to put a care plan into perspective by saying what setting it needs to occur in – delivered in an in-patient setting (ideally a Mother and Baby Unit) or overseen by a community team with a specific intensity of care (e.g. home treatment versus standard community team) and/or specific specialism (e.g. perinatal team if feasible). Give the reasons for your choice. Outline your intent to work in a multidisciplinary fashion with the GP, obstetrics team, and so forth. Note that perinatal teams often work in concert with community mental health teams (CMHTs); they do not always have urgent response capabilities or duty teams, for example.

Further information and investigations

First, say what other information or investigations you need in order to inform the diagnostic formulation and plan: 'I would like to speak to her partner to get more details on X, Y and Z. I am going to organise a physical examination and some tests to rule out an organic cause – bloods tests such as…etc.' Considering the mental state, you will definitely need a collateral to fill in parts of the history, such as the psychiatric history, family history, and so forth. Outline any other investigations you will do to support your upcoming treatment (e.g. an electrocardiogram [ECG] with a view to starting an anti-psychotic). If you are concerned about physical health, consider referring to accident and emergency in the first instance, then speaking with the obstetrics team. Consider things like infection (retained products or others), delirium, medication adverse effects or a thromboembolic event.

- From a medical perspective, consider anti-psychotics with or without other psychotropics if mood is a component. Consider if the mother is breast feeding. If not breast feeding, anticonvulsants and lithium may have a role when manic features predominate. ECT may or may not have a role depending on the facts of the case.
- From a psychological perspective, self-help groups, counselling, formal psychotherapy (CBT) and psycho-education are relevant.
- From a social perspective, practical support for the mother, increased natural support networks and social services are relevant. Provide help enrolling with a support group like the Association for Post Natal Illness, whose members are women with experience of puerperal psychosis or postnatal depression. The Action Postpartum Psychosis Network is also very good for educational resources and avenues of social support.

Risk

Always consider the risk to the mother and the baby.

Rapport and communication

Make eye contact with the team manager and engage; do not spend all of your time looking at or reading from notes. You will need to judge what concerns the team manager may have about the case and how the team can approach treatment, as well as the team manager's personality in terms of how involved they want to be in the collaborative decision making. Remember that you have seen the patient so do not be afraid to outline your judgement in a confident way, and simply present evidence for your approach if challenged. Nonetheless, do not be dismissive of the team manager's concerns; acknowledge them and allow them to inform your views if appropriate. Show that you value this discussion.

Conclusion

Summarise the plan and next steps.

FURTHER READING

National Institute for Health and Clinical Excellence (2014) Antenatal and postnatal mental health: Clinical management and service guidance. http://www.nice.org.uk/guidance/cg192

Taylor, D., Paton, C. & Kapur, S. (2015) *The Maudsley Prescribing Guidelines in Psychiatry*, 12th edn. London: Wiley-Blackwell.

Royal College of Psychiatrists information leaflet: Postpartum psychosis: Severe mental illness after childbirth. http://www.rcpsych.ac.uk/healthadvice/problemsdisorders/postpartumpsychosis.aspx

The examiner's mark sheet

Domain/ percentage of marks	Essential points to pass	✓	Extra marks/comments (make notes here)
1. Rapport and communication 20% of marks	Clear communication Professional attitude Collaborative approach Willingness to listen to and address team manager's concerns		
2. Presentation of assessment 20% of marks	Symptoms History Differential/formulation		
3. Management plan (1) 25% of marks	Investigations Further information Place of care		
4. Management plan (2) 25% of marks	Bio-psycho-social care plan		
5. Risk 10% of marks	Effective risk management		

% **SCORE** _____

___

5

OVERALL IMPRESSION

(CIRCLE ONE)

Good Pass

Pass

Borderline

Fail

Clear Fail

NOTES/Areas to improve

○ SINGLE STATIONS

STATION 3: BIPOLAR DISORDER AND PREGNANCY

INSTRUCTION TO CANDIDATE

Sarah Trimble is a 33-year-old lady with a history of bipolar illness. Her illness has been well controlled over the last 8 years with lithium.

Today, she informs you that she has had a positive pregnancy test and thinks she must be 6–8 weeks pregnant. She has been in a stable relationship with her boyfriend for 4 years and has decided to keep the baby.

As you look through her records, you note that she also takes regular diazepam.

Her medications are: lithium (as Priadel®) 600 mg nocte and diazepam regular 10 mg ter die sumendum (TDS – three times a day).

You are asked to advise on medication management.

ACTOR (ROLE-PLAYER) INSTRUCTIONS

You are currently mentally well; the lithium has kept you well for years, but you know it is 'bad and toxic' in pregnancy.

You have no idea whether diazepam is a problem (and do not mention the latter unless the doctor does); your perspective is that it has kept you 'even and stable' and will only change your mind about this with very good reason.

You have had two manic episodes years ago each lasting approximately 3 months each, with one resulting in detention under the Mental Health Act for treatment against your will; you were restrained a lot during this admission.

You had one depressive episode at age 17 and superficially cut your left arm but did not attempt suicide, nor have you ever done so.

You decide to continue the lithium after hearing both benefits and risks, and ask, 'So what happens now?' and later 'Can I breast feed?'

SUGGESTED APPROACH

Setting the scene

Begin the task by addressing the patient by name and introducing yourself as usual. Acknowledge her current circumstances: 'I understand you're pregnant, is that something you're pleased about? Well, congratulations. It's important that we have this time to talk because we need to try to make sure that your baby stays healthy and, at the same time, try to keep your mental health stable.' Ask if she knows anything about lithium in pregnancy.

Managing the situation

In the first instance, you need to take a brief targeted history:

- Recent mental health.
- Has she had any other pregnancies?

- Confirm current medications – how long she has been on them, indication for benzo-diazepine (BZD), compliance and what has happened during any drug-free periods.
- Natural history of bipolar illness – depressive versus (hypo)manic episodes (number of relapses, when they occurred, triggers, duration, how severe, required Mental Health Act (MHA) detention or not and how it was treated in the acute phase), history of medication and treatment interventions (ECT and psychotherapy) and history of self-harm and/or harm to others when unwell.
- Alcohol/illicit drugs/cigarettes.
- Stressors and supports.

The benefits and risks of lithium in the perinatal period

Lithium can be used in pregnancy if the benefits outweigh the risks; state this clearly. Stopping an effective prophylactic mood stabiliser means that the woman is more likely to relapse. The risk of relapse can be as high as 30%–50% in women with a history of bipolar disorder. Patients who discontinue mood stabilisers are twice as likely to relapse and have a longer duration of illness. The risks of relapse are *often* considered to outweigh the risks of medication.

Start with outlining the benefits of lithium during pregnancy, drawing on elements of your history: 'The key benefit of lithium is that it has kept you well for years and could continue to do so throughout pregnancy and in the postnatal period. You have had at least one serious, risky episode of bipolar disorder in the past, and having that happen in pregnancy could be a serious problem for you and the baby. Having a psychiatric illness during pregnancy is an independent risk factor for death of the baby, congenital malformations and pre-term delivery. In the event of relapse, you might self-harm or attempt suicide, harm others or engage in other risky behaviours. If you became unwell postnatally, the baby might not be well looked after or, at worst, intentionally or unintentionally harmed.' Allow the woman to make comments, provide feedback or ask questions.

Proceed to discussing the potential adverse effects: 'So stopping lithium has clear risks, but there are also risks of continuing it.' The period of maximum risk is 2–6 weeks after conception, which has already passed. Ebstein's anomaly (a disfigurement of the tricuspid valve which can lead to cardiac failure) has a relative risk of 10–20-times that of controls, but in absolute terms, the risk is still only 1:1000 in mothers on lithium. Other risks are neonatal goitre and the *reversible* adverse effects of hypotonia, lethargy, cardiac arrhythmias and respiratory difficulties.

An example of presenting this in lay terms is: 'One risk is something called Ebstein's anomaly, which is a malformation of one of the four valves in the baby's heart. For every 1000 mothers on lithium, only one baby will have it. The primary risk period for this abnormality is in the first 6 weeks of pregnancy, which unfortunately has already passed in your case, as it does in many mothers before they realise they are pregnant. Another risk is an enlargement of the thyroid, a gland in the neck that regulates metabolism. Finally, rare things that can happen (which are generally reversible) are having a lethargic baby or a baby with breathing difficulties or heart rhythm problems.'

You will have to judge how much of this you say at a time while allowing the woman to make comments, provide feedback and ask questions. If she is very confused, say that written information could be provided as well, and that an absolute decision does not have to be made today.

If the woman chooses to stop lithium, you may well have to consult perinatal mental health services. Lithium is normally withdrawn very slowly over months in order to prevent relapse. Should she decide to stop the medication, her mental health team and

GP/midwife should provide regular support and monitoring of her mental state throughout the pregnancy.

Monitoring lithium in the perinatal period

If the woman chooses to hear more or continue lithium (as is likely in the CASC), you need to explain that lithium would be continued at the lowest effective dose and closely monitored. You will do a baseline lithium level now. The pregnancy needs to be booked (if not done already) with an obstetrics team with detailed ultrasound and echocardiography at 6 and 18 weeks. Lithium levels will be done 4 weekly until 36 weeks, and weekly thereafter, as the levels can change. Lithium levels can rise exponentially after birth, so delivery should take place in a hospital, and the dose will likely need reduction with a lithium level within 24 hours of giving birth. Anything that affects fluid balance (hyperemesis, fluid retention and renal problems) can affect lithium levels; monitor urea and electrolytes and levels more regularly if appropriate.

Informing her of alternatives

If she decides to stop lithium, suggest alternative medications and the need for more support from the team. There is limited evidence for most drugs in pregnancy, but an antipsychotic (e.g. olanzapine) could be recommended. Olanzapine has its own risks in pregnancy, however. Lithium is generally considered to be safer than valproate or carbamazepine in pregnancy. Lamotrigine is not recommended, although there is growing evidence that it is also safer than valproate or carbamazepine.

Advising her on the risks of BZD usage

Regular benzodiazepines during pregnancy are not recommended, although they need to be withdrawn slowly in order to prevent seizures. Benzodiazepines are probably not associated with congenital malformations, although there have been variable reports of associations with oral clefts, pylorostenosis and alimentary tract atresia. There is also an association with low birth weight and pre-term delivery. Stopping both lithium and diazepam would leave this woman particularly vulnerable; in the event of a decision to stop both, one drug being gradually withdrawn at a time is sensible. A formal detoxification or admission to hospital for BZD withdrawal may be safer. She also needs to be informed about the withdrawal state from benzodiazepines in new-borns – 'floppy baby syndrome' – characterised by lethargy, irritability, reduced muscle tone and respiratory depression.

Discussing a possible management plan

When it comes to making decisions, you can involve the partner and suggest educational resources (leaflets and Internet sites). You can discuss and document her views on the treatment in the event that she becomes unwell. It is important to communicate and work with multidisciplinary professionals – obstetrics, the GP, the midwife, the perinatal service, and so forth.

Breast feeding

Breast feeding is not recommended in mothers on lithium, as lithium can cause infant toxicity. Any infants who are breast fed need to be closely monitored. BZDs can cause sedation, lethargy and weight loss. Strategies to limit exposure include using the lowest effective doses, using drugs with shorter half-lives or taking the drugs once daily before the baby's longest sleep (usually nocte) in order to avoid peak plasma levels. Small amounts of carbamazepine, valproate and lamotrigine also pass into breast milk.

FURTHER READING

British Association for Psychopharmacology (2009) Evidence-based guidelines for treating bipolar disorder. http://www.bap.org.uk/pdfs/Bipolar_guidelines.pdf

National Institute for Health and Clinical Excellence (2014) Antenatal and postnatal mental health: Clinical management and service guidance. http://www.nice.org.uk/guidance/cg192

Taylor, D., Paton, C. & Kapur, S. (2015) *The Maudsley Prescribing Guidelines in Psychiatry*, 12th edn. London: Wiley-Blackwell.

The examiner's mark sheet

Domain/ percentage of marks	Essential points to pass	✓	Extra marks/comments (make notes here)
1. Rapport and communication 20% of marks	Clear communication Open and closed questions Empathy Demonstrating patience		
2. History 20% of marks	Targeted history		
3. Lithium (1) 25% of marks	Risk of relapse Benefits of lithium Risks of lithium		
4. Lithium (2) 25% of marks	Alternatives Monitoring Breast feeding Reaches a decision		
5. BZD 10% of marks	Benefits Risks Plan		

% SCORE _____

___

5

OVERALL IMPRESSION

(CIRCLE ONE)

Good Pass

Pass

Borderline

Fail

Clear Fail

NOTES/Areas to improve

STATION 4: BABY BLUES

> ## INSTRUCTION TO CANDIDATE
>
> You are going to see Mrs Gray. She is a patient of yours and you have been seeing her in the clinic for anxiety and concerns related to dying and ill health. She has been physically well.
>
> You started her on fluoxetine a year ago; this had a modest effect. She later informed you that she was keen to start a family and had stopped the antidepressant. Her anxiety worsened and you referred her for a course of CBT. She responded well, although she required more sessions than was anticipated and needed several top-up sessions.
>
> She was able to conceive and handled the physical manifestations of pregnancy well.
>
> She had a healthy baby boy 5 days ago and has asked that she see you urgently. Your secretary has squeezed her into your already overbooked clinic.
>
> **Take a brief history and mental state examination and formulate a management plan.**

ACTOR (ROLE-PLAYER) INSTRUCTIONS

You know and like the doctor.

You had a wonderful pregnancy and have given birth to a beautiful baby boy 5 days ago; despite everything going well, however, you have felt intermittently sad, tearful and 'fed up' for 4 days.

At times you are sleepy and confused like a 'zombie', but then bounce back.

You are worried that you will not be a good mother, but have no significant guilt, shame nor any suicidality or thoughts about harming the baby; you still enjoy periods of time with the baby and with your partner, but then start crying again without reason.

Before the baby was conceived (i.e. 1–2 years ago), you had irrational health worries after your mother died of cancer. Fluoxetine helped, but you stopped taking this before conception of the baby. CBT psychotherapy also helped, and these worries are no longer significant concerns; very occasionally, you think an ache or a pain might be 'something serious', but brush it off.

You ask if you need fluoxetine or more CBT.

SUGGESTED APPROACH

Setting the scene

You know the patient, so a simple recognition of seeing her again and greeting is all that is required. Acknowledge her recent delivery and ask if the baby is well. If so, feel free to congratulate her before moving to an open question that is relevant to the task: 'I understand you wanted to see me urgently. Can you tell me a bit about what has been happening?'

Targeted history and MSE

You are asked to review this patient. This may sound 'vague', but it gives you the opportunity to interview in a scenario approximating real life and address her concerns and main problems. Before you even see the patient, you should be considering if her request to see you might have something to do with her prior anxiety issues or be related to 'baby blues' or postnatal depression/psychosis. Allow your history and mental state examination to evolve based on the information she gives you and with this differential diagnosis in mind.

Enquire fully about her prior anxiety symptoms and whether she feels they have worsened since the baby was born. If you identify an area of concern (e.g. anxiety), then probe further (refer to anxiety stations). Take a history of recent events and, in particular, ask how her anxiety and mood have been over the last 2 weeks. Enquire about the delivery and any complications prenatally, perinatally or immediately postnatally – is she still in pain? Has there been any physical illness? Screen for depression and psychotic features – if positive for any, continue as for puerperal psychosis or postnatal depression.

From there, it is important to establish what medications she is taking (prescription or over-the-counter), any alcohol or drug misuse and stressors and supports. Common stressors are simply adjusting to the role of motherhood and breast feeding. Failure to breast feed easily can be associated with guilty feelings and frustration.

Supports to consider are natural networks like family/partner/friends, a health visitor or antenatal peers. The relationship between Mrs Gray and her baby is important.

Risk

Do not forget the risk assessment!

Diagnosis

In baby blues, it is useful to 'normalise'. Acknowledge that many of her anxieties are understandable and that many women experience similar feelings. The actor is primed to give you a history and features of 'blues' in this case – tearfulness, emotional lability (potentially with features of both low and elevated mood) and confusion a few days after delivery. Postnatal depression is different from 'the blues', which is a brief period of low, irritable and fluctuating mood (feeling a bit weepy) occurring approximately 3–5 days after giving birth. It does vary in intensity and duration, but is transient and considered a normal process. Baby blues should not involve hopelessness, worthlessness or suicidality.

Management

You can reassure her that the baby blues usually resolves in a few days and that up to 80% of new mothers are affected. Bearing this in mind, (further) antidepressant treatment is not immediately indicated unless something else is going on. If medications are discussed, the benefits and risks will need to be considered if she is breast feeding.

The best psychological and social care at this stage is supportive with the following options considered: a clinic review or a home visit from a community psychiatric nurse (CPN) or health visitor. You might consider a few sessions with a psychologist, if available.

Make sure you have follow-up arrangements in place in order to make sure that this does not develop into a more serious condition (e.g. postnatal depression). Discuss her natural support networks (friends/family/partner) again and postnatal support groups. You can provide written information on the baby blues and relevant charities.

FURTHER READING

National Institute for Health and Clinical Excellence (2014) Antenatal and postnatal mental health: Clinical management and service guidance. http://www.nice.org.uk/guidance/cg192

The examiner's mark sheet

Domain/ percentage of marks	Essential points to pass	✓	Extra marks/comments (make notes here)
1. Rapport and communication 25% of marks	Clear communication Open and closed questions Empathy Demonstrating patience		
2. History and MSE 20% of marks	Targets history and MSE		
3. Risk 10% of marks	Risk assessment		
4. Diagnosis 20% of marks	Feedback impression Reassurance Education		
5. Management plan 25% of marks	Bio-psycho-social approach		

% **SCORE** _____   ___ **OVERALL IMPRESSION**

5   (CIRCLE ONE)

Good Pass

Pass

Borderline

Fail

Clear Fail

NOTES/Areas to improve

STATION 5: METHADONE IN PREGNANCY

INSTRUCTION TO CANDIDATE

Carla London is a 22-year-old lady who has just found out a few days ago that she is 6–8 weeks pregnant. She briefly considered an abortion but has decided to keep the baby. She has been on methadone 40 mg daily for a long time. She comes to you as she is worried about the effect of methadone on her baby.

Take a targeted history and discuss the options in terms of managing her methadone treatment.

DO NOT PERFROM A MENTAL STATE EXAMINATION.

ACTOR (ROLE-PLAYER) INSTRUCTIONS

You (Carla London) are a curt, matter-of-fact, straightforward lady who does not mince words; you admit frankly that you were a 'druggy' who injected drugs while in a youth offenders' institute for stealing, but do not want the 'drug life' anymore.

Your methadone has been prescribed by the GP for the last 4–5 years and you collect your 'takeaway' every 3 days from the pharmacy; you had a keyworker at the local drug service years ago, but they 'dumped me like everybody else'.

Your mental health has been perfectly fine for years; you believe that people who work in drug and psychiatric services are out-of-touch 'egos', but begrudgingly accept help so that you can be a better mother than yours was to you.

You respond well to a doctor who is honest, straightforward and non-judgemental, and are keen to know the effects of methadone in pregnancy and what you should do; you skipped a day once as a test and 'nearly died', although wonder if for the sake of the baby you should go 'cold turkey', or at least cut it down.

You ask the following questions: 'So is methadone dangerous or what?', 'Will the baby be damaged?', 'Can I stop the methadone or change to something safer?', 'What should I do?', 'Will the baby need methadone when it comes out?' and 'Will I be able to breast feed?'

You (if asked) do not drink alcohol, have the occasional cigarette, have never had an HIV or hepatitis screen and are a single mother of one daughter age 6 who is 'gorgeous' and 'does brilliant at school' – you have not needed the 'shower' at social services for years.

SUGGESTED APPROACH

Setting the scene

Begin the task by addressing the patient by name and introducing yourself. Acknowledge her recent pregnancy and ask if she is happy about this news. If so, feel free to congratulate her before specifying the purpose of your meeting: 'I understand you are on methadone and want to find out more about what this means for your pregnancy. What do you know about methadone and pregnancy?' Allow her to respond. If she starts asking questions, explain that you need some information first: 'Before you leave here today, we will have agreed on a management plan with regards to the methadone. First, however, it's important that I ask a few questions so I can fully understand your situation.' If you park a question for later, make sure you return to it – the actor may not ask again.

The targeted history

The history is essential in order to formulate a management plan and address her questions. You need to allow time for both. Stick to the task; a mental state examination is not requested. Key features of a history in this case include:

- Any recent mental health problems.
- Her perspective on the pregnancy. Has she booked the pregnancy? What input from services does she currently have?
- Psychiatric and medical history (including obstetric history and recent HIV/hepatitis screen).
- Medications and details of methadone prescription (when started, dose and dose changes and who prescribes and monitors).
- History of, and current consumption of, illicit street drugs, alcohol and cigarettes. Screen for (do not assume) past intravenous use.

- Social setup (stressors and supports and the patient's lifestyle in terms of employment/ who is at home/other children/partner).
- Risk assessment.

Methadone in pregnancy

Recommend that she books her pregnancy if she has not done so already with a local obstetric service. You should also consider referrals to drug services and a specialist perinatal mental health team as appropriate. In terms of investigations, you should consider blood tests (HIV and hepatitis screens if not done recently and baseline renal and liver function) and a baseline ECG (for QTc interval). You should advise that methadone levels in the bloodstream may fall in the third trimester of pregnancy, so if she experiences craving or withdrawal symptoms, she should seek advice on increasing the dose immediately.

Is methadone dangerous to the baby? Will the baby need it after birth?

There is no convincing evidence that methadone leads to congenital abnormalities. Neonates may experience neonatal abstinence syndrome (with gastrointestinal, respiratory and autonomic symptoms), and the birth should take place in a centre with access to paediatric services. The neonate may need methadone within 48 hours, particularly if they are not being breast fed.

Should I continue the methadone?

It is recommended that methadone is continued, at the same dose, during pregnancy. Suddenly stopping methadone (or opiates) is *dangerous* and can cause spontaneous abortion (first trimester) and pre-term delivery (third trimester). However, tapering of the dose at a controlled rate is not contraindicated and depends on the woman's wishes; requested detox is safest in the second trimester. The risks of craving and withdrawal (with an ensuing temptation to perhaps use drugs) must be balanced with the benefits of any taper or detox; this should be openly discussed. For methadone reduction in pregnant patients, one should be particularly cautious.

Are there alternatives?

There is limited evidence at present on the safety profile of buprenorphine in pregnancy, so methadone is (at least for now) preferred. There is some evidence that the risk of neonatal abstinence syndrome is less with buprenorphine. If a pregnant patient were to present already on buprenorphine, it can be continued; it does not have to be switched to methadone.

What can I do?

The best approach the patient can take is to discuss any changes to methadone in advance with a healthcare professional, seek help if she feels craving or withdrawal symptoms at any stage in her pregnancy, book her pregnancy with a local obstetric service and engage with drug services and a specialist perinatal mental health service as appropriate. She should avoid drug use, alcohol and cigarette smoking.

Can I breast feed?

NICE guidelines state that breast feeding should be encouraged in mothers on methadone in the absence of HIV or hepatitis or concomitant illicit drug use. Some methadone (2%–3% of the mother's dose) does enter the breast milk.

Rapport and communication

It is important to maintain a non-judgemental attitude towards past drug use, lifestyle and her future intentions, while balancing this with clear and unambiguous advice as appropriate. There should be a sense of equal partnership in collaborating in order to come up with a management plan; to a significant extent, a lot will depend on the patient's informed choices based on the information you provide.

Conclusion

It is important to summarise a management plan as agreed. You can offer further written information on methadone and pregnancy.

FURTHER READING

National Institute for Health and Clinical Excellence (2014) Antenatal and postnatal mental health: Clinical management and service guidance. http://www.nice.org.uk/guidance/cg192

Taylor, D., Paton, C. & Kapur, S. (2015) *The Maudsley Prescribing Guidelines in Psychiatry*, 12th edn. London: Wiley-Blackwell.

The examiner's mark sheet

Domain/ percentage of marks	Essential points to pass	✓	Extra marks/comments (make notes here)
1. Rapport and communication 20% of marks	Clear communication		
	Open and closed questions		
	Empathy		
	Demonstrating patience		
2. History 20% of marks	Targets history		
3. Methadone (1) 25% of marks	Risk of craving/drug use		
	Benefits of methadone		
	Risks of methadone		
4. Methadone (2) 25% of marks	Alternatives		
	Monitoring		
	Breast feeding		
	Reaches a decision		
5. Conclusion 10% of marks	Follow-up		
	Supports		

% SCORE _____

___

5

OVERALL IMPRESSION

(CIRCLE ONE)

Good Pass

Pass

Borderline

Fail

Clear Fail

NOTES/Areas to improve

Chapter 13

Psychotherapy

Dinesh Sinha

O LINKED STATIONS

STATION 1(a): PSYCHOTHERAPEUTIC TECHNIQUES IN PATIENT MANAGEMENT

INSTRUCTION TO CANDIDATE

You have been asked to see Ms Jones, a patient you have seen once since joining the community mental health team (CMHT). She has a diagnosis of anxiety and depression, but is known as a 'difficult patient' by the team. She has worked with several care co-coordinators, although you have not previously met her. It is Friday at 4.45 p.m. and she is insisting on being seen immediately by you and threatening self-harm if you are not available.

Using techniques learnt in psychotherapy, talk to her and see how you are able to help.

ACTOR (ROLE-PLAYER) INSTRUCTIONS

You are in a state of crisis.

You do not recall details of discussions in previous conversations with your care coordinator at the CMHT. You are insistent and agitated, wanting there to be an immediate cure for your distress, although are unable to speak clearly of what you need.

You easily lose your temper and threaten self-harm.

SUGGESTED APPROACH

Setting the scene

Begin the interview by using as many open questions as you possibly can, which will indicate a willingness to listen to your patient. 'Hello, Ms Jones, I was told that you were really struggling at the moment. Please can you tell me about how things are at the moment and how we could help?' Allow the patient to speak her mind and perhaps begin to tell you about what is causing her crisis and try to put her at ease by maintaining a flow of conversation, such as by making it clear that you are hearing what she is saying and trying to understand the issues.

You will need to find out why the patient has demanded to see you. The aim here is to make a robust effort at building a therapeutic alliance and to move her away from a confrontation. If the patient is very angry/abusive, you may have to do some boundary setting, suggesting that she needs to calm down or you need to meet again when she is able to talk. 'Ms Jones, please do try not to shout, as we cannot continue the conversation in that manner. It would be really helpful if we could try and work together, as if we can't talk calmly, then I won't be able to work out how to best help you.' Addressing the patient formally helps by reminding the patient of the setting. If she is anxious and wants to talk, your being able to set the boundary and an enquiry with open questions will help her to start talking to you, as it will indicate your availability. 'OK, Ms Jones, so what is worrying you? Has something happened since you were last seen at the CMHT?'

Treatment

You will need to hear her complaints and anxieties without feeling pushed to solve them instantaneously. What may help is if you are able to hold in mind that a patient who has only recently begun to see you and then finds it hard to let go (at the end of the week) has issues regarding separation. This may then present in a manner with a number of grievances, which will leave you feeling that you are doing something very wrong by leaving her at the start of the weekend. 'Ms Jones, we have spent the last few minutes thinking about how the week has gone and clearly you are feeling very distressed. It seems from what you are saying that quite a significant part of the problem may be the impending weekend, which is leaving you feeling very alone. Is it possible for us to think about this?' You need to talk to her about what is worrying her and point out that she will be meeting her care coordinator early next week. Remaining calm when the patient is clearly in a state of panic/anger will be important. You will have to take her self-harm threats seriously while also coaxing out why she is presenting like that. 'How long has it been since you have been thinking about harming yourself? Have you got any thoughts currently or plans of self-harm? Have you done anything to harm yourself so far?' You need to demonstrate both robustness and openness. An attempt to connect emotionally with her experience of loss will help more than simply providing her with a practical solution.

Patients are often thought about based on their existing diagnosis. The diagnosis may undergo revision over time, but long-term patients who present in a needy way, such as this patient, can be thought of as having prominent attachment difficulties that manifest with separation issues. The interplay of functional symptoms overlying deeper personality issues needs to be kept in mind for such patients.

The emphasis could remain on the patient being able to manage until you meet next time. 'Ms Jones, can you tell me the things you could do over the weekend that could help you to feel better? You have spoken about visiting family and friends and keeping yourself occupied as helpful. Can you give me some idea of how you will manage if things get worse, and do you think you'll be able to keep yourself safe given the things we've already talked about?' However, this may well depend on the history of the patient and the level of risk that she presents with. There is only so much you can offer in the time available. You must attempt to have a discussion with her, which includes issues of risk. If she is not able to offer you an assurance of her capacity to keep herself safe, then you must suggest to her other ways in which she can seek help. 'However, if the sort of plans we are making for the weekend don't work out or things get worse, then I suggest you try making contact with our crisis line to talk things through or then visit the out-of-hours surgery or accident and emergency.'

Rapport and communication

This is an example of talking to a distressed patient in an emotionally disconnected state. The relevant communication skills relate to engaging her in issues of interest to her and thus demonstrating the capacity to talk calmly with an angry and anxious patient. Being able to do this demonstrates some understanding of the patient's needs while managing your own counter-transference. Hence, you need to be able to keep the conversation going without being pushed to terminate the conversation. You will also need to complete a risk assessment regarding threat of self-harm and giving additional follow-up advice. It is also important to do some boundary setting early on in the conversation and to remind Ms Jones of the team's ongoing involvement.

Conclusion

Here you can summarise what you have discussed, any further information you want to give and what the next steps will be. 'Ms Jones, we had a discussion about how you have been feeling and have made a plan to get through the weekend and what to do if things don't seem manageable. I will be able to see you next week and I suggest we keep that appointment to review how things have gone.'

FURTHER READING

Rosenfeld, H. (1987) *Impasse and Interpretation*. London: Tavistock.

Steiner, J. (1992) Patient-centered and analyst centered interpretations: Some implications of 'containment and countertransference'. *Psychoanalytic Enquiry, 14*, 406–22.

The examiner's mark sheet

Domain/percentage of marks	Essential points to pass	✓	Extra marks/comments (make notes here)
1. Communication and empathy 25% of marks	Clear communication Open and closed questions Empathy Sensitivity Ability to put patient at ease and engage in a dialogue		
2. Building a therapeutic alliance 25% of marks	Moves her away from a confrontation Maintains professional boundaries		
3. Interview technique 25% of marks	Engages her in issues of importance to her Understanding transference and counter-transference		
4. Risk assessment 25% of marks	Brief screening and advice		

% SCORE _____

___

4

OVERALL IMPRESSION

(CIRCLE ONE)

Good Pass

Pass

Borderline

Fail

Clear Fail

NOTES/Areas to improve

STATION 1(b): ASSESSMENT FOR PSYCHODYNAMIC PSYCHOTHERAPY

INSTRUCTION TO CANDIDATE

The patient you have just spoken to is discussed in the team meeting. She is very needy and rapidly engages with care workers. However, there can be situations in which people are left feeling very anxious for her and provide a lot of support for her. The patient will often use the intervention and be grateful, but this does not result in any lasting change to her presentation. Her heavy use of alcohol is assumed to account at least in part for this.

The team manager has referred her to psychology for cognitive behavioural therapy (CBT). She only attended some of those sessions, but was appreciative of the help offered. The manager believes a deeper approach, such as psychodynamic therapy, may help her.

Discuss a referral for psychotherapy with Laura, your team manager.

ACTOR (ROLE-PLAYER) INSTRUCTIONS

You have been working with Ms Jones, who has been with your community mental health team (you are its team leader), but you do not feel that the team really understands her needs. You feel she struggles to be by herself and things have become worse since she moved from her previous area 1 year ago to this part of town. She has been misusing alcohol and other substances and you are concerned that this is affecting her presentation.

However, you feel strongly that, having tried some sessions of CBT, which were helpful, the need now is for a more sustained therapeutic intervention of long-term therapy, if there is to be any chance of having a positive effect on Ms Jones.

SUGGESTED APPROACH

Setting the scene

The discussion will be with the manager who has some knowledge of psychotherapy, but perhaps not of its details. She wants to discuss the patient, who she believes requires a psychodynamic intervention. 'Laura, can you tell me what you think about Ms Jones? I know we have been worried about her contact with the team and the repeated crisis.' The information that is conveyed would guide the discussion and decision. 'I agree that the CBT was useful, but it does not seem to have any lasting impact. I think we should consider alternatives and look at the possibility of other psychological interventions, as well as how we could manage the crisis better as a team including doing joint risk assessments.'

Treatment

The manager describes the young woman as being someone who has chronic drug and alcohol difficulties. There is a sense of perpetual chaos evident from the description of the patient, including in her use of services. 'You know, it does seem like she takes what we offer very much on her terms. I think she is really unable to make use of what has been offered so far.' She can make use of the support, but explorative psychotherapy is not an intervention for providing support per se. Such information should alert you to the possibility that this may not be the best time for the patient to be engaging in a psychotherapy intervention. Motivation is a key ingredient in the process of any psychological intervention.

Further questioning of the manager would reveal ongoing and prolific use of substances, including alcohol. The manager admits that the patient at times continues to use crack cocaine, along with the methadone, which she gets from drug services. 'Laura, the problem is that patients such as Ms Jones who are addicted to substances do poorly in therapy, and the difficulty is that the relationship is with the substance rather than with the therapist. Also, as painful issues will come up in the process of therapy, the patient's capacity to manage without drugs will be put increasingly under strain if it is not yet proven that she can manage without them for a sustained period before commencing therapy.'

As part of the discussion, it comes to light that Ms Jones has been resistant to discharge from the team, even when things seem to be going well for her. You could discuss the sense of an underlying narcissism and the patient's apparent neediness. There is a feeling that somehow everyone needs to be available to her and the engagement is often on her terms only. She does not easily tolerate boundaries, and the anxiety that is felt and responded to by professionals is evidence of the rampant projective identification at work. 'Laura, I spoke with her care coordinator and her view was that Ms Jones disengaged whenever their sessions begin to move towards more sensitive areas. Her difficulty with being able to think of her emotional state bodes ill for any deeper explorative work.' Patients need to have some ego strength and curiosity about themselves to engage in long-term work. This patient appears to be able to engage, although this does tend to be as a helpless recipient.

Problem solving

Your colleague may be feeling pressure from the patient and the discussion of the referral could represent a need for a third person to intervene in a stuck relationship. A formulation could be the need for a firm paternal presence in thinking of this patient and to help set the boundaries. In this way, thinking about the needs and motivations of the patient would be beneficial in order to help the manager to separate herself from the projections of the patient. Further risk evaluation (the patient is not currently self-harming or suicidal) would help guide consideration of the alternatives. Ms Jones may currently only be able to use supportive psychological interventions that help her reduce her addiction and promote psychological thinking.

Rapport and communication

Patients being considered for psychodynamic psychotherapy need to be sufficiently motivated and curious. Ego strength and engagement are important considerations for long-term psychodynamic psychotherapy.

In this and similar scenarios, options of supportive versus explorative therapies can be considered. Discussions of difficult clinical scenarios can be a helpful way of promoting enquiry about a patient within the team. Finally, patients with an active dependence on substances are not good candidates for explorative psychological interventions.

Conclusion

Here you can summarise what you have discussed, any further information you want to give and what the next steps will be. 'Laura, we both agree that Ms Jones needs a lot of thought and attention from the team in managing her contact with us better, as it does not feel like she is currently using our help in the best possible way and is causing a lot of anxiety. I agree that CBT was worth a try and it does seem to have been helpful during this period, although there is possibly a need for deeper psychodynamic work. However, I think that now is not the best time for it, and given her issues with motivation and the use of illicit drugs, we will need to wait for some stability before referring her for longer therapy.'

FURTHER READING

Holmes, J. (1991) *Textbook of Psychotherapy and Psychiatric Practice.* Edinburgh: Churchill Livingstone.

Storr, A. (1990) *The Art of Psychotherapy.* New York and London: Routledge.

The examiner's mark sheet

Domain/ percentage of marks	Essential points to pass	✓	Extra marks/comments (make notes here)
1. Communication with a colleague 25% of marks	Clear communication Discusses a clinical scenario Case synthesis		
2. Psychodynamic psychotherapy 25% of marks	Knowledge of psychodynamic psychotherapy Patient motivation Ego strength and engagement considerations		
3. Risk evaluation 25% of marks	General supportive measures Risk to self/others Substance misuse		
4. Answering other questions 25% of marks	Appropriate answers		

% SCORE _____

____

4

OVERALL IMPRESSION

(CIRCLE ONE)

Good Pass

Pass

Borderline

Fail

Clear Fail

NOTES/Areas to improve

STATION 2(a): CBT FIRST SESSION

INSTRUCTION TO CANDIDATE
You are meeting Mr Jones for the first of 12 sessions of CBT.

Determine with the patient what will happen in the therapy and attempt to answer any queries the patient may have.

ACTOR (ROLE-PLAYER) INSTRUCTIONS
You have been assessed and are waiting to start CBT for recurrent problems with anxiety and stress. You have been contacted by the psychotherapy service by a therapist you have never met before to discuss the start of therapy and are meeting her for the first time. You are feeling anxious and stressed about the appointment. There had been a basic discussion about CBT in the assessment, but it was a few months ago and you have forgotten the details. You have done research on the Internet, which has left you feeling concerned about the amount of work you need to do and the result of therapy.

SUGGESTED APPROACH

Setting the scene

The patient will be meeting you for the first time. 'Mr Jones, hello. My name is Dr_____. I understand you have been on the waiting list to start CBT.'

Start by asking what he knows about CBT already. The aim of CBT of enabling the patient to acquire skills with which they can function better can be pursued from the beginning of the meeting, as you could explain to them that you will not be someone who will be simply instructing them on what to do to get better. You will be working alongside them in discovering more about themselves and learning skills that they could then use both inside and outside of the sessions.

You must demonstrate your knowledge of CBT and be empathically responsive to questions from the patient while putting him at ease by engaging him in dialogue about any concerns. In this way, you will quickly begin to build a therapeutic alliance.

Treatment

'Mr Jones, I suggest we agree to an agenda for the session and the things we would like to discuss. I do want to set aside time for us to talk through any questions you may have.' You need to discuss the frame of the sessions, including the length, place, progress since last seen (bridge), current difficulties, aims from therapy, knowledge of CBT, homework/work outside the sessions and summary. Mr Jones may have further questions, which could relate to the anxiety of starting therapy. An acknowledgement of his feelings along with an enquiring and encouraging stance will help the patient feel more at ease with you.

'How have things been since you went onto the waiting list?' This can be followed up by a discussion of how CBT may help him with understanding his difficulties. You should introduce the central role of thoughts with the link to mood/feelings and behaviour. The key is to allow the patient lots of room to ask questions while allowing new information about the duration/structure and possible content of sessions to be introduced in the first session. Drawing a simple diagram linking all of these together with a reinforcement loop can help.

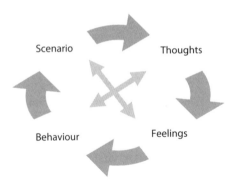

Scenario   Thoughts

Behaviour   Feelings

Problem solving

Some patients could ask if there is any evidence that this therapy works. You could cite NICE guidelines, which are based on systematic reviews of current relevant evidence and make specific recommendations about the use of CBT. Avoid the use of technical jargon and try to present the information to the patient in simple terms. Allowing the patient to express their doubts and reservations as the session progresses will help with setting up a therapeutic alliance. 'Mr Jones, homework is about the work done in therapy continuing outside the sessions. Similarly, behavioural experiments are opportunities for us to allow the skills which are being learnt here to be tested in the real world.'

Rapport and communication

CBT is a here-and-now therapy typically consisting of 8–20 sessions on a weekly basis over a few months. The emphasis is on a collaborative experience, with the patient and therapist working together to resolve the difficulties with which they have presented. Therapy can include tasks like problem solving, diary keeping, homework, and so forth, and this model has been shown to be useful in depression and anxiety.

Weekly sessions involve problem solving and reviewing diary keeping and the homework that was set from the last session.

Conclusion

Here you can summarise what you have discussed, any further information you want to give and what the next steps will be. 'Mr Jones, we have been talking about the period in which you have been waiting to start CBT. We have discussed various concerns about what therapy would bring up and if it would, in the end, be helpful. I think we have covered a lot of ground of what to expect in CBT and discussed the structure of sessions. I suggest now that we confirm that we will meet next week to start the therapy.'

FURTHER READING

Beck, A.T. (1987) Cognitive models of depression. *Journal of Cognitive Psychotherapy*, *1*, 5–37.

Greenberger, D. & Padesky, C. (1996) *Mind over Mood*. New York, NY: The Guildford Press.

The examiner's mark sheet

Domain/ percentage of marks	Essential points to pass	✓	Extra marks/comments (make notes here)
1. Communication and empathy 25% of marks	Clear communication Open and closed questions Empathy Sensitivity		
2. Knowledge of CBT 25% of marks	Explains the principles and what treatment will involve		
3. Building a therapeutic alliance 25% of marks	Puts patient at ease by engaging him in dialogue about his concerns		
4. Answering other questions 25% of marks	Appropriate answers		

% SCORE _____

___ **OVERALL IMPRESSION**

4 (CIRCLE ONE)

Good Pass

Pass

Borderline

Fail

Clear Fail

NOTES/Areas to improve

STATION 2(b): BEHAVIOURAL EXPERIMENT IN CBT

INSTRUCTION TO CANDIDATE

You have now seen your patient for three sessions of CBT and he has explained in some detail his difficulties in social situations. He can find it difficult to function socially and spends much of his free time at home. He feels that his career is also affected. He has often felt a failure when describing past episodes of being in social situations.

Discuss a behavioural experiment with him.

ACTOR (ROLE-PLAYER) INSTRUCTIONS

You have been attending weekly sessions with your CBT therapist and the initial discussions have been about the theoretical model of the therapy. You have explained your problems with anxiety and your particular problems in social situations, which have been making you feel so stressed that you have avoided social occasions. You have felt its impact on your career, as you cannot interact well at work events and this makes you feel like a failure. Talking has been difficult, but you are really not looking forward to an 'experiment' in therapy.

SUGGESTED APPROACH

Setting the scene

The behavioural task is a useful tool in CBT and one of the important ways in which the patient carries on the work outside of the sessions. It enables the patient to translate the theory into practice and provides the therapy with an *in vivo* experiment to discuss and base further work on. It can give the patient a real sense of picking up the skills being discussed and a sense of mastery over the problems for which they have sought therapy.

It captures the need for collaborative work with the patient, and to do this, you need to be able to explain the theory, explore anxieties and engage him in a dialogue. The therapeutic alliance and capacity to listen will help to put the patient at ease while using the opportunity to impart knowledge of CBT as you seek to improve his skills.

Treatment

The rationale for the behavioural task needs to be explained to the patient. He will be understandably anxious, as this is the first such task in the therapy. Allow enough space for questions from the patient. The task for a patient with social anxiety has to be carefully graded to be a step up from what they may be currently able to achieve and yet not too much. 'I suggest that we start small, such as the Friday meeting that you described at work, and see if we can set a small experiment around this situation, such as talking over coffee with a colleague.' Too much too soon can leave a patient feeling more of a failure and ward off attempts at change. Thus, graded exposure to increasingly more difficult tasks provides a sense of mastery over the problem. Later, there may be more challenging tasks that could be set up, which could include different settings and levels of tasks to be achieved. The setting of the task, the people involved, the patient's anxieties and fears and the actual task (talk for 5 minutes over coffee) need to be considered and agreed upon. Making clear notes and encouraging the patient to keep a record of the task also helps, as does imagining and discussing a situation (cognitive rehearsal).

The patient could have catastrophic outcomes in mind and going through this following the model of thoughts, behaviour and consequences in the setting will help him. 'Given your concerns about things going wrong, let's have a think about various strategies you could use to help you finish the task.' This may include using distraction techniques preceding the task to reduce anxiety or cue cards to help carry out the actual task. Role-play (modelling) also helps by providing a taste of the experience in a contained setting where the task can be rehearsed and misgivings addressed.

Problem solving

Adequate contingency planning to anticipate known reasons for avoidance and failure to complete a task is important. After the task, there may be an opportunity to use a feedback survey to properly evaluate task completion. This behavioural feedback can help provide a more balanced report, which can be used to question black-and-white thinking. Further work on automatic thoughts and clarification of rules, assumptions and beliefs will help the patient understand his difficulties.

Rapport and communication

In the discussion, you need to address the patient's anxieties and, using the experience of therapy so far, agree on the details of the behavioural experiment. You would then explore the sequence of events needed to complete the experiment and confirm strategies to tackle issues that may arise. You could also decide how to evaluate completion, such as by agreeing to obtain feedback from colleagues.

Conclusion

Here you can summarise what you have discussed, any further information you want to give and what the next steps will be. 'Mr Jones, we have spent some time today discussing the progress of therapy. We have been talking about the structure of CBT and exploring the details of your problems that have brought you into therapy. That has brought us to behavioural experiments and their crucial role in this kind of therapy. We have looked at starting small and decided on a social behavioural experiment in a social setting at work to start things off, including how we will evaluate its success. I suggest you do give it a go in the next week and we review it in our session next week.'

The examiner's mark sheet

Domain/ percentage of marks	Essential points to pass	✓	Extra marks/comments (make notes here)
1. Communication and empathy 25% of marks	Clear communication Collaborative work with the patient		
2. Patient education 25% of marks	Explains the theory Explores anxieties Imparts knowledge of CBT Discusses the behavioural experiment		
3. Planning for the next session 25% of marks	Summarises what you have discussed, any further information you want to give and plan the next steps		
4. Answering other questions 25% of marks	Appropriate answers		

% SCORE _____

____ **OVERALL IMPRESSION**

4   (CIRCLE ONE)

Good Pass

Pass

Borderline

Fail

Clear Fail

NOTES/Areas to improve

STATION 3(a): OVERDOSE IN ACCIDENT AND EMERGENCY

INSTRUCTION TO CANDIDATE

Ms Jones has presented to accident and emergency (A&E) having taken an overdose. She has an unclear diagnosis, with several being mentioned in records. She initially wanted help, but is now refusing treatment. A&E staff are concerned about her physical state, but she does not allow them to examine her.

Assess this patient and, in particular, the motivation for the overdose. In the next station you will be asked to consider the case psychodynamically; this will help focus your assessment.

You are not expected to complete a full history and mental state examination in the available time.

ACTOR (ROLE-PLAYER) INSTRUCTIONS

You have been feeling very bad since a friend stopped answering your calls. It feels like it is a repetition of events in which everyone you help takes advantage of you and then cuts off contact. This has really upset you and you took an overdose of paracetamol, as you felt that there was no point in going on. You then felt panicky and so went to A&E, but now feel confused about being saved. Perhaps it would be better to die so you do not have to feel so sad?

SUGGESTED APPROACH

Setting the scene

Start by asking the patient, 'Ms Jones, I am one of the A&E doctors. Please can you tell me what has brought you here today?' The emphasis at the beginning needs to be on finding out what has happened using open questions without creating an atmosphere of confrontation, which could be persecuting for the patient. Her responses will guide you into the body of the task. Your interview technique needs to make use of open questions using empathy and managing anxiety in a challenging situation. 'It seems things have felt really hard after this falling out with your friend. Why did you take the overdose of paracetamol? What were you hoping would happen?'

In talking to the patient, you have to be able to try to find out what has happened, including the reason for the overdose, in order to understand why she has presented (her motivation to seek help) and what the problem is regarding accepting treatment, including a risk assessment.

Treatment

'Ms Jones, please can you tell me if this is the first time you have felt like this or have there been difficulties with your mood in the past?' She may report a lifetime of feeling low and repeated self-harm. 'I notice that you did seek help after the overdose, but are now refusing help when it is available. Please can you tell me what you would like to happen?' After this you could present her with options that are available, along with the risks and benefits (in a concise way) of each.

The actor might have instructions to engage with you fleetingly and then ask what you think would help. If you mention the need for an in-patient assessment or community follow-up, she will refuse and try to leave, as she is now in the midst of such intense anxiety that the object quickly shifts from being good to bad. These are features of a paranoid schizoid position, which is a persistent feature in borderline personality disorder, although it can also affect other individuals in situations of stress. 'Ms Jones, it seems like something of what I am suggesting does not meet your expectations. Can you tell me what you think would be helpful at a time like this?' This makes use of your counter-transference, such as feelings of anxiety of how to deal with the situation, followed by a sense of being unsure of what has gone wrong in your conversation with the patient, even feeling that you have done something to provoke the patient to try to leave and being left with feelings of rejection.

Problem solving

This could include having to deal with your own frustration when talking to such a patient, as you need to be calm when the patient is agitated and anxious, without appearing to be detached. While talking to the patient, you would also need to avoid being authoritarian, and instead try to give her a sense of having options. 'Ms Jones, I know it feels like we are struggling to agree on what would help, but actually, you have done something very important by seeking help and we must not let that be forgotten.' Parts of her are acting in opposition. Appealing to the more adult part of her mind is one way to engage with her limited awareness of needing help.

Rapport and communication

The patient will ask questions, which you would need to answer. As the interview progresses, you will also need to ask questions regarding risk relating to suicidal ideation, planning and intent as far as possible. Furthermore, there could be a discussion with the examiner in the next station about the heightened risk if she were to have a diagnosis like personality disorder. An investigation of psycho-social precipitants and their link to a signature in her presentations should be attempted.

Conclusion

Here you can summarise what you have discussed, any further information you want to give and what the next steps will be. 'Ms Jones, we have been talking about the events which led to your overdose with paracetamol earlier today. We have explored the problems that led to the overdose and spent some time thinking about your risk to yourself at a time like this. I think it is important that you have sought help from services at a stressful time for you and agree that you do need further support. You continue to feel unsafe and are unable to assure me of keeping yourself safe. We have agreed that it would help for you to have support with a brief admission to our in-patient unit. I will now arrange your transfer to the ward.'

FURTHER READING

Gabbard, G. (2000) *Psychodynamic Psychiatry in Clinical Practice*. Washington, DC, and London: American Psychiatric Press, Inc.

Steiner, J. (1987) The interplay between pathological organizations and the paranoid–schizoid and depressive positions. *International Journal of Psycho-Analysis, 68*, 69–80.

The examiner's mark sheet

Domain/ percentage of marks	Essential points to pass	✓	Extra marks/comments (make notes here)
1. Communication and empathy 25% of marks	Clear communication Open and closed questions Empathy Sensitivity		
2. Relevant history and mental state to allow a subsequent psychodynamic formulation 25% of marks	History of the events Interpersonal relationships How she handles adversity/ stress/anxiety What she hoped to achieve by the overdose, seeking help and refusing treatment Understanding and awareness of transference and counter-transference		
3. Risk assessment 25% of marks	Considers the key risk issues in this case		
4. Answering other questions 25% of marks	Appropriate answers		

% SCORE _____

___

4

OVERALL IMPRESSION

(CIRCLE ONE)

Good Pass

Pass

Borderline

Fail

Clear Fail

NOTES/Areas to improve

STATION 3(b): BORDERLINE PERSONALITY DISORDER

INSTRUCTION TO CANDIDATE

The patient you have just seen has been admitted to your ward. Her case notes clarify her diagnosis as chronic depression with significant borderline traits along with occasional possible psychotic symptoms, although opinion has been divided regarding their nature (psychosis or pseudo-psychosis). The patient now appears paranoid and talks about hearing voices. Some nursing staff are unimpressed and feel that the bed could be better used. They feel angry towards her (and you for admitting her) and are suspicious that she is here as her benefits are under threat.

Discuss a psychodynamic formulation and case management with the newly appointed consultant, Dr James. He does not know the patient and wonders if she could be discharged.

ACTOR (ROLE-PLAYER) INSTRUCTIONS

You are the consultant on the ward where a patient was admitted from A&E after agreeing that she needed to be in hospital following an overdose. You have not met her before and do not have a previous relationship with her, as she was treated by another colleague until a few months ago, and you have just returned from your summer break.

However, things have become worse after she felt badly treated by nursing staff. You have heard a couple of nurses discussing her, as they felt she was taking up a bed that another patient could have used. They are insisting that she is immediately discharged, as other 'more unwell' patients need to come in. You need to take a decision and are discussing her with your clinical trainee who has been involved in her care.

SUGGESTED APPROACH

Setting the scene

The consultant wants information about the patient and your opinion on what you think may be going on. You need to start the discussion keeping in mind that there are already strong opinions about her. You should summarise the circumstances surrounding her admission and mention the need for more collateral information. 'Dr James, I have known her for the relatively brief period since she has been on the ward, as there was no previous knowledge of her prior to this admission.' In your comments, you need to demonstrate your understanding of transference and knowledge of counter-transference, making links with her defensive manoeuvres. In this way, you would link the psychiatric presentation with a psychodynamic formulation.

Treatment

The difficulty here will be keeping an open mind about the patient. Patients with border-line presentations can arouse deep splits and conflict amongst clinicians involved in their treatment. Indeed, they can often present with a combination of affective and psychotic disturbances, which can coexist, causing additional difficulties in formulation. Along with this, there may be comorbid alcohol and drugs misuse. Think about 'splitting' fairly early on in your discussion, in which the patient tries to manage opposing feelings by lodging them in different members of staff. The good and bad split refers to the inability to hold a whole object and the predominance of part objects in the internal world, while the extreme reactions in the ward staff appear to mirror this problem. This can be linked to in your discussion about the response to such feelings in staff (which includes yourself), which can be understood by the defence of projective identification employed uncon-sciously by the patient. 'Dr James, I do feel that the responses of the various staff members are all part of the presentation of the patient. We need to try to hold these opposing feel-ings together in order to deal with the patient in the most helpful way, which would include evaluation and boundary setting.'

You may then be asked about her possible discharge from the ward and whether you agree with one or other staff members who have strong feelings about the patient being on the ward. 'I think the problem is that she does provoke extreme feelings in all of us. The risk is that we may make an unhelpful decision about her care if we don't think about her needs.' It is known that long periods of in-patient treatment are not helpful for such patients.

Problem solving

You should emphasise the need for risk assessment in managing the patient in the ward and also the importance of the continuity of care into the community setting. If her mental state is stable, discharge should be considered early, along with a clear plan on how to manage crises in the community, preferably with the involvement of a limited and small group of caseworkers. Discussion with care workers in the community helps manage splits and provides the patient with some sense of being thought about, although any sense of being discharged is likely to provoke persecutory responses.

Rapport and communication

You will need to demonstrate your role in helping colleagues avoid splitting and emphasising the need for joined-up thinking. You need to point out the importance of consistent boundary setting, such as in the prescription of additional medication and avoiding a long admission. You need to confirm the importance of treating this as a short-term respite admission rather than a long-term admission in order to avoid excessive dependence and promote rehabilitation in the community. Community management is best done along a clear-cut contract with fixed members of staff.

Conclusion

Here you can summarise what you have discussed, any further information you want to give and what the next steps will be. 'Dr James, thanks, it has been helpful discussing the care of Ms Jones. It seems likely that the strong reactions that have been evident in the ward are connected to her issues and that as a group of clinicians we need to spend more time thinking about our responses. I will speak to the nurses' in charge ward manager about this and we can also discuss our decision about boundaries and the period of in-patient care in the ward round tomorrow.'

FURTHER READING

Bateman, A. & Holmes, J. (2003) *Introduction to Psychoanalysis*. New York and London: Routledge.

Hinshelwood, R.D. (1999) The difficult patient. *British Journal of Psychiatry*, *174*, 187–90.

The examiner's mark sheet

Domain/percentage of marks	Essential points to pass	✓	Extra marks/comments (make notes here)
1. Communication 25% of marks	Clear communication with a senior colleague		

| 2. Psychodynamic formulation | Linking the psychiatric presentation with psychodynamic formulation |
| | |

2. Psychodynamic formulation

   55% of marks

Linking the psychiatric presentation with psychodynamic formulation

Understanding of transference and counter-transference

3. Risk evaluation

   10% of marks

Consideration of risk in the formulation

4. Answering other questions

   10% of marks

Appropriate answers

% SCORE _____

___

4

OVERALL IMPRESSION

(CIRCLE ONE)

Good Pass

Pass

Borderline

Fail

Clear Fail

NOTES/Areas to improve

O SINGLE STATIONS

STATION 4: POST-TRAUMATIC STRESS DISORDER – TREATMENT OPTIONS

INSTRUCTION TO CANDIDATE

This patient, Ms Smith, has a diagnosis of post-traumatic stress disorder (PTSD) and wants help. She has been started on antidepressant therapy by her GP.

Discuss the possible psychotherapeutic options available.

ACTOR (ROLE-PLAYER) INSTRUCTIONS

You are a 22–year-old woman who was a student at a university doing a law course. However, during a night out, you were knocked over while returning home. You were then attacked by the person driving the vehicle and sustained injuries, although the physical trauma has now resolved.

However, you increasingly feel too frightened to leave home and have missed a lot of classes. You are suffering from nightmares and even when awake can see the events of the night before your very eyes, as if you were reliving them. You have been jumpy and afraid at home and have begun to drink a little more alcohol than usual to cope. You are keen on psychodynamic psychotherapy.

SUGGESTED APPROACH

Setting the scene

The need is to reach a collaborative decision following an explanation of the theory and choices. The patient could present in a helpless and anxious manner or she may confront you with her research that she conducted on the Internet and want a particular type of therapy. 'Ms Smith, please can you tell about the difficulties for which you have been referred here today? It looks like the problems of nightmares, flashbacks and anxiety around going outside and avoiding situations outside are becoming worse. Let's talk about the various options that may be available. I note that your GP has already started you on antidepressants which are likely to help with these problems. There are types of therapy which could also be helpful.' You have to be mindful of the need to discuss options and try to help the patient arrive at a decision without pushing a decision onto the patient.

You need to explain best practice based on the NICE guidelines and explore her anxieties while answering questions. This will help engage her in a dialogue and demonstrate empathy.

Treatment

Ask what she knows about the talking therapies that have been recommended. Guidelines need to be considered, but not necessarily adhered to rigidly. 'Ms Smith, there is a choice of psychological treatments such as cognitive behavioural therapy or eye movement desensitisation and reprocessing for the sort of difficulties that you are having. It is quite common to consider a combination of medication and psychotherapy to help with PTSD.' The level and timing of intervention will depend on the period since the trauma. 'At the beginning, we usually suggest that people wait and see if the problems resolve on their own over time. However, in your case, there has already been a period of 4 weeks and so this period of what we call watchful waiting is past.' If the symptoms have lasted for over 3 months, then trauma-focussed psychological treatment should be carried out using trauma-focussed CBT or eye movement desensitisation and reprocessing (EMDR), while treatment beginning within 3 months of symptom onset can be briefer.

The treatment centres on psycho-education, exposure and cognitive restructuring. The exposure can be *in vivo* (previously avoided situations) or imaginal. The model for treatment-focussed CBT therapy is somewhat along the lines of any anxiety disorder, incorporating feedback loops, anticipatory anxiety, avoidance behaviours and misperceptions/misunderstandings of (physical and emotional) cues. 'Ms Smith, the therapy will try to reduce anxiety by working to increase your confidence in situations that are currently causing you to avoid going out, for instance.' When the symptoms have lasted for a longer duration, a much longer period of treatment may be required than the usual 8–12 sessions. This is particularly important as CBT sessions will have to be focussed on over the longer term in order not to forget the treatment aims. This restructuring aims to target unhelpful thinking and uses thought records in order to identify automatic thoughts.

The patient is already using pharmacological therapy, which is not usually a first-line treatment. The use of specific antidepressants (like paroxetine and mirtazapine) is advocated and can also be given in combination or as adjuncts to the psychological intervention. Presenting all of the available options and encouraging discussion will also help soothe the patient.

Problem solving

Discussion of alternatives and weighing up the options can help with the patient's engagement with the eventual treatment, and the decision a patient may then reach should be respected. 'Ms Smith, I know that you think the current issues are probably related to your early childhood and that you have researched psychodynamic therapy. However, there are reasons why this treatment is not indicated for the sort of problems that you are having at the moment. The need is for you to understand the basis of these difficulties in the here and now and to work out ways to overcome your problems, such as not avoiding going out altogether.' You could speak of the evidence base (quality of evidence) used for the recommendations (e.g. for CBT) whilst making it clear that there are options to choose from.

Rapport and communication

CBT attempts to modify cognitions, assumptions, beliefs and behaviours and aims to influence disturbed emotions. Through the identification of irrational thoughts and beliefs leading to negative emotions and maladaptive behaviours, the aim is to replace them with more realistic and positive alternatives. You must be able to convince Ms Smith that there is likely to be the potential for benefits from the therapy and that there is reasonable proof for this, but that you are unable to predict the outcome of therapy.

EMDR is a method of psychotherapy that is designed to treat trauma and anxiety-related disorders. It combines therapeutic methods, including imaginable exposure, cognitive restructuring and self-control techniques into specific structured protocols, which are modified to meet the unique needs of each person.

Conclusion

Here you can summarise what you have discussed, any further information you want to give and what the next steps will be. 'Ms Smith, we have spent some time in our meeting today talking about the awful incident that led to your difficulties with post-traumatic stress disorder. We have also considered your questions about the best mode of therapy and your interest in psychodynamic psychotherapy. You have told me about the extent of your ongoing problems and we have thought about how the CBT therapy could help you gain some mastery over these issues and give you more of a sense of control and relief. I think we are agreed that the treatment of choice for your problems currently would be CBT.'

FURTHER READING

Bisson, J. & Andrew, M. (2005) Psychological treatment of post-traumatic stress disorder (PTSD). *Cochrane Database of Systematic Reviews* (2), CD003388.

National Institute for Health and Care Excellence (2005) Post-traumatic stress disorder: Management of post-traumatic stress disorder in adults in primary, secondary and community care. https://www.nice.org.uk/guidance/cg26

The examiner's mark sheet

Domain/ percentage of marks	Essential points to pass	✓	Extra marks/comments (make notes here)
1. Communication and empathy 25% of marks	Clear communication		
	Open and closed questions		
	Empathy		
	Sensitivity		

⬆ 2. Psychotherapeutic   Collaborative decision taken
     treatment options   with patient

     50% of marks   Explaining the theory and
                         choices

                         Explaining best practice

3. Answering other   Appropriate answers
    questions

    25% of marks

% SCORE _____

                                                 ___   **OVERALL IMPRESSION**

                                          3   (CIRCLE ONE)

                                                   Good Pass

                                                   Pass

                                                   Borderline

                                                   Fail

                                                   Clear Fail

                                                   NOTES/Areas to improve

STATION 5: PSYCHODYNAMIC PSYCHOTHERAPY

INSTRUCTION TO CANDIDATE

You are seeing Mr Jones for the first time. He has been on the waiting list for psychotherapy for a year. He has a history of having been in multiple foster placements. He seems hesitant and gives practical reasons for not being able to commence therapy.

Conduct the business meeting to discuss the start of psychotherapy.

ACTOR (ROLE-PLAYER) INSTRUCTIONS

You were referred, assessed and offered psychodynamic therapy. After being on the waiting list for some time, you are now meeting the potential therapist. However, you have become increasingly concerned that therapy will bring up very difficult memories for you. You found it disturbing after the assessment, as it reminded you of many childhood events that had not previously been on your mind. Hence, when the call for starting the therapy came, you felt very anxious and concerned and did not sleep well before the appointment today. Now you are completely unsure if therapy is the best way forward.

SUGGESTED APPROACH

Setting the scene

Introduce yourself and acknowledge that the patient has been on the waiting list for some time. You should explain that the meeting is not a therapy session, but instead aims to agree to start therapy with you as the therapist (i.e. a business meeting). This will be particularly important for such a patient who has a history of being recurrently moved on and thus experiencing possible difficulties regarding attachment and separation.

'Mr Jones, I know that you have been waiting for a long time to begin therapy. As we discussed in my letter, I now have a space for therapy and wanted to meet so we can agree to the therapy. This is not the start of therapy, but more about agreeing on the plan and structure for the sessions, such as times and the length of therapy. How have things been since you were seen for your last review?' Your interview technique must focus on the use of open questions to elicit your patient's current feelings of anxiety.

The patient tells you that he is not sure now is the best time for him to start, saying that he is likely to be starting a new job. Your aim may be to understand his ambivalence without being persecutory or dismissive. 'Mr Jones, I wonder if the possibility of therapy starting has brought up some difficult feelings. Please can we talk about how this feels?' In opening up the possibility of talking openly about his concerns, you are helping the patient with a difficult decision, as the final decision of commencing therapy remains with him.

Treatment

The business meeting gives the therapist the opportunity to learn about the person, to understand the current situation and to formulate ideas about treatment. 'Mr Jones, the sessions will be once weekly at a fixed time and day and the length of the therapy will be approximately 12 months.' It is within this context that positive changes in the patient's outlook and behaviours are able to unfold. The therapist maintains a consistently neutral and accepting stance and is trained to listen objectively without criticism.

The patient is likely to have had a prolonged assessment (usually two to three sessions) with another therapist when he was entered onto the waiting list and there could be feelings of resentment about having been moved again onto yet another person to actually commence therapy. He may insist that he does not need therapy any longer. He could also say that he is now working or hoping to begin work and so can only do therapy if it is offered to him in the evenings. 'We do sometimes have out-of-hours therapy available, but as discussed at the assessment, most spaces are during working hours. I do think we need to consider what else may be posing problems for you entering therapy when you have been waiting for such a long time.' The aim throughout is to encourage a dialogue and acknowledge feelings of anxiety or anger. All of this needs to be done whilst not converting the business meeting into a therapy session. The discussion needs to consider the balance of claustrophobic anxiety (the patient feels trapped when therapy is available) and agoraphobic anxiety (he does not want to be left out, hence remaining on the waiting list).

The patient may then tell you that he is afraid of what he will find out about himself in the therapy. He may have feelings of anxiety about being picked up and then left by you. As you continue to talk, the patient may then seem to become less dismissive. Acknowledging the patient's anxieties while at the same time pointing out that he has been waiting for a long time for therapy and opening up further dialogue about this will help him to make a decision. Be mindful that while you can help him to think about what may be difficult, the decision of whether to start or not is his in the end.

Rapport and communication

This is not an easy station. The patient and you have to struggle with feelings of anxiety and rejection. The manner in which you handle this situation will be crucial, as he may be uncontained or dismissive. Such a patient could bring up powerful feelings of wanting to get him into therapy or, if he persistently refuses, to get rid of him and go along with his stated wish of not commencing therapy. Awareness of counter-transference is thus very important to convey to the examiner, as well as that you are emotionally involved with the patient's dilemma while at the same time not being caught up in an enactment.

Psychodynamic psychotherapy aims to help find relief from emotional pain. It is similar to psychoanalysis in attributing emotional difficulties to unconscious motives and conflicts. Psychodynamic psychotherapy is employed for a variety of problems including mood difficulties, relational issues, and so forth. Sessions can take place on 1–3 days per week, with greater frequency allowing for more in-depth treatment, and they usually last for 45–50 minutes. Most NHS-based services will now offer no more than 1 year (approximately 40 sessions) of therapy.

Conclusion

Here you can summarise what you have discussed, any further information you want to give and what the next steps will be. 'Mr Jones, we have met to discuss the possibility of you starting your treatment of psychodynamic therapy after the period you have spent on the waiting list. However, you did have some serious concerns about any future work interfering with you being able to attend therapy. I think in our discussion we worked out that some of these concerns were also linked to the worry that therapy would be disturbing and may make things worse. However, having thought about the possible benefits, you have decided to give it a go, and so I suggest we meet next week at this time for the first session of therapy.'

FURTHER READING

Bateman, A. & Fonagy, P. (2004) *Psychotherapy for Borderline Personality Disorder*. Oxford: Oxford University Press.

Hughes, P. (1999) *Dynamic Psychotherapy Explained*. London: Radcliffe Medical Press.

The examiner's mark sheet

Domain/ percentage of marks	Essential points to pass	✓	Extra marks/comments (make notes here)
1. Communication and empathy 30% of marks	Clear communication Open and closed questions		
2. Business meeting 30% of marks	Explaining the principles and practicalities Maintaining the session's focus – not a therapy session		
3. Psychodynamic knowledge 30% of marks	Understanding transference and counter-transference Helping the patient with ambivalence without being persecutory or dismissive Helping the patient with a difficult decision		

⇧ 4. Answering other   Appropriate answers
     questions

     10% of marks

   % SCORE _____

                                      ___   **OVERALL IMPRESSION**

                                    4   (CIRCLE ONE)

                                          Good Pass

                                          Pass

                                          Borderline

                                          Fail

                                          Clear Fail

                                          NOTES/Areas to improve

STATION 6: MANAGING ANGER

INSTRUCTION TO CANDIDATE

You are seeing Ms Jones, a patient with bipolar affective disorder who has been known to the team for several years. She is very angry with the consultant who admitted her to the ward earlier that year under a section of the Mental Health Act and is refusing to see him. She is seeing you in the clinic for the first time as she is threatening to stop all of her medication and to terminate contact with the team.

Speak to this patient and attempt engagement and discussion regarding the future.

ACTOR (ROLE-PLAYER) INSTRUCTIONS

You have been affected by a mental illness for many years and have repeated episodes of becoming very unwell. However, you do not think you have an illness that requires you to be admitted to hospital, even though this has repeatedly happened over many years. You believe that you have knowledge about your illness and that your consultant does not respect your wishes sufficiently, as happened when he forced your admission under the Mental Health Act earlier this year. You are very angry with him and feel like cutting off all contact with him and the rest of the community team. You are seeing a new doctor in the same team after refusing to meet with the consultant. If adequately handled, you settle down. You also tell the doctor that you wish to start a family and want to stop medication.

SUGGESTED APPROACH

Setting the scene

This is a potentially challenging station involving managing a patient who is very angry and ready to have a fight with you regarding her medication and her recent treatment. She believes that she should not have been admitted to hospital against her wishes. You will need to demonstrate empathy and develop rapport while not reacting to provocation.

'Ms Jones, I know that you have been distressed and upset by your recent treatment and I wonder if we can talk about your concerns.'

Her insistence on and belief in her understanding of her illness have led to her anger. This could become a point of disagreement involving her insistence that she comes off all of her medication and your anxiety that this does not happen, as there is a history of relapse on stopping treatment. It is important that you start with an open statement such as acknowledging that she has a lot to talk about with you and allowing her to have her say without seeming to be ready to disagree.

Treatment

She may launch into a provocative account of how she feels she was 'put' into hospital by the consultant who did not know her well. The actor would then tell you that she is planning to start a family, how she feels completely well and that all your team has done is to leave her in more difficulty. A lot of this is an evacuation of her resentment, which you simply need to be able to bear and make some sense of. However, there is a lot in the content and process of what is being said which could be helpful in this consultation. She intends to stop her medications and withdraw from the team. She will not be coming to any more of these 'useless' clinic appointments. 'Ms Jones, I recognise that the last few months have been difficult. I wonder how this leaves you feeling about your care and the team.'

The anger could also mask anxiety about what might happen with you and an attempt to avoid mourning the effect of her illness. There may be an unconscious fantasy of a successful union with you (unlike that with the consultant recently) and the birth of a shared understanding. 'I do understand what you are saying about your knowledge through experience and research of bipolar disorder.' Good listening is key. Do not dismiss her thoughts about wanting to start a family, which should be explored. In addition, this discussion would feel more hopeful if it is led away from the point of contention (the argument about the medication). This may help her begin to talk about plans and think about her needs. Clearly, there is an aspect of the patient that does want to be thought about (she has turned up for the appointment after all), and that is the aspect you need to try to engage. When the patient begins to talk to you, you could begin to explore the disruption that falling ill causes to her life and the need to be mindful of this given her plans for the future.

Problem solving

Depending on your handling of the initial stages of the station, you may see a calmer period in the conversation in which her ambivalence regarding accepting her illness and the effects of this upon her can be talked about. On the other hand, she could well turn back onto the grievance and demonstrate ambivalence in her interaction. The further you can progress into the conversation and address the future while acknowledging her grievance and also her wish for care, the better are the chances of engaging with her more concerned aspect.

The mother and feeding baby dyad could be one way of thinking about this interaction psychodynamically. The baby needs a feed in order to survive and at the same time experiences fury at not having control of the breast. The rage is expressed in the initial biting of the breast until a persistent and containing mother soothes the infant to feed.

Rapport and communication

The aim must be to focus on forming an alliance to inform her care for the future, including her wishes to have a family. You should check whether she has already stopped the medication due to her wish to have a baby (and if she is in a supportive relationship), rather than getting caught up in any provocation or conflict. 'Ms Jones, it's really great that you are thinking about the future and have some clear ideas of what you would like. Perhaps we could discuss what could be helpful for you to get there and how we could best support you?'

It will be helpful to consider your counter-transference. The rage from the patient and your feeling trapped with her could be an experience of her difficulty with emotional states in which she has to process a lot by herself, like a hungry infant that has to manage hunger until the withholding breast returns.

Focus on the future so that the hopeful aspects of the patient's interaction can begin to be thought about, even if some of the plans may seem unrealistic.

Conclusion

Here you can summarise what you have discussed, any further information you want to give and what the next steps will be. 'Ms Jones, we have been talking about your concerns about the care you previously received from the team. We spent some time thinking about the impact of the recent admission and your wish to stop your medication. However, I thought what really did seem important were your wishes and plans for the future. It is really important that we do help you to get there and consider the support we can offer you. We agreed that you will continue your medication for now, and we will continue to meet in order to review your treatment.'

FURTHER READING

Steiner, J. (2006) Seeing and being seen: Narcissistic pride and narcissistic humiliation, international. *Journal of Psychoanalysis*, 87, 939–51.

The examiner's mark sheet

Domain/ percentage of marks	Essential points to pass	✓	Extra marks/comments (make notes here)
1. Communication and empathy 30% of marks	Clear communication Open and closed questions Empathy Sensitivity		
2. Managing her anger 30% of marks	Not reacting to provocation Manages hostile projections Considers own counter-transference		
3. Management 20% of marks	Focusses on future plans Offer of support from team		
4. Answering other questions 20% of marks	Appropriate answers If she wishes to complain, informing her of the process – she is within her rights to do so		

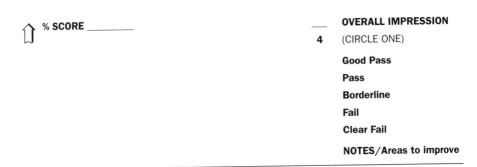

STATION 7: PSYCHODYNAMIC INTERPRETATION

INSTRUCTION TO CANDIDATE

This patient, Ms Patel, is a senior executive in an advertising firm. In the records, you note that she has once-weekly private therapy. She tells you that things have been well despite a hectic life. She has a diagnosis of depression with a history of self-harm attempts a long time ago. She was brought up by her father after her mother left when she was 6 years old. She had no contact with mental health services for a year, but the GP believes she is now less well.

Speak to this patient and use your experience of psychodynamic psychotherapy to interpret her presentation.

ACTOR (ROLE-PLAYER) INSTRUCTIONS

You are a busy advertising executive working in an important and busy post with a large company. You have had periods of depression, but none in the past year. You have also been having once-weekly therapy privately, and this has been helpful. In the past, you were much more disturbed, with periods in which you had self-harmed, but this is not currently a problem. However, your GP has been concerned that signs of strain are beginning to show, as you have complained repeatedly of fatigue and difficulties with your sleep. You have also been having many difficulties with colleagues at work.

SUGGESTED APPROACH

Setting the scene

'Ms Patel, how have things been recently for you?' She is likely to respond by giving you a lot of detail of her busy life. She has been busy travelling abroad with her work. She goes on to mention that she has been puzzled as to why she is not able to get out of bed on some days. 'Ms Patel, it seems like on the one hand things are going rather well. Yet there are problems that are harder to understand and seem to need some further thought. Have you any idea of why your sleep has been disturbed?' You need to highlight the discrepancy and ask her more about this, otherwise she might continue to dazzle you with her 'functioning' aspects, which may present a false picture.

In conversing with the patient in a more general way with open questions, you demonstrate the establishment of rapport. 'Ms Patel, it feels like it's harder for us to stay with what you are finding difficult at the moment, as I notice you keep moving back to talking about the busy events of your life, such as work. However, even here it seems from what you said that there have been some problems.' If she dismisses your attempt to understand her difficulties, you may respond thoughtfully to it rather than being provoked into an irritable response. In this way, you will explore current issues including risk and maintain empathy for a defensive patient while exploring the need for the defence.

Treatment

It is important to make an emotional link with this patient who herself seems to function in a cut-off way, making a manic flight away from her more depressive feelings. 'Ms Patel, you say there have been days when you are unable to get out of bed. I wonder if you have a sense of everything not being well.' She says this has only happened now for the past 2–3 months. 'What have been the recent stresses?' She mentions an incident 2 weeks ago in which she had gone into the shop to buy some medication for a cold and instead bought several packets of paracetamol. She had never thought much about this and had certainly not wanted to or planned an overdose. You might now feel anxious, a shift away from the slightly cut-off and even irritated feeling at the beginning while she discussed her work. Despite the task that has been set, you will need to consider a risk screen. 'Ms Patel, please can you tell me about why you bought the paracetamol. What were you planning to do with it? Have you thought of self-harm or attempting suicide? What stops you or prevents you?'

Ask about what is coming up in therapy for her and if she has been going to her therapy sessions. It transpires that she has been so busy in the past few months that she has missed several sessions. This is another example of the scotomisation of her needs by moving away from the space where her experience of loss could be considered. The patient is struggling to process her loss, seeming to be stuck in a stage of denial about it. This is acting out of her background in which she achieved a lot early on while seemingly managing the loss of her mother, who left home when she was very young. The problem with this is that her feelings of rage and hurt are ignored and instead turned inwards, as captured in her faltering motivation to work and the purchasing of tablets.

You could now have a discussion about her blocking out and highlight that there is a process going on in which the frame that is available to help her think of her emotional state is being left behind. Perhaps in leaving her therapist waiting, she is acting out how left behind and messed about she feels, although this is only a fleeting triumph.

Problem solving

The patient might ask for more medication, as this is what has helped her in the past. She thinks this is what will help her and she lapses back into telling you of all the meetings which are coming up and the plans for travel which are a part of this.

You could feel very controlled by this patient, and when you try to direct to her therapy, she seems to have shifted the discussion to something intellectual. She bristles when you suggest her feelings of loss and her controlling you in the consultation are further examples of her method of seeking to ensure distance from the object that makes her feel needy. 'Ms Patel, I wonder if we need at the moment to stay with your need for the therapy that you have been missing, rather than moving on to medication.' You could also point out that you are now also available for monitoring her in out-patient appointments.

Rapport and communication

The task captures the difficulty of engaging a patient in discussing topics that may be pertinent to her current mental state and not getting swept up in doing something concrete. In this way, you will be helping her challenge her cut-off state of denial. This is not easily done, as her response to making emotional contact is to seek to control the emotion/object. Scotomisation is a defensive process by which the person fails (consciously) to perceive circumscribed areas of their environmental situation or of themselves (as in a visual scotoma – a blank area in the visual field).

Conclusion

Here you can summarise what you have discussed, any further information you want to give and what the next steps will be. 'Ms Patel, we have been talking about how you have been doing more recently. We agreed that while things may appear fine with work and so on, there may be some things that are becoming concerning, such as your sleep and thoughts of suicide. We discussed the care you were receiving from your GP and in your therapy. We agreed that it may be best for you to have some more support and this could well be from regularly attending your therapy, instead of the number of sessions that have recently been missed. I also think that the medication increases mentioned by your GP will be helpful. I will speak with your GP, if that's OK, and see you in another 2 weeks to see how things have progressed.'

FURTHER READING

Rosenfeld, H. (1971) A clinical approach to the psychoanalytic theory of the life and death instincts: An investigation into the aggressive aspects of narcissism. *International Journal of Psycho-Analysis*, 52, 169–78.

The examiner's mark sheet

Domain/ percentage of marks	Essential points to pass	✓	Extra marks/comments (make notes here)
1. Communication 45% of marks	Establishes rapport Responds thoughtfully to dismissal		
2. Offering psychodynamic interpretations 45% of marks	Able to explain in lay terms to the patient credible psychodynamic interpretations		
3. Risk screen 10% of marks	Considers risks based on the role-player's comments		

% SCORE _____

___ **OVERALL IMPRESSION**

3 (CIRCLE ONE)

Good Pass

Pass

Borderline

Fail

Clear Fail

NOTES/Areas to improve

STATION 8: COGNITIVE DISTORTIONS

> ## INSTRUCTION TO CANDIDATE
>
> Mr Cole, a footballer, presents with depression. He underperformed in a recent key match. He has various cognitive errors, including minimisation, maximisation, selective abstraction and catastrophic thinking.
>
> **Assess him and identify these distortions.**
>
> **Discuss psychological treatment options.**

ACTOR (ROLE-PLAYER) INSTRUCTIONS

You are a successful footballer who has performed well in local leagues and have been progressing well in your career. However, your last match was a disaster. It was the most important match of your career, as talent scouts were there to watch and a good game could have meant career progress and a move to a professional level. You were sick earlier in the morning and then felt exhausted for much of the game, with the result that your performance was lacklustre. You did not score any goals and your team drew the game.

You have been devastated since and have felt upset, exhausted and unable to continue practice. You are sure that this means the end of your career and your family has become so concerned that they insisted you seek help, although you are very unsure of whether anything can be of use.

SUGGESTED APPROACH

Setting the scene

In conversing with the patient in a more general way with open questions, you demonstrate the establishment of rapport. 'Mr Cole, please tell me what has brought you here today. What are your concerns?' You will need to engage a rather ambivalent patient who is unsure about the benefits of talking. 'I understand you are a footballer and it seems like there have been problems with your work. Please can you tell me some details of what happened?' In talking with such a patient, you may notice that he struggles to speak or to describe his difficulties.

Treatment

You can help by reassuring him about the usefulness of the meeting. 'Mr Cole, it may be useful to talk, as your coming here, even though you are unsure about how much use it will be, suggests that there are things that need more thought. It's perfectly normal to feel anxious or unsure about talking in the beginning, and perhaps we could start by discussing what concerns you have about talking.' He goes on to describe how the game was lost due to him not scoring and that this means he has let everyone down.

Cognitive distortions describe flaws and errors in the cognitive processing of information that lead to incorrect conclusions, which cause and maintain disturbances in feelings. 'Mr Cole, please can you tell me about what was happening earlier that day in the lead up to your match.' He speaks about feeling unwell but is insistent that his poor game was the problem. 'Mr Cole, I notice that you completed the game in spite of being unwell and prevented goals being scored against your team. Was this not important?' Minimisation is a cognitive distortion in which the patient minimises the importance of a success incorrectly, while in maximisation, a minor issue is considered to hold importance out of proportion as responsible for the event, often to the exclusion of other contributory factors. In this scenario, the patient may present the sickness before the game as seemingly of little importance, which increases his sense of guilt and responsibility for subsequent events.

Losing the game may mean the end of everything, overshadowing all previous or future achievements. The patient may show catastrophic thinking if he says that not scoring and being picked by the talent scouts means the end of his career. 'I wonder if it's inaccurate that your not being at your best in a single game will mean that you will have no chances of progressing your career in the future.'

By challenging the evident cognitive distortions, you enter into a dialogue with the patient about events, understand the errors in cognitive processing and determine whether they are more widespread, affecting other areas of the patient's life. 'Mr Cole, it seems to me that you are underplaying the importance of being part of a team that held its place and drew. Would you consider other players on the team as also not pulling their weight if they were unwell?'

Another distortion can be selective abstraction in which the patient takes an isolated aspect of an event and makes conclusions based entirely on it while ignoring the broader context. 'Mr Cole, it seems like not getting a goal in that one match, even if others in your team praised your resilience, has come to define you as a player and as a person for everyone who knows you.'

The aim is to demonstrate the distortions and involve the patient in this discussion.

Rapport and communication

The task addresses a whole gamut of psychological skills that you need to have as a clinician and a therapist. There is a need to engage a patient who has recently had an experience that has left him with a confusing mixture of powerful feelings that are made worse by various cognitive distortions. You will need to demonstrate sensitivity and empathy in probing the distortions, which need to be discussed for you to complete the task. The patient may present as either unwilling to speak about his thoughts or becoming overwhelmed with the depth of his feelings.

Conclusion

Here you can summarise what you have discussed, any further information you want to give and what the next steps will be. 'Mr Cole, we have been talking about the recent episode in your game, which has left you very upset and distressed. In talking about this experience, it is clear that this has set off painful feelings. As we discussed, I feel that the sort of thoughts linked to these feelings are making things worse, and this is where CBT could be of use. In CBT, we can explore and work on the thoughts being set off in situations such as what has happened to you and their links to feelings and behaviours. Hence, you are likely to benefit from a course of CBT.'

FURTHER READING

Beck, A. T. (1976) *Cognitive Therapies and Emotional Disorders*. New York, NY: New American Library.

The examiner's mark sheet

Domain/ percentage of marks	Essential points to pass	✓	Extra marks/comments (make notes here)
1. Communication 25% of marks	Clear communication Open and closed questions Empathy Sensitivity		
2. Explaining cognitive distortions 25% of marks	Minimisation Maximisation Selective abstraction Catastrophic thinking (in lay terms)		
3. Treatment options 25% of marks	Psychological therapy discussion – should include CBT		
4. Answering other questions 25 % of marks	Appropriate answers		

% SCORE _____

OVERALL IMPRESSION

___

4   (CIRCLE ONE)

Good Pass

Pass

Borderline

Fail

Clear Fail

NOTES/Areas to improve

STATION 9: PATIENT EXPERIENCING TRANSFERENCE REACTION IN PSYCHODYNAMIC THERAPY

INSTRUCTION TO CANDIDATE

Mr Jones, a patient, is experiencing a transference reaction in psychodynamic therapy and wishes to discontinue. You are not the regular therapist, but the patient has asked to meet another doctor, as he is considering ending treatment.

Explore his experience of therapy from a psychodynamic perspective that is understandable to the patient.

ACTOR (ROLE-PLAYER) INSTRUCTIONS

You have been attending therapy for the past 3 months (it is meant to continue for a period of 1 year). You sought therapy after dissatisfaction in relationships and work. You became very upset when you felt others were critical and unsupportive. In the assessment, you had been reassured to find that your initial thoughts about the reasons for your problems were sufficiently explored and understood. You had grown up in a family where your father ruled with an iron fist and was highly critical and punishing. Your mother had been unable to protect you or your siblings and had instead supported your father or had become another victim of his rules and punishments.

However, you have become increasingly irritated with your therapist, who refuses to reveal anything about herself, while seeming to set harsh and cold rules for the sessions. She does not greet you warmly, say very much or even ask you enough questions, which means you have to do all of the talking. This has left you feeling that she is disinterested and controlling. You are considering leaving the therapy, but have agreed to see another doctor in the service.

SUGGESTED APPROACH

Setting the scene

This situation is problematic, as the patient is not with you in therapy, but is meeting you as he is unwilling to return to see his therapist. 'Mr Jones, I understand there have been some issues with your treatment. Please can you tell me a little about them?' He may speak with some hesitation about his concerns with his therapist. He complains that she does not greet him or say much during the sessions. He has found that the past 3 months have achieved little, with her behaviour remaining unchanged.

Treatment

'Mr Jones, it is concerning that things are not going as well as we would like, but it could be useful for us to think further about these difficulties. Was the process of therapy discussed with you at assessment and before it started?' He may concur that it was, but that the experience in therapy was still disturbing for him. 'Mr Jones, there can sometimes be problems between patient and therapists, but I noticed in the assessment notes that some of these issue have appeared in other settings, such as work.' He may agree and talk about what brought him into therapy, including the difficulties with various bosses and colleagues. He had previously left jobs after he felt badly treated by employers and agrees that he may be sensitive to such experiences, although he still insists that the issues in therapy would not be there if his therapist could just behave differently.

You need to continue to link the past with his current issues. 'Mr Jones, given what you have said so far about these problems happening repeatedly, I wonder if there could be a connection with these coming up in therapy with your therapist.' At this point, he may become more open to thinking about this or continue to resist the idea of the problems being connected to the past. 'It may be that the problems and feelings we are discussing are what brought you into therapy and they need more space for exploration, rather than stopping therapy early.'

Rapport and communication

The task captures the problem of engaging a patient who is having a negative therapeutic reaction as a result of transference. You are not his therapist, but your role is crucial in the task of sensitively helping someone recognise that the problems in therapy do not mean that the therapy itself is at fault, but that it is bringing up issues which need further exploration. This is a crucial interaction, as he is facing a decision of continuing or not with the longer 1–year commitment to the therapy.

Conclusion

Here you can summarise what you have discussed, any further information you want to give and what the next steps will be. 'Mr Jones, we have been talking about the problems that have come up in therapy, which you have attended over the past few months. It's clear that your relationship with your therapist is under strain. You have helpfully spoken about your experiences in therapy and we have explored these and other issues within this and other relationships. We have explored the links between these issues and your early experiences and there was some agreement that this could do with more analysis. Hence, I suggest that you return to the therapy and bring up these issues with your therapist so that you may both explore them.'

FURTHER READING

Sandler, J.J. (1976) Countertransference and role-responsiveness. *International Review of Psycho-Analysis, 3*, 43–7.

Seinfeld, J. (2002). *A Primer for Handling the Negative Therapeutic Reaction.* Lanham, MD: Jason Aronson, Inc.

The examiners mark sheet

Domain/ percentage of marks	Essential points to pass	✓	Extra marks/comments (make notes here)
1. Communication and empathy 25% of marks	Clear communication Open and closed questions Empathy Sensitivity		
2. Exploring the difficulties the patient has been experiencing 25% of marks	Active listening Psychodynamic explanation – considering transference – relating to previous relationships		
3. Management 25% of marks	Agreeing with the next steps in therapy with original therapist		
4. Answering other questions 25% of marks	Appropriate answers Acknowledging the unusual circumstances, as this would normally be worked through with the therapist		

⇧ **% SCORE** _____

___

4

OVERALL IMPRESSION

(CIRCLE ONE)

Good Pass

Pass

Borderline

Fail

Clear Fail

NOTES/Areas to improve

Physical examinations

O GENERAL POINTS FOR ALL PHYSICAL EXAMINATION STATIONS

A structured approach to the physical stations will help you pass well.

Tell the patient that you normally ask if they would like a chaperone, but ask if they are happy to proceed.

Optimally expose the patient whilst maintaining their decency at the start of the physical examination.

Ideally, examine from the patient's right.

Always dress and thank the patient.

Do not make up physical signs. Be honest if unsure of your findings and say that you would ask for further advice (e.g. medical referral).

Use alcohol gel before and after physical examination. The gel will be placed in a prominent position within the station.

STATION 1: ALCOHOL EXAMINATION

> **INSTRUCTION TO CANDIDATE**
>
> You have been asked to see Mr Howard in your clinic. He has been drinking alcohol for many years and would now like help. He has stopped meeting his friends as they also drink heavily and he would like to be 'dry' so that he can get his life back on track.
>
> He saw his GP, who has given him information on local alcohol services and also Alcoholics Anonymous.
>
> As part of your assessment, you want to undertake a physical examination.
>
> **Examine him for the physical stigmata of chronic alcohol misuse.**

ACTOR (ROLE-PLAYER) INSTRUCTIONS

You have been drinking a bottle of vodka a day for the last year. You are happy to be examined and are pleasant and appropriate throughout. You want to stop drinking and acknowledge the need for help.

SUGGESTED APPROACH

Setting the scene

Introduce yourself: 'Hello, my name is Dr_____, it's nice to meet you. I'm glad you've decided to come and talk to me today about the drinking. First of all, would it be OK if I examined you? Please feel free to ask me any questions you have as I go along.'

Completing the tasks

Examine him for the physical stigmata of chronic alcohol misuse.

Gastrointestinal

Abdominal examination is important, as gastritis and peptic ulcer disease are common. Liver disease is common (fatty liver, alcoholic hepatitis, cirrhosis, portal hypertension and carcinoma). Alcohol is also the most common cause of chronic pancreatitis.

Inspection:

- Ask the patient if you can examine his/her 'stomach or tummy.'
- Tell the patient: 'If at any point you are uncomfortable or want me to stop, tell me.'
- Expose the abdomen (and chest if male).
- Look for any obvious abnormalities/clinical signs (e.g. spider naevi, gynaecomastia, tattoos, jaundice [sclera], pigmentation or abdominal distension [ascites]).
- Examine the hands for clubbing, palmar erythema, Dupuytren's contracture or flapping tremor.

Palpation:

- Ask if the patient is comfortable lying flat. Ask that they put their arms by their side.
- Feel the neck and supraclavicular fossae for enlarged lymph nodes (they may be enlarged in carcinoma of the stomach, particularly on the left side).
- Conduct light palpation in all four quadrants. Look at the patient's face and ask if there is any tenderness.
- Deeper palpation: as above, and also in the midline for possible aortic aneurysm.
- Then examine the main organs individually.
- Liver (start in right lower quadrant and work upwards).
- Spleen (start in right lower quadrant and move across to left upper quadrant).
- Kidneys (bilateral palpation of lateral abdomen).

Percussion:

- From the level of the nipple downwards, percuss out both the size of the liver and the spleen.
- The edges of both organs should become apparent.
- Shifting dullness should be demonstrated if ascites is suspected.

Auscultation:

- Bowel sounds
- Renal artery bruits

Musculoskeletal

Chronic alcoholic myopathy affects proximal muscles more prominently. Look at muscle bulk and for evidence of wasting (e.g. thigh muscles).

Cardiovascular (refer to cardiovascular station)

Examine for alcohol associated:

Hypertension

Arrhythmias

Cardiomyopathy and related heart failure

Neurological

Ask some screening questions for cognitive impairment and observe his gait.

Wernicke–Korsakoff syndrome (confusion, ataxia, ophthalmoplegia, nystagmus and peripheral neuropathy)

Alcoholic dementia

Cerebellar degeneration (cerebellar signs – intention tremor, dysdiadochokinesis, nystagmus, dysarthria and broad-based gait)

Dermatological
There are a number of skin changes associated with alcohol:

Facial erythema (alcohol-induced vasodilation)

Psoriasis (mainly of the hands and feet)

Problem solving
As part of a comprehensive physical examination, one would also want to examine the male external genitalia and rectum – you could mention that, ordinarily, this should be done and that his GP could do this.

ADDITIONAL POINTS

Alcohol-related changes occurring in the following areas consist of:

Face:	Scleral icterus, telangiectasia, xanthelasma, Cushingoid facies
Hands:	Clubbing, leukonychia (white nails), palmer erythema, Dupuytren's contracture, hepatic flap (indicating liver cell failure)
Skin:	Spider naevi, loss of axillary hair, jaundice
Abdomen:	Hepatomegaly (a cirrhotic liver may be dull to percussion and small), splenomegaly (in portal hypertension), ascites
Endocrine:	Gynaecomastia, atrophic testes

FURTHER READING
Kelleher, M. (2006) Drugs and alcohol: Physical complications. *Psychiatry*, 5(12), 442–5.

The examiner's mark sheet

Domain/ percentage of marks	Essential points to pass	✓	Extra marks/comments (make notes here)
1. Rapport and communication 25% of marks	Clear communication Open and closed questions Empathy Sensitivity Explanation		
2. Examination 1 35% of marks	Gastrointestinal examination		
3. Examination 2 20% of marks	Other systems (e.g. Neurology)		
4. Addressing other concerns 20% of marks	Appropriate responses		

⬆ **% SCORE**_____

___ **OVERALL IMPRESSION**

4 (CIRCLE ONE)

Good Pass

Pass

Borderline

Fail

Clear Fail

NOTES/Areas to improve

STATION 2: EATING DISORDER

> ### INSTRUCTION TO CANDIDATE
>
> Ms Gordon has been referred with concerns about her nutritional status. She has been an out-of-work model for some time. As a teenager, she was told that she was too fat to ever be successful.
>
> She has had a difficult relationship with food for a number of years and heavily restricts her calorific intake.
>
> Her GP has an interest in mental health and believes she has anorexia nervosa. She has been referred to your out-patient clinic.
>
> **Examine this patient for the physical manifestations of starvation.**

ACTOR (ROLE-PLAYER) INSTRUCTIONS

You feel weak and have only come along at your GP's request. You are anxious at first, but then helpful and allow the doctor to examine you. You wonder if you have cancer.

SUGGESTED APPROACH

Setting the scene

Introduce yourself: 'Hello, my name is Dr_____, it's nice to meet you. I've had a letter from your GP. Do you know why your doctor has referred you to see me today? As part of my assessment, I would like to check you physically. This will include listening to your heart and examining your tummy. Is that OK?'

Mention a chaperone.

Completing the tasks

Examine this patient for the physical manifestations of starvation
If possible, you should weigh her and measure her height.

In anorexia nervosa (AN), body weight is 15% lower than expected, or there is a body mass index (BMI) of 17.5 or less (BMI = weight [kg]/height [m]^2)

Cardiovascular (refer to cardiovascular station)

There is decreased cardiac muscle, chamber size and output. Examine her cardiovascular system and her pulse and lying and sitting blood pressure.

Bradycardia: <60 bpm in 80% of patients

Tachycardia

Hypotension: <90/60, often due to chronic volume depletion

Ventricular arrhythmias: electrolyte disturbances from diuretic/laxative abuse

Cardiac failure: may be terminal event

Electrocardiogram (ECG) changes include sinus bradycardia, ST depression and a prolonged QT interval. Regular ECG monitoring is recommended, especially if severely undernourished.

Cachexia

Examine for loss of body fat and reduced muscle mass (proximal myopathy – ask about difficulty climbing stairs). Ask the patient to squat and then rise again to an upright position – this will be difficult for her if present.

Examine for oedema – this may be present as part of malnutrition, although it may also be due to electrolyte imbalance.

Ask about cold intolerance.

Gastrointestinal (refer to alcohol station)

Conduct an abdominal examination.

Ask specifically about or examine for: enamel and dentine erosion if vomiting frequently.

Benign enlargement of the parotid gland

Mouth – angles of mouth and nutritional deficiency.

Oesophagitis, erosions and ulcers.

Oesophageal rupture (Boerhaave's syndrome) is a complication associated with vomiting after meals (i.e. after binging).

Constipation from inadequate food intake and fluid depletion from diuretics/ laxatives.

Diarrhoea from stimulating laxatives.

Reproduction

Ask her about amenorrhoea and delayed sexual maturation. Absence of menses is a defining feature of AN.

Skin

Examine her for dry skin, Lanugo hair or hirsutism, calluses on her hands (from repeated vomiting), bruising and purpura.

Problem solving

The patient is unlikely to complain of anorexia or weight loss. She may be uncooperative, at least initially. Be supportive and clear as to why you are asking to examine her. Asking about any problems she has been having (e.g. abdominal pain, bloating or constipation) may be a good way to engage her in a dialogue.

ADDITIONAL POINTS

Investigations can be helpful as part of the assessment in anorexia nervosa.

Full blood count (FBC): a pancytopenia is common in severe AN. Leucopoenia is present in up to two-thirds. Mild anaemia and thrombocytopenia can occur in up to a third of patients.

Blood film: there can be morphological changes in red blood cells – acanthocytes (spur cells).

Urea and electrolytes (U&Es): hypokalaemic, hypochloraemic alkalosis and hypomagnesaemia.

Thyroid: reduced thyroid metabolism (low T3 syndrome).

Sex hormones: low luteinizing hormone (LH) and follicle stimulating hormone (FSH).

Osteoporosis: bone density scan (dual energy x-ray absorptiometry [DEXA]).

FURTHER READING

Patrick, L. (2002) Eating disorders: A review of the literature with emphasis on medical complications and clinical nutrition. *Alternative Medicine Review*, 7(3), 184–202.

The examiner's mark sheet

Domain/ percentage of marks	Essential points to pass	✓	Extra marks/comments (make notes here)
1. Rapport and communication 30% of marks	Clear communication		
	Open and closed questions		
	Empathy		
	Sensitivity		
2. Physical examination 30% of marks	Signs of malnutrition		
	Signs of purging		
3. Systems examination 30% of marks	Cardiovascular		
	Gastrointestinal		
	Endocrine		
4. Additional questions 10% of marks	Appropriate responses		
% SCORE _____		___ 4	**OVERALL IMPRESSION** (CIRCLE ONE) **Good Pass** **Pass** **Borderline** **Fail** **Clear Fail** **NOTES/Areas to improve**

STATION 3: EXTRAPYRAMIDAL SIDE EFFECTS

INSTRUCTION TO CANDIDATE

This 28-year-old patient, Mr Brown, began hearing voices 2 months ago. He was seen by the local community psychiatric service and diagnosed with schizophrenia.

The consultant psychiatrist prefers prescribing the older traditional drugs. He will often quote new research indicating that the atypical anti-psychotics have no advantages and are much more expensive.

Having been given 100 mg of chlorpromazine daily, Mr Brown stopped taking it after complaining of uncomfortable legs, stiffness and a feeling of 'unease'. The community psychiatric nurse is concerned that the patient is refusing further treatment and asks you to see him.

Assess this patient for extrapyramidal side effects.

Explain to the patient what has happened and how you will manage him.

ACTOR (ROLE-PLAYER) INSTRUCTIONS

You are restless and a little bit agitated, but allow the doctor to examine you. Your legs in particular feel uncomfortable, and you find it difficult to sit still. You think the medicine has caused these side effects and do not wish to try any further treatment. You do not feel suicidal.

SUGGESTED APPROACH

Setting the scene

Introduce yourself: 'Hello, my name is Dr_____, I'm one of the psychiatrists. I'm sorry to hear that you've been having some problems with your legs and some stiffness. Can you tell me a little bit more about this? That sounds very uncomfortable. So that I can try to help you, would you mind if examined you?'

Mention a chaperone.

Completing the tasks

Physical examination
The patient should be seated, but may be too restless.

Talk the examiner through your examination (based on the Simpson–Angus scale and the Abnormal Involuntary Movement scale).

Start with a general inspection and then move from the face down the body.

Global
Observe for restlessness, inability to sit/stand still and anxious/tense state.

Face

Inspect the following areas:

Expression:	Movements of forehead, eyebrows, periorbital area, cheeks, frowning, blinking and smiling or grimacing
Lips/peri-oral:	Puckering, pouting and lip smacking
Jaw:	Biting, clenching and lateral movements
Tongue:	Increased movement in and out
Salivation:	Look under tongue for increased/pooling of saliva
Glabellar tap:	Tap forehead gently with index finger. Parkinsonian patients continue to blink instead of accommodating after several taps

Upper limbs

Inspect for abnormal resting movements (choreic/athetoid movements):

- Arm dropping: Ask the patient to stand and put arms out to the side, then let them drop. You should demonstrate for the patient. In unaffected individuals, the arms fall freely with a slap and rebound
- Elbow rigidity: Place one hand on the forearm and the other at the elbow. Move back and forth. Feel for stiffness and resistance (lead pipe rigidity)
- Wrist rigidity: As above, except examine flexion, extension, lateral, medial and rotational movements (cog wheeling if tremor is superimposed)
- Legs: Observe the resting legs (e.g. restlessness). If possible, examine the patient on a couch so that the feet do not touch the ground. Ask the patient to swing their legs (demonstrate if necessary). Look to see if legs swing freely or if there is resistance
- Gait: Ask the patient to walk five to ten paces away and then back again. Is there reduced arm swing, stiff gait or a stooped, shuffling gait (Parkinsonian features)?

Explain what has happened

'This is very likely to be a side effect of the medication, which can sometimes happen.' Acknowledge that this can feel very unpleasant. The medication that he has been taking works on brain receptors (dopamine, D2) that help with their illness, and is also involved in controlling movements. Thank the patient for telling the nurse because it is something you can help with. Explain that the newer medications have less activity against this receptor and are less likely to produce this side effect. Arrange for the nurse to follow up closely over the next few weeks and arrange to see the patient again in out-patients soon.

Management

Further management depends on the type of side effect. It is important to discuss treatment options with the patient.

Dystonic reactions

Unlikely here (usually in early stages of treatment)

Includes oculogyric crisis and torticollis

Anticholinergic treatment (per os/intramuscularly/intravenously)

Withdraw anti-psychotic

Pseudo-Parkinsonism
Tremor, rigidity and bradykinesia

Can be treated with anticholinergics

Change to an atypical anti-psychotic

Akathisia
Reduce anti-psychotic or switch to an atypical such as olanzapine or quetiapine

Responds poorly to anticholinergics

Other treatment options might include propranolol, benzodiazepines, cyproheptadine and clonidine

Seek senior advice if no improvement

Tardive dyskinesia
Think of risk factors (e.g. female or elderly)

Withdraw any antimuscarinic

Consider withdrawing anti-psychotic or changing to an atypical

Consider clozapine if appropriate

Vitamin E, clonazepam and propranolol

Problem solving
Have a discussion about alternative anti-psychotics.

It is important to discuss continued engagement with psychiatric services as the patient will need monitoring.

Ask the patient how they feel about these symptoms and enquire about risk (to self/others).

It is important that any agitation is not simply attributed to akathisia, but that psychosis is considered. Ask how his thoughts have been since stopping the chlorpromazine and whether the voices he used to hear have returned.

ADDITIONAL POINTS

Tardive dyskinesia is difficult to treat and its aetiology is more complex than it appears. Anyone treated with anti-psychotics is at risk of developing this condition, although greater risk may occur in those with an affective illness, diabetes, learning disability (LD), females and the elderly.

FURTHER READING

Gervin, M. & Barnes, T.R.E. (2000) Assessment of drug-related movement disorders in schizophrenia. *Advances in Psychiatric Treatment*, 6, 332–4.

Taylor, D., Paton, C. & Kerwin, R. (eds) (2007) *The Maudsley Prescribing Guidelines*, 9th edn. London: Informa.

The examiner's mark sheet

Domain/percentage of marks	Essential points to pass	✓	Extra marks/comments (make notes here)
1. Rapport and communication 25% of marks	Clear communication Open and closed questions Empathy Sensitivity		
2. Examination for extrapyramidal side effects 35% of marks	Appropriate examination		
3. Explanation of symptoms 15% of marks	In lay terms Medication side effects		
4. Management plan 15% of marks	Alternative treatment Risks versus benefits		
5. Other queries 10% of marks	Appropriate responses		Ask about low mood, thoughts of self-harm or suicide

% SCORE _____

___

5

OVERALL IMPRESSION

(CIRCLE ONE)

Good Pass

Pass

Borderline

Fail

Clear Fail

NOTES/Areas to improve

STATION 4: THYROID DYSFUNCTION

INSTRUCTION TO CANDIDATE

Mrs Lloyd has been taking lithium for 12 years. She is an intensive care unit charge nurse working in a busy teaching hospital. Her bipolar illness had been poorly controlled prior to this and she was admitted to a psychiatric ward where lithium was commenced. Mrs Lloyd is keen to continue with the lithium treatment as she has been on various treatments which she could not tolerate or were ineffective. Recently, she has noticed that her neck has become more prominent and has questioned whether the lithium could be causing this.

She has had some blood tests:

Blood test	Result	Reference range/value
Thyroid stimulating hormone (TSH)	3.56	0.34–5.6
Free T4	0.9	0.6–1.6
Free T3	2.9	2.5–3.9
Anti-thyroperoxidase (TPO)	435	<35
Parathyroid hormone (PTH)	29	12–65
Calcium	9.3	8.3–10.5
T3: total	1.0	0.9–1.8

Conduct an appropriate physical examination, explain her blood results and discuss how you intend to manage her.

ACTOR (ROLE-PLAYER) INSTRUCTIONS

You are an intelligent and inquisitive individual. You understand the terminology and basic principles relating to thyroid function and you would like a clear management plan. You are a no-nonsense type.

SUGGESTED APPROACH

Setting the scene

Introduce yourself: 'Hello, my name is Dr_____, it's nice to meet you, I'm one of the psychiatrists. I understand you've noticed that your neck has changed. When did you first notice this? Would it be OK if I examine you and then we could talk about your blood results?'

Remember to mention a chaperone.

Completing the tasks

Physical examination
Inspection:

> Patient should be sitting with their neck in a neutral or slightly extended position.
>
> Ask the patient if you can examine her neck.
>
> Expose the neck.
>
> Make a show of looking at the thyroid from the front. A goitre or enlarged thyroid nodule may be visible.
>
> To enhance visualisation of the thyroid, one can extend the neck.
>
> Look at the eyes from the sides and from above.
>
> Next, ask the subject to 'Take a sip of water and hold it in your mouth.'
>
> Looking at the neck, say 'Now swallow.'
>
> Watch for any goitre moving upwards as they swallow.

Palpation:

Ask the patient if you can feel her neck.

Stand behind her and to the right. This is less threatening than standing directly behind.

With the fingers of both hands, feel the left and right lobes of the thyroid. Ensure the neck is slightly flexed to ease palpation.

Attempt to locate the thyroid isthmus by palpating between the cricoid cartilage and the suprasternal notch.

Move your hands laterally to try to feel under the sternocleidomastoids for the fullness of the thyroid.

Assess hard or soft texture and the presence of any nodules.

Assess the extent of any enlargement.

Again, ask the patient to swallow some water whilst feeling a possible goitre move beneath the examining fingers.

Examine local lymph nodes as the carcinoma (CA) thyroid can spread to local lymphatics.

Percussion:

If able to, percuss the manubrium sterni to see if a goitre extends downwards (dullness) into the chest.

Auscultation:

If a stethoscope is available, listen to both lobes of the thyroid for bruits.

Thyroid status:

Examine their hands for tremor (hyperthyroidism), sweaty palms, erythema and thyroid acropachy.

Pulse: rate and rhythm (atrial fibrillation [AF] and sinus bradycardia).

Examine for brisk/slowly relaxing tendon reflexes (hyper/hypothyroid, respectively)

Examine their eyes specifically for lid retraction (sclera visible above cornea) and lid lag, exophthalmos (sclera visible above the lower lid is a sign of Graves' disease and not related to thyroid status).

Comment on any hair loss, dry flaky skin, lateral loss of eyebrows, hoarse croaky voice or carpel tunnel syndrome (hypothyroidism).

Enquire about intolerance to heat/cold, weight change and appetite.

Ask about increased agitation (hyperthyroid).

Problem solving

Interpretation of results

Feed back to the patient about your findings from the physical examination if you have not already done so. Do not make up findings; if the thyroid feels normal, then say so.

You will need to explain to her that her thyroid function tests are all within the normal range. However, her thyroid antibodies are high. As a professional colleague, ask her if she has heard of Hashimoto's thyroiditis. It is an autoimmune disease of the thyroid that is often associated with normal or hypothyroid function. Suggest to her that she needs to be seen by an endocrinologist as a first step. Certainly you would not be suggesting that she discontinues the lithium at this point.

She may need thyroid medication, but you will be asking the endocrinologist to advise on further management.

She might ask you about alternative treatments should the physician advise that lithium is withdrawn. This would demand a discussion about the mood stabilisers, including the anticonvulsants and also the anti-psychotics.

ADDITIONAL POINTS

You can talk to the patient in order to describe the physical examination as it is being performed or summarise when the examination is completed. When finished, thank the patient.

Note: an enlarged thyroid is referred to as a goitre. There is no direct correlation between size and function – a person with a goitre can be clinically euthyroid or hypo- or hyper-thyroid.

A normal thyroid is estimated to be 10 g with an upper limit of 20 g or 2–4 teaspoons.

Thyroid nodules are common (prevalence 4%). Half of the thyroid glands examined by ultrasound or direct visualisation (surgery or autopsy) have nodules. Less than 5% of all nodules are cancerous.

Differential diagnosis for an enlarged thyroid gland

- Multinodular goitre
- Graves' disease
- Familial goitre
- Hashimoto's thyroiditis
- Painless postpartum thyroiditis
- Malignancy
- Iodine deficiency goitre
- Iodine excess

FURTHER READING

Epstein, O., Solomons, N., Perkin, G.D., Cookson, J. & De Bono, D.P. (2003) *Clinical Examination,* 3rd edn. London: Mosby – Year Book Europe Ltd.

The examiner's mark sheet

Domain/ percentage of marks	Essential points to pass	✓	Extra marks/comments (make notes here)
1. Rapport and communication 25% of marks	Clear communication		
	Open and closed questions		
	Empathy		
	Sensitivity		

2. Thyroid examination
   20% of marks

   Inspection

   Palpation

   Percussion

   Auscultation

3. Enquiry about thyroid status
   20% of marks

   Symptoms and signs of thyroid dysfunction

4. Blood test results
   25% of marks

   Explanation of blood test results

5. Management plan
   10% of marks

   Options based on findings

% SCORE_____

_____ **OVERALL IMPRESSION**

5 (CIRCLE ONE)

Good Pass

Pass

Borderline

Fail

Clear Fail

NOTES/Areas to improve

STATION 5: LOWER LIMBS

INSTRUCTION TO CANDIDATE

Mr King is reporting having lost the ability to walk. There was a recent 'incident' and, since this time, he has been reporting a loss of function.

The GP made an urgent referral to the neurologist who saw him within 10 days. The neurologist reported that the patient showed 'no obvious course for his functional loss. The pattern of paralysis was not typical and plantar reflexes were present and down going. There is no evidence of muscular atrophy. Of note, I believe that the muscles are capable of reacting when the patient's attention is directed elsewhere.' Nerve conduction studies are reported as normal.

Examine this gentleman's lower limbs.

ACTOR (ROLE-PLAYER) INSTRUCTIONS

You cannot walk and report weakness in your legs; you need a wheelchair to mobilise. You do not believe the psychological explanation for your symptoms, but do not deny that the onset followed your redundancy after 20 years in the same company.

SUGGESTED APPROACH

Setting the scene

Introduce yourself: 'Hello, my name is Dr_____, I'm one of the psychiatrists.' Be prepared for some hostility as it is clear that he is not keen on seeing a psychiatrist.

'Thank you for seeing me today. I understand from your GP that you've had some difficulties with your legs. Could you tell me what's been happening? Could you tell me about the 'incident' which happened recently? Would it be OK if I examine your legs?'

Mention that you would normally offer a chaperone, but ask whether he is happy to proceed without this today.

Completing the tasks

What to do next

The subject should ideally be on an examination couch.

Expose the legs and remove any socks.

By explaining what you are doing at each step, you are letting the examiner know you are competent.

Inspection

Look for any obvious abnormalities/deformities.

Skin colour/rashes.

Muscle bulk (wasting).

Muscle fasciculation (motor neuron disease).

Restlessness (extrapyramidal side effects; ask about any medication).

Tone
'I'm just going to move your legs; let them go all floppy.'

Examine each leg by moving it passively at the hip and knee joints. Roll the leg sideways and bend the knees backwards and forwards on the couch/bed. Lift the knee and let it drop. With the legs hanging over the side of the bed, lift the leg and let it drop. Observe natural swing at the knee.

Look in particular for increased/decreased tone and evidence of cog-wheeling or lead pipe rigidity.

Power
Ask the subject to:

1. 'Lift your leg straight up, don't let me push it down' (L1, L2)
2. With his knee bent, ask to 'push against my hand' (L3, L4)
3. 'Bend your knee, don't let me straighten it' (L5, S1, S2)
4. 'Point your toes up towards your face, don't let me push them down' (L4, L5)

Coordination
Ask the subject to place his heel just below his knee and run it down his shin then back up and down once more. Ask to repeat with the other foot.

Reflexes

Knee jerk (L3, L4)

Ankle jerk (L5, S1)

Plantar response (start at outer part of sole, move inwards towards big toe)

Sensation

Ideally, one should test light touch and pinprick in the following areas. Test the same dermatomes on each leg:

Outer thigh (L2)

Inner thigh (L3)

Inner calf (L4)

Outer calf (L5)

Inner foot (L5)

Outer foot (S1)

Vibration sense can be tested in the medial malleoli (if tuning fork is present), as can joint position sense (up and down).

Gait

Ask if the subject is OK to walk for you (he is likely to decline)

Observe his normal gait

Then ask him to walk heel to toe (ataxia)

Romberg's test

Ask the patient to put his feet together, stretch out his arms and close his eyes

Stand in front of the patient with your own arms outstretched to ensure they do not fall

Problem solving

For the purposes of the examination, you will probably not be expected to examine pinprick sensation. Light touch using either cotton wool or asking the patient to close their eyes and say 'yes' when they feel you touching them with a finger should suffice.

ADDITIONAL POINTS

Romberg's test is only positive if the subject is more unsteady with their eyes closed.

A positive Romberg's test indicates a loss of proprioception (e.g. subacute combined degeneration of the cord and tabes dorsalis).

FURTHER READING

Epstein, O., Solomons, N., Perkin, G.D., Cookson, J. & De Bono, D.P. (2003) *Clinical Examination*, 3rd edn. London: Mosby – Year Book Europe Ltd.

The examiner's mark sheet

Domain/ percentage of marks	Essential points to pass	✓	Extra marks/comments (make notes here)
1. Rapport and communication 30% of marks	Clear communication Open and closed questions Empathy Sensitivity		
2. Examination 30% of marks	Tone Power Reflexes		Bilateral
3. Further examination 30% of marks	Coordination Sensation Gait		Bilateral He may refuse, but asking secures the marks
4. Functional assessment 10% of marks	Asks about recent stressors and life events and their meaning		

% SCORE_____

___ **OVERALL IMPRESSION**

4 (CIRCLE ONE)

Good Pass

Pass

Borderline

Fail

Clear Fail

NOTES/Areas to improve

STATION 6: UPPER LIMBS

INSTRUCTION TO CANDIDATE

Mrs Kleiner was admitted to the clinical decisions unit at her local hospital. She was brought in by her family, who have become concerned that she is unable to move her left arm. The accident and emergency doctor has examined her and performed routine blood tests and a computed tomography brain scan, which are all within normal parameters. You are the psychiatrist on call and have been asked to assess her. Although you are aware that she has already been examined, you are keen to assess her yourself.

Perform a neurological examination of her upper limbs.

ACTOR (ROLE-PLAYER) INSTRUCTIONS

You are perplexed as to the loss of function in your left arm. It happened suddenly 48 hours ago. Your daughter, with whom you have always been close, has decided to move to Australia in the next month. You deny that this is upsetting for you. There are no other stressors.

SUGGESTED APPROACH

Setting the scene

Introduce yourself: 'Hello, my name is Dr_____, I'm one of the psychiatrists. I know that you've already seen one of the doctors, but could I ask you to briefly tell me what has been happening with your arm? Would it be OK if I examine you? Has anything stressful happened recently?'

Mention a chaperone.

Completing the tasks

The subject should ideally be on an examination couch and optimally exposed.

By explaining what you are doing at each step to the patient, you are letting the examiner know you are competent.

Inspection

Look for any obvious asymmetry/deformities in the arms and hands.

Skin colour.

Muscle bulk (wasting).

Muscle fasciculation (motor neuron disease).

Tremor (extrapyramidal side effects or Parkinson's disease).

Tone

'I'm just going to move your arms; let them go floppy.'

Examine each arm by passively bending the elbow joint to and fro. Flex and extend the hand at the wrist and rotate the hand to detect cog-wheel rigidity (Parkinson's disease).

Power

Demonstrate movements to make instructions easier.

Ask the patient to:

1. Put arms at right angles to their body, 'Don't let me push them down' (deltoid, C5)
2. Bend elbow, 'Don't let me straighten it' (biceps C5/6)
3. Push each arm out straight against your resistance (triceps C7)
4. 'Squeeze my fingers,' offer two fingers (C8, T1)
5. Keep fingers straight, 'Don't let me bend them' (motor C7/radial)
6. Spread your fingers out, 'Don't let me push them together' (dorsal interossei – ulnar)
7. Point your thumb to the ceiling, 'Don't let me push it down'
8. Put your thumb and little finger together, 'Don't let me pull them apart'

Coordination

1. 'Tap quickly on the back of your hand' (demonstrate)
2. 'Touch my finger touch your nose' (test)

Reflexes

Biceps jerk (C5, C6)

Triceps jerk (C7)

Supinator (C5, C6)

Sensation

Ideally, one should test light touch and pinprick in the following areas (although for the purposes of the exam, a light touch using either cotton wool or a finger should be adequate). Ask the patient to close their eyes and tell you when they feel something. Reassure them that you will be gentle.

Shoulder (C4, C5)

Upper arm (C5, C6)

Forearm (C6, C7, T1)

Hand (C6, C7, C8)

Vibration and joint position sense can also be tested.

Problem solving

Once the physical examination is complete, help the patient get dressed, thank her and explain your findings. If your examination is normal and there is time, a conversation about psychological contributory factors may ensue. Take care not to upset the patient if possible, as this will be an unsatisfactory end to the station. Establish whether she believes her presentation could have a psychological component. The use of normalisation here is very helpful.

ADDITIONAL POINTS

A discussion related to management may follow and you should explain that you have only had time to conduct a physical examination. You would want to look at her health records, speak to the GP and invite her back for a consultation where you would take a thorough history of recent and past events that could account for her presentation.

FURTHER READING

Epstein, O., Solomons, N., Perkin, G.D., Cookson, J. & De Bono, D.P. (2003) *Clinical Examination*, 3rd edn. Elsevier Health Sciences.

The examiner's mark sheet

Domain/ percentage of marks	Essential points to pass	✓	Extra marks/comments (make notes here)
1. Rapport and communication 30% of marks	Clear communication Open and closed questions Empathy Sensitivity		

⇧ 2. Examination	Tone	Bilaterally
30% of marks	Power	
	Reflexes	
3. Further examination	Coordination	Bilaterally
30% of marks	Sensation	
4. Appropriate questioning	Asks about recent stressors/ life events	
10% of marks		

% SCORE_____

___

4   OVERALL IMPRESSION
(CIRCLE ONE)

Good Pass

Pass

Borderline

Fail

Clear Fail

NOTES/Areas to improve

STATION 7: CRANIAL NERVES

INSTRUCTION TO CANDIDATE

Whilst trying to get out of a chair on the ward, Michael, a 78-year-old depressed gentleman, lost his footing and fell over. The fall was witnessed by nursing staff who observed him hit his head. He was difficult to rouse at first but soon became re-orientated. He has a haematoma to his left temple and is complaining of a headache. The staff also report that he appears to be more irritable following the fall.

Examine this gentleman's cranial nerves.

Do not examine:

• **Smell**

• **Pinprick to face**

• **Gag reflex**

• **Corneal reflex**

ACTOR (ROLE-PLAYER) INSTRUCTIONS

You are a little confused following the fall, but reasonably orientated. You are downplaying the incident and think a fuss is being made over nothing. You would like to go to your room and back to bed, but you allow an examination by the doctor. You do not have any abnormal symptoms or signs.

SUGGESTED APPROACH

Setting the scene

Introduce yourself: 'Hello, my name is Dr_____, it's nice to meet you. Can I ask your name? I was told about your fall. Can you remember what happened? How is your head now? Do you have any concerns at the moment? Do you feel confused, or sick at all? I would like to examine you. This will involve looking at your eyes and testing your hearing, would that be OK?'

Completing the tasks

What to do next

Ask the patient if you can examine him.

Tell him to 'let you know if he's uncomfortable at any point.'

The patient should be sitting.

Mention a chaperone.

Cranial nerves (CN)

(I)	'Do you have any problems with your sense of smell?'
(II)	'Do you have any problems with your eyesight?'
	Ask to put on glasses if he normally wears them
	'Can you see that clock on the wall?' (or similar distant object)
	'What does it say?'
(II)	Visual fields
	Use your finger or red-headed pin if available
	'Keep looking at my nose.' Ask the subject to cover one eye
	'Tell me when you see the pin.' Map out their field of vision
	Light reflex and accommodation – convergence reflex (with your finger close to their nose, ask them to look at an object in the distance and then at your finger)
	Fundoscopy (refer to eye station)
(III, IV, VI)	Eye movements (keep the head still)
	'Can you see my finger? Keep looking at it whilst it moves'
	Move in the shape of a cross
	At the extremes of their gaze, ask whether they can see one or two fingers (i.e. double vision). Also look for nystagmus
(VII)	Facial movement
	'Raise eyebrows, screw eyes up tight, puff out cheeks, whistle, show me your teeth'
(V)	'Clench your teeth.' As they do, feel masseter and temporalis
	'Open your mouth and stop me closing it.' Gently try to close chin
(IX, X)	Palate and gag reflex
	'Open your mouth and say 'aah'.' Look at the back of the throat

Gag reflex – touch the back of throat on both sides with an orange stick*

(XII)   Tongue

Ask to stick tongue out. Observe for deviation to left/right

Observe resting tongue for wasting and fasciculation

(XI)   Accessory nerve

'Shrug your shoulders and don't let me push them down'

'Turn your head to the right' (feel left sternomastoid) 'And to the right' (feel right side)

(VIII)   Hearing

'How is your hearing?'

Can they hear you rubbing your index finger against your thumb in each ear?

(V)   Trigeminal – sensation

'Can you feel me when I touch here?' Use finger/cotton wool. Examine ophthalmic, maxillary and mandibular territories (corneal reflex*)

Problem solving

Should be able to assess all nerves within 7 minutes.

ADDITIONAL POINTS

- Smell and taste (I, VII, IX)
- Visual acuity (II)
- Visual field (II)
- Eye movements (II, IV, VI)
- Nystagmus (VIII and cerebellum)
- Ptosis (III, sympathetic)
- Pupils (III)
- Discs (II)
- Facial movements (V, VII)
- Palatal movements (IX, X)
- Gag reflex (IX, X)
- Tongue (XII)
- Accessory (XI)
- Hearing (VIII)
- Facial sensation (V)
- Corneal reflex (V)

FURTHER READING

Epstein, O., Solomons, N., Perkin, G.D., Cookson, J. & De Bono, D.P. (2003) *Clinical Examination*, 3rd edn. London: Mosby – Year Book Europe Ltd.

---

* Will often be asked to omit pinprick, corneal and gag testing, but be able to do them in practice.

The examiner's mark sheet

Domain/ percentage of marks	Essential points to pass	✓	Extra marks/comments (make notes here)
1. Rapport and communication 25% of marks	Clear communication Open and closed questions Empathy Sensitivity		
2. Examination 65% of marks	Shows competency in demonstrating knowledge of cranial examination (CN I–XII)		
3. Clinical management 10% of marks	Although not specifically requested, in view of the clinical scenario, the need for a medical/ neurological assessment of further investigations should be considered		

% SCORE _____

___

3

OVERALL IMPRESSION

(CIRCLE ONE)

Good Pass

Pass

Borderline

Fail

Clear Fail

NOTES/Areas to improve

STATION 8: CARDIOVASCULAR SYSTEM

INSTRUCTION TO CANDIDATE

You are called to the psychiatric intensive care unit. This patient, detained under the Mental Health Act, was restrained following aggressive and threatening behaviour that was putting other patients and staff at risk. He has subsequently settled somewhat with a time out and oral olanzapine and clonazepam, but is now complaining of chest pain. You are called to see him.

Examine this patient's cardiovascular system.

ACTOR (ROLE-PLAYER) INSTRUCTIONS

You have calmed down, but are still upset as to how you were treated earlier on. You have central, crushing chest pain. You are a smoker. You ask if you are having a heart attack. You do not feel sick. You do not have pain radiating anywhere else. You do not have a known cardiac history.

SUGGESTED APPROACH

Setting the scene

Introduce yourself: 'Hello, my name is Dr_____, I'm one of the doctors. I understand you've had some chest pain, when did it start? Can you tell me what it feels like? Where is the pain now? Is the pain travelling anywhere or is it only in your chest? I need to examine your heart, would that be OK?'

Mention that you normally offer a chaperone, but ask whether it would be OK to proceed without.

Completing the tasks

Remember inspection, palpation and auscultation.

Expose the patient's chest while he is lying at 45° on the bed.

Explain that if he feels uncomfortable at any point to let you know.

Whilst explaining the above, look for features of anxiety or shortness of breath.

Hands:	Sweaty, hot/cold and erythematous/cyanosed. Nails for splinter haemorrhages/clubbing
Radial pulse:	Rate and rhythm (tell patient; e.g. 80 bpm is regular)
Blood pressure:	Sitting (tell patient reading)
Jugular venous pulse (JVP):	Lie patient at 45° and observe
Face:	Look at face, eyes, tongue and mouth
Inspection:	Chest: inspect for any abnormalities. Observe breathing pattern
Palpate:	Feel for the apex beat and for any heaves or thrills.
Auscultate:	Listen to the heart sounds. Try to pick up any abnormal flow murmurs at the apex (mitral – fourth intercostal space). Listen at second intercostal (IC) space (pulmonary artery – left, aortic – right). Listen over the carotids
Lungs:	Listen to the lung bases for any inspirational crepitations (congestive cardiac failure [CCF])
Oedema:	Check ankle for pitting oedema. If present, determine its extent. Press gently

Problem solving

The patient may be anxious or distressed and need reassurance. A discussion about how you intend to manage him is possible. Offer some analgesia/aspirin if appropriate. If you believe the pain to be cardiogenic, explain the need for further investigations (bloods, ECG and chest x-ray [CXR]). If you are concerned that he has had a myocardial infarct, immediate management and emergency transfer will need to be organised.

ADDITIONAL POINTS

Remember to dress the patient and thank them when you have finished your physical examination. Explain your findings.

FURTHER READING

Epstein, O., Solomons, N., Perkin, G.D., Cookson, J. & De Bono, D.P. (2003) *Clinical Examination*, 3rd edn. London: Mosby – Year Book Europe Ltd.

The examiner's mark sheet

Domain/ percentage of marks	Essential points to pass	✓	Extra marks/comments (make notes here)
1. Rapport and communication 25% of marks	Clear communication Open and closed questions Empathy Sensitivity		
2. Examination 1 25% of marks	Inspection		
3. Examination 2 25% of marks	Palpation Auscultation		
4. Management 15% of marks	Reassurance Explains plan		
5. Answering additional questions 10% of marks	Appropriate responses		

% SCORE_____

___

5

OVERALL IMPRESSION

(CIRCLE ONE)

Good Pass

Pass

Borderline

Fail

Clear Fail

NOTES/Areas to improve

STATION 9: EYE EXAMINATION

INSTRUCTION TO CANDIDATE

Mr Khan has come back to see you in your out-patient clinic. She has bipolar affective disorder and has been commenced on carbamazepine, as she has a rapid cycling condition and could not tolerate lithium. She is anxious as she has developed blurred vision and occasional diplopia.

Examine her eyes.

ACTOR (ROLE-PLAYER) INSTRUCTIONS

You are anxious that you have experienced a change in your vision and wish to know whether it relates to your medication. You cooperate with the examination.

SUGGESTED APPROACH

Setting the scene

Introduce yourself: 'Hello, nice to see you again. I'm sorry to learn you've had some problems with your eyes. Could you tell me how your vision has been since we last met? I would like to examine your eyes. Would that be OK? Part of the examination will involve shining a light into your eyes, so let me know if it is uncomfortable at any point.'

Mention the chaperone.

Completing the tasks

You are asked to examine her eyes, so remember to perform a complete eye examination (i.e. CN II–VI, not just fundoscopy).

Visual acuity
Monocular (i.e. test each eye individually) finger count: 'How many fingers do you see?'

Visual fields
Monocular: ask the patient to cover one eye; you cover your eye on the opposite side so that you are comparing the patient's visual fields to your own. 'Keep looking at my eye.'

Test the patient's upper and lower temporal quadrants by moving your wagging finger from the periphery to the centre. Ask them to say 'yes' when they see your finger moving. To test their nasal fields, you need to swap hands. Any area of field defect will become obvious by comparing the patient's visual fields to your own. Do the same for the other eye.

Eye movements (ocular palsy, nystagmus and lid lag)
Binocular (i.e. both eyes together): 'Follow my finger with your eyes. Keep your head still.'

Move your finger in the shape of an 'H' from side to side, then up and down at the extremes. Ask if they can see one finger clearly, and ask whether the image changes.

Reflexes
First accommodation – convergence reflex: 'Look into the distance. Now look at my finger.' Place your index finger close to the patient's nose; if normal, pupils will constrict.

Light reflex: pick up the ophthalmoscope, switch it on and check that it works. Shine the light into each eye twice to check direct and consensual reflexes.

Fundoscopy
Hold on to the ophthalmoscope to examine the patient's fundi. 'I'm going to look at the back of your eyes now. I will need to get quite close – please let me know if it is too uncomfortable and I will stop.' Tell the patient to fixate on a distant target. Examine the patient's right eye with your right eye and then his left eye with your left eye. Sit at arm's length opposite the patient. Aim to find the optic disc and comment on this and the appearance of blood vessels around it. Come away from the fundus once you have had a good view.

Optic disc
Locate and bring it into focus. Look for size, blurred disc edge, cupping (glaucoma), new vessels (diabetic retinopathy) and a pale disc (e.g. optic atrophy).

Blood vessels
Arteries are narrower and brighter and have a reflective, pale streak.

Start at the disc and follow the vessels out to look for hypertensive changes (A-V nipping) and atherosclerotic changes.

The fundus

Look for haemorrhages, exudates, cotton wool spots, new vessel formation and micro-aneurysms.

Ask the subject to look straight at the light in order to examine the macula.

Be familiar with the basic appearance of:

Papilloedema: blurred disc edge, haemorrhages, hard exudates (late feature) and cotton wool spots (due to retinal infarction)

Diabetic retinopathy: micro-aneurysms, small haemorrhages, exudates, cotton wool spots and new vessel formation (proliferative diabetic retinopathy)

Hypertensive retinopathy: silver wiring, A-V nipping, haemorrhages, cotton wool spots and disc swelling if malignant

Glaucoma: optic disc enlargement, undermining of the disc margins and blood vessel bowing (advanced)

Photocoagulation (laser) scars

Optic atrophy

Problem solving

If faced with a mannequin in the examination, treat it as you would a real patient.

ADDITIONAL POINTS

Describe any features with reference to a clock face and optic disc size (i.e. 'There are soft exudates at 3 o'clock, two disc diameters away from the disc').

Explain that, ideally, you would like to examine the retinas in a dark room or dilate the pupils to get a better view (1% cyclopentolate).

FURTHER READING

Epstein, O., Solomons, N., Perkin, G.D., Cookson, J. & De Bono, D.P. (2003) *Clinical Examination*, 3rd edn. London: Mosby – Year Book Europe Ltd.

The examiner's mark sheet

Domain/ percentage of marks	Essential points to pass	✓	Extra marks/comments (make notes here)
1. Rapport and communication 25% of marks	Clear communication		
	Open and closed questions		
	Empathy		
	Sensitivity		
2. Examination 1 20% of marks	Visual acuity		
3. Examination 2 20% of marks	Eye movements		

⇧ 4. Examination 3   Reflexes
       25% of marks
    5. Examination 4   Fundi
       10% of marks
    % SCORE_____

___

5

OVERALL IMPRESSION

(CIRCLE ONE)

Good Pass

Pass

Borderline

Fail

Clear Fail

NOTES/Areas to improve

STATION 10: BASIC LIFE SUPPORT

INSTRUCTION TO CANDIDATE

You are on call. A nurse bleeps you asking if you could attend to a patient who has collapsed on the ward. When you arrive, you are told that he is unconscious and does not appear to be breathing. There is no equipment/defibrillator available.

Manage this situation.

ACTOR (ROLE-PLAYER) INSTRUCTIONS

There will be a mannequin (patient) and a nurse at this station.

SUGGESTED APPROACH

Setting the scene

The patient is unconscious and non-responsive. There is also a member of staff in this scenario.

'Hello, I'm the on-call doctor, Dr_____, could you quickly tell me what happened and how long he's been like this?'

Completing the tasks

You will most likely be presented with a Resuscitation Annie. Do not stop to have a chat with the nurse, but talk to her as you are assessing the patient (based on the Basic Life Support algorithm, Resuscitation Council UK, 2005)

1. Ensure the safety of the patient and yourself.
2. Check the patient and see if they respond.

   Gently shake shoulder and ask loudly 'Are you OK?'

3. If he does not respond:

   Shout for help from a nurse.

   Turn the patient onto his back and open the airway by gently tilting the head back and chin lift.

4. Keeping the airway open and look, listen and feel for breathing.

   Look for chest movement and listen for breath sounds.

   Feel for air on your cheek.

   Spend no more than 10 seconds deciding whether the patient is breathing normally.

5. If unresponsive and not breathing normally:

   Send someone for help (999, crash team, resus trolley and antiepileptic drug [AED]).

   If on your own, do not leave the patient.

   Start chest compressions.

   Do not apply pressure over the lower tip of the sternum or upper abdomen. Depress the sternum by 4–5 cm during a compression.

   After each compression, release all of the pressure on the chest, but do not let go of your hands.

   Repeat at a rate of approximately 100 times a minute (a little less than two compressions a second).

6. Combine chest compression and rescue breaths.

   After 30 compressions, open the airway again using head tilt and chin lift.

   Give two slow, effective rescue breaths, each of which should make the chest rise and fall.

   Ensure head tilt and chin lift.

   Pinch the nose closed with the finger and thumb of the hand on the forehead.

   Open the mouth a little (maintain chin lift).

   Take a deep breath, place lips around their mouth and make sure you have a good seal.

   Blow steadily for approximately 2 seconds and watch chest rise.

   Continue with chest compressions and rescue breaths at a ratio of 30:2.

   Stop to recheck the patient only if he starts breathing normally; otherwise, continue resuscitation.

7. Continue resuscitation until:

   Help arrives and can take over.

   Victim starts breathing.

   You become exhausted.

Problem solving

Ideally, you would want to protect yourself by using a reservoir bag and mask for ventilation, rather than 'mouth to mouth'. Ask the nurse whether the patient has any known infectious diseases.

Dilated pupils are an unreliable sign, so continue cardiopulmonary resuscitation if present.

Mouth to nose ventilation can be used if, for example, mouth obstruction cannot be relieved.

Ask the nurse if there is any resuscitation equipment available. Explain that you want to use the resus trolley to get a cardiac tracing and start defibrillation if required.

Ask the nurse to call for help early on in the scenario, especially if no equipment is available.

ADDITIONAL POINTS

Once you establish that the person is not breathing and is unresponsive, start immediate resuscitation.

Get as much history from the nurse as possible; for example, is this a drug overdose or suicide attempt? Can you initiate pharmacological treatment (e.g. flumazenil in benzodiazepine overdose)? Ask about other vital signs.

Ask if the nurse has been trained in cardiopulmonary resuscitation, as this could allow you to examine the patient more thoroughly whilst she continues chest compressions.

If the cervical spine is damaged, as in a hanging attempt, care must be taken to maintain the alignment of the head, neck and chest. Use minimal head tilt when opening airway.

FURTHER READING

Resuscitation Council (UK) (2005) www.resus.org.uk. Check this website for more information and any updates to guidelines.

The examiner's mark sheet

Domain/ percentage of marks	Essential points to pass	✓	Extra marks/comments (make notes here)
1. Communication 25% of marks	Clear communication and instructions (e.g. requesting assistance and resuscitation protocol)		
2. Information gathering 25% of marks	Points from the nurse Background history		
3. Risk/safe resuscitation 50% of marks	Ensures a safe environment		
	Use of resuscitation equipment and automatic external defibrillator if present		
	Basic life support (BLS) algorithm		

⇧ % **SCORE** _____

Good Pass

Pass

Borderline

Fail

Clear Fail

NOTES/Areas to improve

Chapter 15

Russell Foster

Investigations and procedures

O SINGLE STATIONS

STATION 1: ADVISING IVDU ON INJECTION TECHNIQUE AND RISK MINIMISATION

INSTRUCTION TO CANDIDATE

You are the ward doctor on an acute adult in-patient ward. You have been asked to see a 30-year-old university student who has a history of cannabis abuse, but recently tried injecting himself with heroin. He was found collapsed in the street and was transferred to the psychiatric ward after being stabilised medically.

He is worried about the risks of injecting and is seeking further advice. He is anxious and has a number of questions for you.

Answer his questions and give him information on harm minimisation and injection techniques should he continue to use.

ACTOR (ROLE-PLAYER) INSTRUCTIONS

You are genuinely surprised to find yourself in hospital. You are anxious about what happened to you.

You want to know what infections you might get from intravenous heroin use.

You want to know if there any medical conditions associated with intravenous heroin use.

You want to know what would happen if you continue with intravenous heroin use.

SUGGESTED APPROACH

Setting the scene

Explain that you have been asked to see him. Try to get some background history of the events leading up to his collapse. Explain that you have not been able to speak to the nursing staff as yet or had access to his notes or other sources of information. Try to briefly get an idea of his current and recent history of illicit drug use.

Completing the tasks

What infections may be associated with intravenous heroin use?

You would need to explain the following in lay terms, perhaps explaining the risks at the injection site and those affecting the 'whole body'.

These may be divided into systemic and local.

Systemic infections may result from direct transmission into the bloodstream of a number of organisms, for example:

Type of organism	Name of organism	Notes
Bacteria	*Clostridium* spp.	May cause myonecrosis; tetanus is relatively uncommon due to vaccination
	Mycobacterium tuberculosis	Tuberculosis may occur in malnourished/ immunosuppressed individuals
	Staphylococcus aureus	Causes tricuspid (right-sided) endocarditis, especially in patients with HIV
	Streptococcus spp.	Can cause septicaemia and endocarditis, especially left-sided
Fungi	*Candida* spp.	Can cause endocarditis, CHS infections, endophthalmitis and disseminated candidiasis
	Aspergillus spp.	Pulmonary aspergillosis may occur
	Rhizopus spp.	Mucormycosis may occur, especially in neutropenic patients. May present with orbital cellulitis, pain and vascular thrombosis
Parasites	*Malaria* spp.	More common in temperate areas of the world
Viruses	Hepatitis A	May be spread via contaminated drugs themselves or water used in injection
	Hepatitis B, hepatitis C	Viruses transmitted via shared needles
	HIV	May be asymptomatic for many years and then present with opportunistic infections (e.g. tuberculosis or pneumocystic carinii pneumonia)

Note that atypical pathogens may be implicated, as can the effects of 'poly-infection' with a number of pathogens. Systemic infections may also affect the nervous system, producing cerebral abscess, infarction or meningitis.

Local infections may result from skin flora such as *Staphylococcus* species (e.g. *S. aureus* or *S. epidermidis*) and include abscesses, cellulitis, necrotising fasciitis, thrombophlebitis or tissue necrosis ('gas gangrene'). Infections may also result from foreign bodies such as broken needles remaining *in situ* or following the use of contaminated drugs/water. Infections of joints and bones have also been reported, and chronic use can lead to 'stigmata' such as fibrosis, bruising, skin discolouration, granulomata and chronic phlebitis.

What other medical conditions may be associated with intravenous heroin use?
These may be divided into drug-related and non-drug-related factors. Examples of the former include sequelae of the drug itself (such as irritant effects leading to thrombophlebitis and thromboembolism), injection with adulterants added to the drug mixture (with variable effects), drug overdose (such as heart failure, pulmonary embolism and respiratory arrest) or drug withdrawal.

Medical effects of intoxication include the following:

System	Condition	Notes
Cardiovascular	Cardiac arrhythmia	Bradycardia may occur in intoxication and tachycardia may occur in withdrawal
	Endocarditis	May be right- or left-sided
Dermatological	Abscesses, cellulitis, necrotising fasciitis, thrombophlebitis or tissue necrosis; 'stigmata' may also be seen with chronic use	Common findings, see above
Endocrine	Hyperglycaemia	Rare, but may occur in heavy, chronic use
	Hyperprolactinaemia	Rare, but may occur in heavy, chronic use or following head trauma or seizures
	Thyroid dysfunction	Raised T4 levels may occur, but may not be clinically significant
Gastrointestinal	Abnormal liver function	Non-specific changes in LFTs may be seen
	Pancreatitis	May occur following the consumption of large doses
Haematological	Eosinophilia	May occur in up to a quarter of addicts
	Lymphocytosis	Common occurrence
	Thrombocytopenia	May occur due to contaminants
Metabolic	Hypocholesterolaemia	Decreased cholesterol levels sometimes seen
	Hypoxia	Occurs with high/toxic doses
Musculoskeletal	Rhabdomyolysis	May occur in infection or in toxic doses
Neurological	Acute transverse myelitis, cerebral infarction, encephalopathy and Parkinsonism	May arise due to hypoxia and increased blood pressure
	Peripheral neuropathies	May be related to trauma
Pulmonary	Emboli	May be secondary to injected, non-dissolved substances
Pulmonary	Pneumonia	Usually bacterial
	Pulmonary granuloma	May be secondary to injected, non-dissolved substances
Renal	Myoglobinuria	Occurs in association with rhabdomyolysis
	Nephropathy	May be due to contaminants

What non-medical risks are associated with intravenous heroin use?

These can be classified as risk to self and risk to others. Amongst risk to self are:

- Violence associated with drug use
- Psychiatric sequelae (lability of mood, personality changes, cognitive impairment, psychosis and mania)
- Economic and social costs (debt, homelessness, loss of employment and relationship difficulties)

Risks to others include:

- Violence
- Social costs (disruption of relationships)
- Economic costs (increased crime and increased costs of policing and providing healthcare)

Harm minimisation

Harm minimisation involves recognising that certain individuals cannot or will not stop using drugs and therefore aiming to minimise the harmful sequelae of drug taking. A number of interventions have been described, including:

Methadone maintenance programmes

Counselling

Supplying clean equipment (e.g. alcohol swabs, sterile containers or filters for mixing drugs, sterile needles and sterile water)

Educating users in order to try to minimise risk of infection

Using non-injecting means of administration

Supervised injection (controversial)

Discouraging poly-substance use

Administering drug in the presence of others

Education regarding safer injecting techniques

Education regarding disposal of used equipment

Using low initial 'test dose' to gauge strength of drug

What advice regarding injection technique can you provide?

- Try to inject when sitting or lying down.
- Try to inject in the presence of others.
- Use of sterile, single-use only needles and syringes.
- Never share needles.
- Pay attention to hygiene, such as washing hands and injection site, possibly by using alcohol wipes.
- Use of sterile water for injection, or, failing this, tap water that has been boiled for at least 5 minutes.
- Allowing heated drug mixture to cool prior to injecting.
- Avoiding use of lemon juice to dissolve heroin and using safer alternatives such as citric or ascorbic acid.
- Filtering drug mix prior to injection via use of sterile, single-use filters.
- Use a small-bore needle.
- Use a vein that is less likely to be painful or inaccessible; the cubital fossa is generally recommended.
- After drawing up drug, tap the syringe to remove air bubbles.
- Gently push syringe plunger to expel air.
- Rotate injection sites to allow veins to heal.
- Do not over-tighten tourniquet or leave in place for too long.
- Ensure that the needle faces the same direction as the blood flow.
- After the needle is in the vein, pull back to ensure blood appears in the syringe to confirm that the needle is actually in the vein.
- Remove tourniquet prior to injecting.

- After removing the needle, apply a clean tissue or cotton wool to puncture site to stop bleeding.
- Dispose of used needles and syringes carefully.

ADDITIONAL POINTS

Clinical features of opiate intoxication/complications

Mental effects: anorexia, decreased activity, diminished libido, drowsiness, euphoria and personality change.

Physical effects: bradycardia, constipation, meiosis, nausea and pruritus.

Features of withdrawal

Abdominal cramps, agitation, craving, diarrhoea, diaphoresis, mydriasis, piloerection, restlessness, tachycardia and yawning.

FURTHER READING

Foster, R. (2008) *Clinical Laboratory Investigation and Psychiatry: A Practical Handbook.* London: Informa.

Hutin, Y., Hauri, A., Chiarello, L. et al. (2003) Best infection control practices for intradermal, subcutaneous, and intramuscular needle injections. *Bulletin of the World Health Organization, 81*(7), 491–500.

Theodorou, S. & Haber, P.S. (2005) The medical complications of heroin use. *Current Opinion in Psychiatry, 18*(3), 257–63.

Zollner, C. & Stein, C. (2007) Opioids. *Handbook of Experimental Pharmacology, 177,* 31–63.

The examiner's mark sheet

Domain/ percentage of marks	Essential points to pass	✓	Extra marks/comments (make notes here)
1. Communication and empathy 25% of marks	Clear communication Open and closed questions Empathy Sensitivity		
2. Recognition or risks of injecting 25% of marks	Relevant risks Physical – infection Psychiatric Environmental/personal		
3. Patient education 25% of marks	Preferable to cease habit Advice on methadone Harm minimisation advice if likely to continue		
4. Answering other questions 25% of marks	Appropriate answers		

STATION 2: ABNORMAL BLOOD RESULTS IN AN ALCOHOLIC PATIENT

INSTRUCTION TO CANDIDATE

In your role as a liaison psychiatrist, you have been asked to see a man who was admitted for treatment of delirium tremens. The 50-year-old homeless man is thought to be mentally unwell and you have been asked to transfer him to the local psychiatric hospital. During your initial review of the hospital notes, you note the following blood results taken earlier today:

Albumin = 21 g/L	(35–50 g/L)
Bilirubin = 250 µmol/L	(3–20 µmol/L)
GGT = 600 IU/L	(<60 IU/L)
ALP = 300 IU/L	(30–130 IU/L)
ALT = 55 IU/L	(0–45 IU/L)
AST = 170 IU/L	(10–50 IU/L)
MCV = 150 fL	(80–100 fL)

You have an extremely inquisitive fourth-year medical student with you who asks you a number of questions.

ACTOR (ROLE-PLAYER) INSTRUCTIONS

You are a very interested and keen medical student and have a lot of questions in relation to this case, specifically:

1. How do you interpret the liver function tests?
2. What other validated markers of alcoholism are there?
3. What are the clinical signs and symptoms of alcohol withdrawal?
4. What are you going to say to the ward staff?

SUGGESTED APPROACH

Setting the scene

Introduce yourself. Ask if the medical student has ever seen anyone with delirium tremens before. You could go on to explain that when seeing any patient in a liaison setting, it is helpful to determine first what has been done to investigate and treat the patient, given that delirium tremens is a medical emergency and often patients can be sedated or be in receipt of ongoing medical treatment and thus may not be immediately amenable to proper psychiatric assessment. You can explain that it is useful to check whether the PLN has seen the patient and whether the patient is medically stable or requires further input.

Completing the tasks

How do you interpret the above results?

All results are above the normal range, suggesting that they are abnormal. Looking at the liver function tests, the raised GGT is consistent with chronic alcohol use, as it is raised in approximately two-thirds of such patients. Although ALP and AST are non-specific markers of liver disease, the ratio of AST/ALT is >2, confirming liver disease – a ratio >3 is suggestive of myocardial infarction. The ration of GGT/ALP is 2, suggesting alcoholic liver disease – a ratio >3.5 is considered by some authorities to be diagnostic. The raised bilirubin suggests an obstructive pattern, such as that found in cirrhosis, and the decreased albumin is probably due to decreased synthesis, as occurs in liver disease. ALP is a non-specific marker of liver disease.

What other validated markers of alcoholism are there?

Carbohydrate-deficient transferrin (normal range approximately 1.9–3.4 g/L) is increasingly being used, especially in the monitoring of abstinence from alcohol. It is a form of iron-transport protein that also increases in liver diseases such as chronic active hepatitis, autoimmune hepatitis and primary biliary cirrhosis.

Mean cell volume is a measure of the average size of red cells (normal range approximately 80–100 fL) and increases in alcoholism and various forms of anaemia. Mood stabilisers such as carbamazepine, lamotrigine and valproate may cause an increased MCV.

Alcoholic cirrhosis may be monitored by measuring a specific plasma peptide (procollagen type III), although raised levels are also seen in infection, inflammation and tissue necrosis.

What are the clinical signs and symptoms of alcohol withdrawal?

Withdrawal syndromes may be considered depending on the period of time elapsed from the last use of alcohol.

Short-term (within 24 hours of stopping use): there are a wide range of possible signs and symptoms, including convulsions (grand mal), depression, diaphoresis, hallucinosis (auditory, transient), hyperacusis, itching, muscle cramps, nausea, tinnitus and vomiting, and these can last for several days.

Medium-term (within 1–3 days of stopping use): delirium tremens – agitation, autonomic overactivity, confusion, delusions and hallucinations (visual) and sleeplessness. Delirium tremens constitutes a medical emergency and patients should be treated in a medical facility which has appropriate resuscitation facilities as mortality is approximately 10%.

Longer-term (variable length of time after stopping use): Wernicke–Korsakoff syndrome.

Alcoholic hallucinosis: auditory hallucinations in clear consciousness. This usually resolves within a week, but rarely may progress to amnesic, cognitive impairment or schizophreniform syndromes.

What are you going to say to the ward staff?

After reviewing the notes and seeing the patient (where you perform a full history, mental state examination and, if possible, a physical examination), you will decide whether the patient is acutely unwell psychiatrically or remains physically unwell with liver cirrhosis. You might need to discuss the case with a senior colleague and then explain to the ward staff that the patient does/does not merit admission to an acute psychiatric ward. If not, you will agree to continue to provide liaison psychiatric input as required.

ADDITIONAL POINTS

The clinical associations of chronic alcohol use

These are numerous, including:

Cardiovascular: angina, arrhythmias and cardiomyopathy

Endocrine: pseudo-Cushing's syndrome and hypogonadism

Gastrointestinal: alcoholic cirrhosis, hepatitis, gastritis and carcinoma pancreatitis

Haematological: anaemia (macrocytic, iron deficiency and sideroblastic)

Musculoskeletal: myopathy

Neurological: Korsakoff's syndrome and seizures

FURTHER READING

Foster, R. (2008) *Clinical Laboratory Investigation and Psychiatry: A Practical Handbook.* London: Informa.

Mannelli, P. & Pae, C.U. (2007) Medical comorbidity and alcohol dependence. *Current Psychiatry Reports, 9*(3), 217–24.

Marshall, W.J. (1995) *Clinical Chemistry,* 3rd edn. London: Mosby.

The examiner's mark sheet

Domain/ percentage of marks	Essential points to pass ✓	Extra marks/comments (make notes here)
1. Communication 25% of marks	Clear communication with a more junior colleague Encouraging Professional	
2. Knowledge of basic liver function tests 25% of marks	Clear explanation to a colleague	

3. Knowledge of clinical features of alcohol use/withdrawal

25% of marks

Short term

Medium tern

Longer term

4. Answering other questions

25% of marks

Appropriate responses to questions arising

% SCORE _____

___ **OVERALL IMPRESSION**

4 (CIRCLE ONE)

Good Pass

Pass

Borderline

Fail

Clear Fail

NOTES/Areas to improve

STATION 3: PHYSICAL EXAMINATION AND LABORATORY INVESTIGATION OF EATING DISORDERS

INSTRUCTION TO CANDIDATE

You are on call in the local accident and emergency (A&E) department and are asked to see a 'difficult' 18-year-old patient who was brought in by her parents, whom she lives with. Her worried mother had informed the A&E doctor that her daughter had not been eating for some time. The mother further stated that her daughter, a ballet dancer, spends hours doing exercises and appears to have stopped menstruating. You note from the A&E clerking that no physical examination has been performed, as the patient is refusing both a physical examination as well as blood tests.

You are about to meet her mother, a university lecturer, who believes her daughter has anorexia nervosa and has a number of questions for you.

Explain anorexia nervosa to the mother and discuss the differential diagnosis.

ACTOR (ROLE-PLAYER) INSTRUCTIONS

You are a no-nonsense, practical person who will press for precise answers. You are curt but polite. You should include the following questions.

1. What eating disorders are there and what are their features?
2. What are the differential diagnoses of anorexia nervosa?
3. What symptoms may be reported in anorexia nervosa?
4. What are the possible medical complications of anorexia nervosa?

Ask for clarification if the doctor is too technical or uses medical jargon.

SUGGESTED APPROACH

Setting the scene

Introduce yourself. Explain that you understand that she must be extremely concerned about her daughter. Find out what she knows about eating disorders. Make sure that you consider issues of patient confidentiality if you discuss issues relating to her daughter. Has the daughter consented to her case being discussed with her mother?

Completing the tasks

Remember to discuss matters in lay terms.

What eating disorders are there and what are their features?

Although there is some disagreement, five major groupings of eating disorders may be identified: obesity, anorexia nervosa, bulimia nervosa, pica and eating disorder not otherwise specified.

Obesity:

Obesity may be defined as a body weight exceeding 120% of the accepted average for age, gender and height in a given culture or setting. It may be further defined using the Quetelet's body mass index: weight (kg)/height (m)^2.

Anorexia nervosa (ICD code F50.0):

The time frame of anorexia nervosa is non-specific.

Features:

1. Weight loss of at least 15% below the expected weight for height and age
2. Weight loss is self-induced
3. Perception/dread of being too fat, leading to a self-imposed desire for low weight
4. Multiple endocrine effects on hypothalamic–pituitary–gonadal axis, leading to alterations in sexual potency and amenorrhoea

Bulimia nervosa (ICD code F50.2):

The time frame of bulimia nervosa consists of specific features (recurrent overeating) at least twice a week for at least 3 months.

Features:

1. Recurrent episodes of overeating (large amounts of food eaten in short periods of time)
2. Preoccupation with eating, with compulsion/craving to eat
3. Manoeuvres are undertaken by the patient to counteract the effects of eating by at least one of self-induced vomiting/purging, alternating episodes of fasting/starvation and use of drugs such as appetite suppressants, thyroid preparation, diuretics and insulin
4. Fear of and self-perception of being fat

What are the main differential diagnoses of anorexia nervosa?

Important differentials include:

Psychiatric:	Depression, obsessive compulsive disorder, psychotic disorders and schizophrenia; note that individuals with eating disorders may have comorbid personality disorders.

Medical:

Endocrine:	Diabetes mellitus, hypopituitarism and thyrotoxicosis.
Gastrointestinal:	Malabsorption.
Other:	Neoplasia and reticulosis.

What symptoms may be reported in anorexia nervosa?

Often patients do not complain of symptoms, although they universally report thinking they are fat. Careful questioning may elicit the following:

Psychiatric symptoms: biological symptoms of depression, compulsions, low mood, obsessions and psychotic symptoms.

Physical symptoms: abdominal pain (possibly secondary to acute pancreatitis), amenorrhoea/menstrual dysfunction, constipation, erectile dysfunction/loss of libido (males), hypothermia, increased urinary frequency (may be secondary to diabetes insipidus or renal failure), muscle cramps, tiredness and vomiting.

What are the possible metabolic complications of anorexia nervosa?

There are many of these, including:

Domain	Condition
Metabolic	Acid–base disturbance (metabolic acidosis/alkalosis)
	Azotaemia
	Hypercholesterolaemia
	Hypertriglyceridaemia
	Hypoglycaemia
	Hyponatraemia
	Hypokalaemia
	Hypoalbuminaemia
	Hypocalcaemia
	Hypomagnesaemia
	Hypophophataemia
	Osteoporosis
Endocrine	Diabetes insipidus
	Thyroid abnormalities (e.g. hypothyroidism, sick euthyroid syndrome, decreased T3)
	Menstrual disturbance/amenorrhoea
	Increased GH and cortisol
Haematological	Anaemia
	Coagulopathies
	Leukopoenia
	Lymphocytosis
	Thrombocytopenia
Gastrointestinal	Abnormal LFTs (hepatitis and steatohepatitis)
	Pancreatitis (increased plasma amylase)
	Nutritional deficiencies

ADDITIONAL POINTS

Eating disorders, especially anorexia nervosa, are complex conditions that require a multidisciplinary perspective due to the large number of associated medical, metabolic and psychiatric complications.

The disorder is more common in females (female:male = 10:1), and young females appear more susceptible. Higher social classes are over-represented, as are athletes, ballet dancers and gymnasts.

Comorbid psychiatric diagnoses are common (especially major depression and possibly personality disorders).

Laboratory investigations should be guided by clinical presentation and it is always advisable to seek expert advice when requesting these.

Management involves the correction of medical/metabolic complications with efforts to promote weight gain being important. Cognitive and insight-orientated approaches are often utilised, but pharmacological approaches have a more limited role.

Prognosis is usually worse with an older age of onset, comorbid personality disorders, long duration of illness (>5–6 years), male gender and previous history of obesity.

FURTHER READING

Berkman, N.D., Bulik, C.M., Brownley, K.A. et al. (2006) Management of eating disorders. *Evidence Report/Technology Assessment (Full Report), 135*, 1–166.

Herzog, W., Deter, H.C., Fiehn, W. & Petzold, E. (1997) Medical findings and predictors of long-term physical outcome in anorexia nervosa: A prospective, 12-year follow-up study. *Psychological Medicine, 27*(2), 269–79.

Van Binsbergen, C.J., Odink, J., Van den Berg, H., Koppeschaar, H. & Coelingh Bennink, H.J. (1988) Nutritional status in anorexia nervosa: Clinical chemistry, vitamins, iron and zinc. *European Journal of Clinical Nutrition, 42*(11), 929–37.

The examiner's mark sheet

Domain/ percentage of marks	Essential points to pass	✓	Extra marks/comments (make notes here)
1. Communication and empathy 25% of marks	Clear communication Open and closed questions Empathy Sensitivity		Clarifies patient confidentiality
2. Knowledge of eating disorders 25% of marks	Clear explanation of the various eating disorders and how these can manifest		
3. Metabolic changes in AN 25% of marks	Physical parameter changes associated with AN and malnourished state		
4. Answering other questions 25% of marks	Relevant risks		

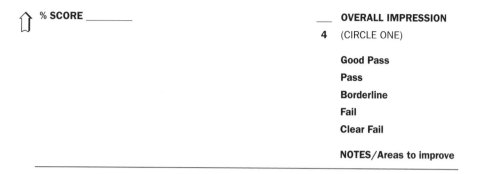

STATION 4: BASIC ELECTROCARDIOGRAM INTERPRETATION

INSTRUCTION TO CANDIDATE

As part of the clerking of a newly admitted patient on the ward you are covering on your week of nights, you have been asked to perform an electrocardiogram (ECG) and report your findings to the notoriously pedantic but supportive on-call consultant. You note that the patient, a 55-year-old female, who has a history of anxiety in the context of a dependent personality disorder, is cooperative, has a GCS of 15/15, appears slightly anxious and sweaty but is otherwise unremarkable. The patient is not on any regular medication. Unfortunately, the nurse on the ward has not done the ECG course and is therefore unable to help you.

You manage to perform the ECG by following the instructions on the machine. You note that the ECG print-out reports the following parameters:

'Sinus rhythm but otherwise normal ECG.'

HR	110
PR	150
QTc	429

Look at this ECG and prepare to report your findings back to the consultant.

ACTOR (ROLE-PLAYER) INSTRUCTIONS

You introduce yourself to the candidate and ask them what the ECG shows.

You then decide to test the candidate's knowledge on ECG interpretation and ask the following questions:

1. What anatomical positions do the different leads of the ECG represent?
2. How do you know that the electrodes have been correctly applied to the patient and that the ECG trace is accurate?
3. How is sinus rhythm represented on the ECG?

4. What is the QTc interval? What psychotropics may be associated with prolongation of the QTc interval?
5. If the patient were being treated on clozapine, what ECG changes might you see?

SUGGESTED APPROACH

Setting the scene

Introduce yourself. You can explain to the consultant why you decided to perform the ECG and what your findings are.

Completing the tasks

What anatomical positions do the different leads of the ECG represent?
Standard leads:

The *left lateral surface* of the heart is looked at by leads *VL, I* and *II*.

The *inferior surface* of the heart is looked at by leads *VF* and *III*.

The *right atrium* is looked at by *VR*.

'V' leads:

The *right ventricle* is looked at by *V1* and *V2*.

The *intra-ventricular septum* and *anterior wall of the left ventricle* are looked at by leads *V3* and *V4*.

The *anterior and lateral walls of the left ventricle* are looked at by leads *V5* and *V6*.

How do you know that the electrodes have been correctly applied to the patient and that the ECG trace is accurate?
Many machines now give real-time interpretations, but with older machines, the following rules of thumb are helpful for confirming correct lead placement in a normal ECG:

Lead	Overall direction of QRS complex
I	Mainly *upwards*
II	Mainly *upwards*
III	Mainly *upwards*
VR	Mainly *downwards*

How is sinus rhythm represented on the ECG? What conditions may be associated with a sinus tachycardia (heart rate >100 bpm)?
Sinus rhythm is indicated by a P wave occurring before a QRS complex. Sinus rhythms may be fast (>100 bpm = tachycardia) or slow (<40 bpm = bradycardia).

Sinus tachycardia may be associated with medical and non-medical conditions, for example:

Medical: anaemia, bleeding, cardiac failure, catecholamine-secreting tumours (rare; e.g. pheochromocytosis), fever, hypovolaemia, pain and thyrotoxicosis.

Non-medical: anxiety, drug intoxication/withdrawal, exercise, extreme emotion (release of catecholamines), fear and psychotropics.

What is the QTc interval? What psychotropics may be associated with prolongation of the QTc interval?

The QTc interval is the time between the initial deflection of the P wave and the end of the T wave that is corrected for heart rate. It is normally less than 450 ms in men, although may be slightly higher in women (up to 470 ms).

Psychotropics commonly associated with QTc prolongation include chloral hydrate, chlorpromazine, citalopram, haloperidol, lithium, pimozide, sertindole, TCAs and ziprasidone.

If the patient were being treated on clozapine, what ECG changes might you see?

Clozapine may cause myocarditis or cardiomyopathy, which may be heralded by non-specific symptoms such as chest pain, fever, shortness of breath, sweating and tachycardia. In some cases there may be no changes, although the following may occur:

On ECG, myocarditis may cause a tachycardia and non-specific, transient ST waves. It may also resemble an motivational interviewing (MI), with Q waves and a lack of R waves in the anterior leads.

Cardiomyopathy may show non-specific ST and T wave changes in association with arrhythmias, such as atrial fibrillation or ventricular tachycardia.

ADDITIONAL POINTS

If asked to report the ECG, it should be done systematically. You should have a scheme in mind, such as the following:

This is the ECG from [name of patient], a 55-year-old [ethnicity] female who was admitted with [brief history].

The ECG was taken on [date] and [time].

The rate is...

The axis is [normal, shows right/let axis deviation].

The rhythm is [sinus rhythm, atrial fibrillation, atrial flutter, etc.].

The PR interval is [normal, shows first/second/third-degree heart block].

The QRS width is [normal, prolonged].

The QRS height is [normal, high].

There are/are no Q waves.

The QT interval is [normal, prolonged].

The ST segment is [normal, elevated/depressed in leads...].

The T waves are [normal, peaked, flattened].

There are/are no U waves.

In summary, this is a 12-lead ECG of a 55-year-old which is normal/shows the following abnormalities...

Interpreting an ECG is often difficult, and if there is any doubt, the opinion of an experienced physician should be sought. When performing an ECG, the patient is instructed to remain still during the recording in order to minimise any artefacts. Note that serial ECGs may be required, and that most modern ECG machines will try to interpret the trace, often inaccurately.

⇧ As you may have forgotten how to interpret an ECG, perusal of a suitable reference text (e.g. *The ECG Made Simple*) is suggested. Despite being a basic investigation, its interpretation is complex and, if uncertain, it is always best to be honest and admit this!

FURTHER READING

Demangone, D. (2006) ECG manifestations: Noncoronary heart disease. *Emergency Medicine Clinics of North America, 24*(1), 113–31.

Goodnick, P.J., Jerry, J. & Parra, F. (2002) Psychotropic drugs and the ECG: Focus on the QTc interval. *Expert Opinion on Pharmacotherapy, 3*(5), 479–98.

Hampton, J.R. (1994) *The ECG Made Easy*, 4th edn. London: Churchill Livingstone.

Mackin, P. (2008) Cardiac side effects of psychiatric drugs. *Human Psychopharmacology, 23*(Suppl. 1), 3–14.

Merrill, D.B., Dec, G.W. & Goff, D.C. (2005) Adverse cardiac effects associated with clozapine. *Journal of Clinical Psychopharmacology, 25*(1), 32–41.

Taylor, D., Paton, C. & Kapur, S. (2015) *Maudsley Prescribing Guidelines in Psychiatry*, 12th edn. Chichester: Wiley Blackwell.

The examiner's mark sheet

Domain/ percentage of marks	Essential points to pass	✓	Extra marks/comments (make notes here)
1. Communication skills 25% of marks	Clear professional communication		
2. Basic ECG interpretation 25% of marks	Key points explained to the consultant		
3. Knowledge of psychotropics that alter specific ECG parameters 25% of marks	Knowledge of medications/ groups that can interfere with heart rhythm		
4. Answering other questions 25% of marks	Appropriate responses to further questions		

% SCORE _____

___ **OVERALL IMPRESSION**

4 (CIRCLE ONE)

Good Pass

Pass

Borderline

Fail

Clear Fail

NOTES/Areas to improve

STATION 5: INITIATION AND MONITORING OF CLOZAPINE

INSTRUCTION TO CANDIDATE

You are the junior doctor on a busy, general adult ward and have been asked by the departing locum consultant to commence clozapine on a 29-year-old patient with newly diagnosed schizophrenia. The patient has been on olanzapine for 8 months, but this was changed to modecate (fluphenazine) depot due to variable compliance, which the patient attributed to side effects.

A student nurse in the team wants to know more about clozapine.

ACTOR (ROLE-PLAYER) INSTRUCTIONS

You are an inquisitive nurse and want to know the answers to the following questions:

1. When should clozapine be considered?
2. What are the life-threatening side effects of clozapine?
3. What other adverse effects of clozapine are there?
4. What blood tests are needed for clozapine and when?
5. What are the grounds for discontinuing clozapine?
6. Are there any protocols when commencing clozapine?

SUGGESTED APPROACH

Setting the scene

Introduce yourself. Ask whether they have ever seen clozapine used before, and if so, what they know about it. Explain that you will need to obtain appropriate background information about the patient, including details of all previous treatments, how long the patient was on them and why they were stopped. The views of the patient should also be canvassed.

Completing the tasks

When should clozapine be considered?

Clozapine is an 'atypical' anti-psychotic that is used in the treatment of schizophrenia in patients who have either not responded to two full courses of other anti-psychotics (one of which should be an 'atypical') or who are intolerant of conventional anti-psychotic agents (e.g. suffer from severe extrapyramidal side effects or severe tardive dyskinesia).

Clozapine is contraindicated in patients with myeloproliferative disorders, active/progressive cardiac, hepatic and renal disease, individuals with uncontrolled epilepsy and in those patients who are unwilling to tolerate blood tests.

What are the life-threatening side effects of clozapine?

Important life-threatening side effects of clozapine	
Agranulocytosis	Incidence approximately 0.8%, risk of fatal agranulocytosis estimated at 1 in 5,000; female sex/older age may be risk factors
Pulmonary embolism	Rare, risk estimated at 1 in 2,000–6,000; may be more likely in early stages of treatment (first 3 months)

⇧	Myocarditis/ cardiomyopathy	Risk variable (from 1 in 1300 up to 1 in 67,000) and may be more likely in early stages of treatment (first 2–3 months)
	Seizures	Incidence approximately 3%, risk is dose-related and may require use of prophylactic valproate

What other adverse effects of clozapine are there?

Agranulocytosis, which occurs in approximately 1% of patients, requires regular, mandatory monitoring of FBC.

What blood tests are needed for clozapine and when?

Blood tests should be done prior to and following initiation. As agranulocytosis (white cell count $<2 \times 10^9$/L) is a major risk, FBC should be regularly monitored. Weekly full blood counts are required for the first 18 weeks, then 2-weekly until 1 year; if blood counts remain stable, then 4-weekly counts are needed thereafter (including 4 weeks post-discontinuation). There is a traffic light system for clozapine FBC monitoring: red = stop clozapine immediately; amber = repeat FBC and proceed with caution; green = safe to continue.

Regular laboratory monitoring of laboratory parameters is suggested below:

Additional laboratory monitoring of clozapine	
Regular monitoring	FBC
3-monthly	HbA$_1$C, lipid panel
6-monthly	U&Es, LFTs, lipid panel*
Other	CPK (if neuroleptic malignant syndrome [NMS] suspected); other parameters as based on clinical suspicion (see table below)

What are the grounds for discontinuing clozapine?

If white cell count $<2 \times 10^9$/L

Suspected myocarditis or other cardiovascular dysfunction

Suspected neuroleptic malignant syndrome

Eosinophilia (above 3.0×10^9/L)

Thrombocytopenia when platelet count $<50 \times 10^9$/L

Are there any protocols when commencing clozapine?

All patients should be registered with a clozapine monitoring service. Prior to commencing clozapine, the patient should be warned about the risk of side effects and should be instructed to notify their key worker in the event of any signs of infection (sore throat, fever, etc.). Close collaboration between the patient, the GP and secondary mental health services is important and may be incorporated into a formal 'shared care' agreement.

ADDITIONAL POINTS

The accepted reference range for clozapine is *350–500* µg/L. Blood should be collected for *trough* levels (i.e. just before the dose) in a plain tube. It should ⇩

---

* Especially advised when specific risk factors are present.

be noted that the time to steady state is approximately 3 days, and levels may be lower in males, especially those who are younger and who smoke.

FURTHER READING

Foster, R. (2008) *Clinical Laboratory Medicine and Psychiatry: A Practical Handbook.* London: Informa.

Raggi, M.A., Mandrioli, R., Sabbioni, C. & Pucci, V. (2004) Atypical antipsychotics: Pharmacokinetics, therapeutic drug monitoring and pharmacological interactions. *Current Medicinal Chemistry*, 11(3), 279–96.

Rostami-Hodjegan, A., Amin, A.M., Spencer, E.P., Lennard, M.S., Tucker, G.T. & Flanagan, R.J. (2004) Influence of dose, cigarette smoking, age, sex, and metabolic activity on plasma clozapine concentrations: A predictive model and nomograms to aid clozapine dose adjustment and to assess compliance in individual patients. *Journal of Clinical Psychopharmacology*, 24(1), 70–8.

Taylor, D., Paton, C. & Kapur, S. (2015) *Maudsley Prescribing Guidelines in Psychiatry*, 12th edn. Chichester: Wiley Blackwell.

The examiner's mark sheet

Domain/ percentage of marks	Essential points to pass	✓	Extra marks/comments (make notes here)
1. Communication 25% of marks	Clear communication with a junior colleague		
2. Knowledge of clozapine pharmacology 25% of marks	Rationale for use Potential adverse effects, including life-threatening effects		
3. Aware of laboratory aspects of clozapine 25% of marks	Therapeutic blood monitoring Metabolic side effects NICE guidelines		
4. Answering other questions 25% of marks	Gives appropriate responses to other questions arising		

% SCORE _____

___

4

OVERALL IMPRESSION

(CIRCLE ONE)

Good Pass

Pass

Borderline

Fail

Clear Fail

NOTES/Areas to improve

STATION 6: INTERPRETING THYROID FUNCTION TESTS

INSTRUCTION TO CANDIDATE

You have been asked to review some blood results for a patient in her fifties who was recently admitted after concerns from her husband that she had become increasingly listless and 'odd'. She has stopped going out for walks, become increasingly forgetful and complained of feeling tired all of the time.

The ward doctor noted that she had no previous psychiatric or medical history and had been gaining weight and complaining of constipation. He also noted she had a hoarse voice and a slow heart rate.

Her husband is a psychologist and wants to understand her test results. He asks:

1. **What blood tests are done and why?**
2. **You perform a number of tests and find that the serum TSH is 120 mU/L (normal range approximately 0.3–0.4 mU/L) and the serum-free T4 is 4 pmol/L (normal range approximately 9–26 pmol/L). How do you explain these results to the husband?**
3. **In general terms, how will she be managed?**
4. **What are the clinical signs and symptoms of hypothyroidism?**

ACTOR (ROLE-PLAYER) INSTRUCTIONS

You are concerned about your wife, who you have seen deteriorate gradually over time. You feel she is also low and not her usual self.

You would like answers to the questions as stated above.

You want to know about hypothyroidism and how it can affect mental state.

SUGGESTED APPROACH

Setting the scene

Introduce yourself to her husband. Remember to consider issues of patient confidentiality and whether the patient has capacity and consents to your discussing her case. In order to understand the blood results, further information about the patient is needed. This can be obtained from ward staff and reading the hospital notes. You will be particularly interested in the history of presenting complaints and medication history, further details of which may be obtained from the husband or GP.

Completing the tasks

What blood tests are done and why?

The above information suggests a possible organic disorder, although a full history, mental state examination, physical examination and appropriate, additional investigations need to be performed.

Suitable first-line screening tests will be guided by the important differentials; in this case, hypothyroidism. Thus, thyroid function tests, a full blood count and urea and electrolytes will be the usual first-line tests.

You perform a number of laboratory investigations and find the following abnormal results

MCV = 106 fL (normal range approximately 76–96 fL)

Serum TSH = 120 mU/L (normal range approximately 0.3–0.4 mU/L)

Serum-free T4 = 4 pmol/L (normal range approximately 9–26 pmol/L)

How do you explain these results to the husband?

The high TSH is suggestive of a diagnosis of hypothyroidism, as is the low serum-free T4. The presence of macrocytic anaemia is consistent with this diagnosis.

In general terms, how will she be managed?

The main treatment for hypothyroidism is with thyroxine replacement, which should be initiated by either the GP or after referral to an endocrinologist. Although the main treatment is with thyroxine (T4) replacement, T3 may be used in patients with ischaemic heart disease. An open and clear dialogue with the patient and her husband will be helpful in order to allay possible fears or concerns.

Psychiatric manifestations of hypothyroidism?

Symptoms that have been reported include anhedonia, delirium (rare), dysphoria, irritability, mania, personality changes, psychomotor agitation or retardation, psychosis (rare, may occur in long-standing, untreated individuals), slowing of cognitive function, sleep disturbance and suicidality.

Clinical signs and symptoms of hypothyroidism?

Clinical signs include bradycardia, cerebellar ataxia (rare), congestive cardiac failure, dry/cool skin, facial swelling, goitre, hair loss, hoarse voice, non-pitting oedema, slowed muscle reflexes (pseudomyotonia), slowed speech, tongue thickening and weight gain.

Clinical symptoms include cold intolerance, constipation, cramps, deafness, fatigue, menstrual disturbances, muscle pain and weakness.

ADDITIONAL POINTS

Psychiatric manifestations of hyperthyroidism

Psychiatric symptoms include anxiety, cognitive decline, delirium, depression, emotional lability, feeling of apprehension, irritability, nervousness and psychosis (rare).

Clinical signs and symptoms of hyperthyroidism

Clinical symptoms include fatigue, heat intolerance, menstrual irregularities and weakness.

Clinical signs include agitation, atrial fibrillation, dermopathy (pretibial myxoedema and pruritus), diaphoresis, diarrhoea, dyspnoea, eye signs (exophthalmos and 'lid lag'), goitre, hair loss, palpitations, tachycardia, thyroid bruit, tremor and weight loss.

Both hyper- and hypo-thyroidism are associated with changes in mental state and many signs and symptoms may be elicited, not all of which are clinically significant. It is always advisable to seek the advice of a physician in order to provide optimal management for such patients.

FURTHER READING

Costa, A.J. (1995) Interpreting thyroid tests. *American Family Physician*, 52(8), 2325–30.

Davis, D. & Tremont, G. (2007) Neuropsychiatric aspects of hypothyroidism and treatment reversibility. *Minerva Endocrinology*, 32(1), 49–65.

Foster, R. (2008) *Clinical Laboratory Investigation and Psychiatry: A Practical Handbook.* London: Informa.

The examiner's mark sheet

Domain/ percentage of marks	Essential points to pass	✓	Extra marks/comments (make notes here)
1. Rapport and communication 25% of marks	Clear communication Open and closed questions Empathy Sensitivity		Mentions patient confidentiality, as this is not the patient
2. Knowledge of thyroid function tests 25% of marks	Explanation of test results		Treatment of hypothyroidism
3. Thyroid dysfunction 25% of marks	How thyroid activity and specifically underactivity can influence mental state		Physical effects of hypothyroidism
4. Answering other questions 25% of marks	Appropriate responses to additional questions		

% SCORE _____

OVERALL IMPRESSION

___ 4 (CIRCLE ONE)

Good Pass

Pass

Borderline

Fail

Clear Fail

NOTES/Areas to improve

STATION 7: INTERPRETATION OF LITHIUM LEVELS

INSTRUCTION TO CANDIDATE

One of the local GPs has referred a 32-year-old lawyer with a history of bipolar affective disorder to your hospital out-patient clinic after recently commencing him on lithium. The patient had previously been discharged from an out-of-area psychiatric hospital and is reported to be intelligent, insightful and willing to

> comply with treatment so that he can get back to work. He is also said to be interested in learning more about lithium, and has been told by the GP that you are the expert on this! The GP has done blood levels and noted that the level after 4 days was 0.2 mmol/L. No other information has been supplied.
>
> **You are about to meet the patient, who has a number of questions in relation to lithium treatment and monitoring. You are asked to address his concerns.**

ACTOR (ROLE-PLAYER) INSTRUCTIONS

You meet the doctor and want to know about lithium treatment. You are accepting of your diagnosis and want to concentrate on the following:

1. What are the clinical uses of lithium?
2. What are the main side effects of lithium?
3. What is the plasma reference range of lithium?
4. What are the signs of toxicity and how do these relate to plasma level?
5. Are there any additional blood tests that should be done in a patient on lithium?

SUGGESTED APPROACH

Setting the scene

Introduce yourself to the patient. Briefly try to obtain some details about the patient's history. Ask what if anything he knows about lithium and how he has been in himself since commencing this treatment.

Completing the tasks

Remember to talk in lay terms.

What are the clinical uses of lithium?

1. Prophylaxis and treatment of bipolar affective disorder
2. Prophylaxis of recurrent depression, especially as an adjunct in refractory depression
3. As an adjunct to anti-psychotics in the treatment of schizoaffective disorder
4. In the treatment of aggressive or self-mutilating behaviour

What are main side effects of lithium?

Early side effects of lithium are dose-related and include gastrointestinal side effects (nausea, vomiting and diarrhoea), tremor (may manifest as intention tremor) and dry mouth.

Later side effects that are amenable to laboratory measurement are more numerous and appear at higher plasma concentrations.

Later side effects of lithium that may affect laboratory parameters

System	Condition	Laboratory tests
Endocrine	Hypothyroidism	TFTs
	Hyperparathyroidism	Calcium, parathyroid hormone (both increased)
	Nephrogenic diabetes insipidus	U&E
	Raised levels of ADH	U&E, urine osmolality, urine sodium

Haematological	Leucocytosis	FBC
	Thrombocytosis	
Metabolic	Hypercalcaemia (may cause cardiac arrhythmias)	Calcium
	Hypokalaemia (may cause cardiac arrhythmias)	U&E
Renal	Nephropathy	eGFR, U&E, urinalysis
	Renal failure	
	SLE	Autoantibody screen
	Myasthenia gravis	Acetylcholine receptor antibodies; Tensilon (edrophonium) test

What is the plasma reference range of lithium?

The plasma reference range of lithium is approximately 0.6–1 mmol/L.

What are the signs of toxicity and how do these relate to plasma levels?

Severe toxicity may occur at levels >1.5 mmol/L and death may occur at higher levels (>2.0 mmol/L), although toxicity has also been reported at only mildly elevated serum concentrations.

Lithium has a narrow therapeutic index and has a number of important adverse effects in overdose, which may be fatal; these include neurological effects (tremor, ataxia, nystagmus, convulsions, confusion, slurred speech and coma) as well as renal impairment.

Are there any additional blood tests that should be done in a patient on lithium?

Prior to commencing lithium, the following baseline tests should be considered:

Baseline laboratory measurements for patients initiating lithium	
Clinical biochemistry	eGFR, U&E, calcium, creatinine, TFTs
Haematology	Full blood count

Additional, regular laboratory monitoring of laboratory parameters is suggested below:

Additional laboratory monitoring with lithium	
After 7 days	Plasma lithium levels, then *weekly* until the required level is reached (between 0.6 and 1.0 mmol/L)
3-monthly	U&Es, plasma lithium levels
6–12 monthly	eGFR, U&Es, calcium, TFTs
Other	CPK (if NMS suspected)
	Calcium if hyperparathyroidism suspected
	U&Es if patient is dehydrated/vomiting/having diarrhoea
	Other parameters as based on clinical suspicion

ADDITIONAL POINTS

NICE recommends the following laboratory monitoring for lithium:

NICE-recommended reviews in medicated patients following initial screening

Time	Medication	Laboratory parameter	Notes
3-monthly	Lithium	Lithium levels	Three times over 6 weeks following initiation of treatment and 3-monthly thereafter
		U&E	U&Es may be needed more frequently if the patient deteriorates or is on ACE inhibitors, diuretics or non-steroidal anti-inflammatory drugs
		TFTs	Thyroid function for individuals with rapid-cycling bipolar disorder; thyroid antibodies may be measured if TFTs are abnormal
		Glucose	As based on clinical presentation

FURTHER READING

Foster, R. (2008) *Clinical Laboratory Investigation and Psychiatry: A Practical Handbook.* London: Informa.

Bazaire, S. (2003) *Psychotropic Drug Directory 2003/04.* Salisbury: Fivepin Publishing Limited.

Taylor, D., Paton, C. & Kapur, S. (2015) *Maudsley Prescribing Guidelines in Psychiatry*, 12th edn. Chichester: Wiley Blackwell.

The examiner's mark sheet

Domain/ percentage of marks	Essential points to pass	✓	Extra marks/comments (make notes here)
1. Rapport and communication 25% of marks	Clear communication Open and closed questions Empathy Sensitivity		
2. Knowledge of lithium 25% of marks	Indications Side effects and plasma concentrations		
3. Knowledge of guidance on treatment and monitoring 25% of marks	NICE guidance or similar international guidelines		
4. Answering other questions 25% of marks	Appropriate responses to matters arising		

STATION 8: INTERPRETATION OF LABORATORY RESULTS (METABOLIC SYNDROME)

INSTRUCTION TO CANDIDATE

You are phoned by a work colleague who is the on-call psychiatrist. He has been called by the A&E registrar concerning an obese 44-year-old man who has presented to A&E saying he feels 'unwell', though only describes vague physical symptoms.

Although apparently stable from a mental state point of view, the registrar wants a review as the patient is known to have a diagnosis of schizophrenia and has been on olanzapine for some years. He also wants the patient transferred to the local psychiatric hospital as soon as possible. He has not performed any blood tests and has only done a brief physical examination as the patient is 'psychiatric' and 'bizarre'. The registrar does not further define this, but feels that the patient is acutely psychiatrically unwell and in urgent need of sectioning.

A urine dipstick suggested microalbuminuria, but the registrar does not feel that this was significant. There was also evidence of hypertension, but again this was dismissed.

Your colleague calls for help as he thinks the patient might have metabolic syndrome and wants your thoughts on the matter.

ACTOR (ROLE-PLAYER) INSTRUCTIONS

You are a medical colleague. You discuss the case and seek answers to the following questions:

1. What important metabolic side effects of anti-psychotics do you know about?
2. What are the clinical symptoms of metabolic syndrome?
3. What are the clinical signs of metabolic syndrome?
4. What is the major differential diagnosis of metabolic syndrome?
5. What general approaches may be used to manage metabolic syndrome in a patient receiving anti-psychotics?

SUGGESTED APPROACH

Setting the scene

Introduce yourself. You will need to obtain any additional appropriate background information about this patient, including details of all previous treatments, how long the patient was on them and why they were stopped.

Completing the tasks

What important metabolic side effects of anti-psychotics do you know about?

Anti-psychotics have a number of metabolic side effects, including those comprising metabolic syndrome; these include disturbed glucose metabolism (raised fasting plasma glucose), abnormal insulin metabolism (hyperinsulinaemia) and dyslipidaemia (reduced high-density lipoprotein and hypertriglyceridaemia). Microalbuminuria may also occur, but this is variable.

What are the clinical symptoms of metabolic syndrome?

Frequently, there may be none in the early stages, while in later stages, there are those of underlying disorder, such as glucose intolerance/diabetes mellitus or hyperlipidaemia.

What are the clinical signs of metabolic syndrome?

These may include obesity, hypertension and signs of associated disorders such as acanthosis nigricans, haemochromatosis or polycystic ovary syndrome.

What is the major differential diagnosis of metabolic syndrome?

The major differential is diabetes mellitus.

Are there any other medications associated with metabolic syndrome?

Apart from anti-psychotics, stavudine, steroids and zidovudine have been associated with the development of metabolic syndrome.

What general approaches may be used to manage metabolic syndrome in a patient receiving anti-psychotics?

This will depend on both clinical presentation and severity and may include general and specific interventions. Interventions will require a multidisciplinary focus. General interventions may include lifestyle modification (increased exercise and weight loss) and dietary changes, while specific interventions may include aspirin prophylaxis for pro-thrombotic states, anti-hypertensive treatment, pharmacological treatment aimed at lowering blood cholesterol and oral hypoglycaemics or insulin.

Regular monitoring of blood sugar via urine dipstick, 'near patient' blood sampling or laboratory testing (fasting glucose and HbA1c) is required, and it may be appropriate to switch to another class of anti-psychotic. In all cases, expert advice is required.

Problem solving

The first task is to try to find out any additional information about the patient. Advise that your colleague obtains collateral information from the CMHT (if there is one) or the GP. He will need to perform a proper history, mental state examination and physical examination in order to determine whether this man is acutely psychiatrically unwell or is in need of immediate medical attention. In his history, he will need to specifically ask about any psychiatric history, medical history and medication history, as you are concerned about the microalbuminuria, which you recall may be associated with the renal toxicity of some medications.

He will need to ask the A&E team to perform a thorough physical examination and request appropriate blood tests in order to rule out an organic cause of this man's presentation.

Laboratory features of metabolic syndrome

Feature	Laboratory investigation	Notes
Disturbed glucose metabolism	Random blood glucose, HbA1c, glucose tolerance test, plasma insulin	May manifest as any of hyperinsulinaemia, impaired glucose tolerance, insulin resistance or diabetes mellitus
Disturbed insulin metabolism		
Obesity	Non-specific	Particularly abdominal distribution
Dyslipidaemia	Plasma cholesterol/ triglycerides	Decreased high-density lipoprotein cholesterol and/or hypertriglyceridaemia
Hypertension	Non-specific	May not have any obvious clinical manifestations in the early stages
Microalbuminuria	Urinalysis	May not be present, but absence does not preclude the diagnosis

ADDITIONAL POINTS

Definition: metabolic syndrome, also called syndrome of insulin resistance, syndrome X and Reaven's syndrome, consists of the association of central obesity with two or more of the four key features of the disorder (hypertension, hypertriglyceridaemia, raised fasting plasma glucose and reduced high-density lipoprotein). The World Health Organisation guidelines also include the feature of microalbuminuria.

Incidence: controversial; in schizophrenic patients treated with anti-psychotics, the published ranges vary between 22% and 54.2%.

Psychiatric associations: psychotic illnesses (especially schizophrenia) – treatment with anti-psychotic medication (especially atypicals); note that other medications have been associated with the development of metabolic syndrome, including some antiretroviral agents (stavudine and zidovudine) and steroids.

FURTHER READING

De Hert, M.A., van Winkel, R., Van Eyck, D. et al. (2006) Prevalence of the metabolic syndrome in patients with schizophrenia treated with antipsychotic medication. *Schizophrenia Research*, 83(1), 87–93.

Grungy, S.M., Cleeman, J.I., Daniels, S.R. et al. (2005) Diagnosis and management of the metabolic syndrome. *Circulation, 112*, 2735–52.

Haddad, P., Durson, S. & Deakin, B. (eds) (2004) *Adverse Syndromes and Psychiatric Drugs – A Clinical Guide.* Oxford: Oxford University Press.

Taylor, D., Paton, C. & Kapur, S. (2015) *Maudsley Prescribing Guidelines in Psychiatry*, 12th edn. Chichester: Wiley Blackwell.

The examiner's mark sheet

Domain/ percentage of marks	Essential points to pass	✓	Extra marks/comments (make notes here)
1. Rapport and communication 30% of marks	Clear communication with a clinical colleague		
2. Knowledge of a diagnosis of metabolic syndrome 35% of marks	Symptoms Screening laboratory tests Management		
3. Answering other questions 35% of marks	Preventing inappropriate psychiatric admission Seeking more information (collateral)		

% SCORE _____

___ **OVERALL IMPRESSION**

3 (CIRCLE ONE)

Good Pass

Pass

Borderline

Fail

Clear Fail

NOTES/Areas to improve

STATION 9: DIAGNOSIS AND MANAGEMENT OF NEUROLEPTIC MALIGNANT SYNDROME

INSTRUCTION TO CANDIDATE

During a night on call, you are called to one of the wards to see a patient whom the nurses are worried about. This is a 35-year-old man who was recently recommenced on anti-psychotic treatment, with lithium having been recently added due to an apparent history of bipolar affective disorder. The nurses inform you that the patient looks 'unwell' and is agitated and sweaty, although not aggressive or hypomanic. He has a temperature, but is not complaining of any pain.

They have done some basic observations and let you know that his pulse rate is 120 per minute, his respiratory rate is 24 per minute and his blood pressure is 160/110.

You are concerned and call the on-call medical team. They want to know more about his presentation and likely diagnosis.

ACTOR (ROLE-PLAYER) INSTRUCTIONS

You are the medical registrar and want to know more about this patient before you consider accepting him as a medical admission.

You want to know what the doctor considers the diagnosis to be.

The doctor should mention NMS and this will be the prompt for the following questions:

1. What are possible differential diagnoses?
2. What is NMS?
3. What are the clinical signs and symptoms?
4. What medications are implicated in NMS?
5. What immediate action needs to be taken on the ward?
6. What additional measures may be useful in the treatment of NMS?
7. What laboratory tests, if any, are useful for the diagnosis and monitoring of NMS?
8. What is the prognosis of NMS?

SUGGESTED APPROACH

Setting the scene

Introduce yourself. It is important to let the medics know that this is a possible case of NMS, which is a medical emergency. Let them know that he needs transferring to a medical setting for further management. Remember to talk in clear, calm and polite terms and be prepared to explain how you intend to manage the situation acutely. If your colleague refuses to accept the patient, you should explain that you will have to call for an ambulance as there is a significant mortality associated with this condition.

Completing the tasks

What are possible differential diagnoses?

Medication-related:	Lethal catatonia, lithium toxicity, malignant hyperthermia, serotonin syndrome and severe extrapyramidal side effects
Drug-related:	Acute intoxication (amphetamine and cocaine), toxicity (anaesthetics, anticholinergics and MAOIs) and withdrawal (alcohol, anti-Parkinsonian medications and benzodiazepines)
Organic:	Cerebral tumours, CVA, dehydration, delirium, heat exhaustion, myocardial infarction, pheochromocytoma, seizures, sepsis (encephalitis, encephalomyelitis, HIV and systemic), SLE, thyrotoxicosis and trauma
Psychiatric:	Mania and severe psychosis

What is NMS?

NMS is a rare, idiosyncratic and life-threatening condition that is thought to be related to the use of medications that block dopamine receptors and thereby induce sympathetic hyperactivity.

What are the clinical signs and symptoms?

Core features:	Behavioural change, diaphoresis, hyperthermia, impaired consciousness, labile blood pressure and tachycardia
Associated features:	Akinesia, dystonia, sialorrhoea, tachypnoea and tremor

What medications are implicated in NMS?

Antidepressants:	(e.g. monoamine oxidase inhibitors and tricyclic antidepressants)
Anti-psychotics:	All, possible increased risk with clozapine and risperidone
Others:	Metoclopramide, reserpine, tetrabenazine and lithium, especially in combination with anti-psychotics
Discontinuation of:	Amantadine, bromocriptine and levodopa

What immediate action needs to be taken on the ward?

Ensure patient and staff safety.

Perform rapid primary survey, ensuring adequate airway, breathing and circulation.

Stop putative offending agent.

Insert Venflon.

Monitor observations (temperature, pulse, respiratory rate, blood pressure and O_2 saturation).

Perform ECG if possible.

If in any doubt, transfer patient to general hospital.

Ensure good communication with ward staff, on-call senior and receiving hospital.

Once patient is stabilised:

Ensure that appropriate documentation occurs

Ensure that ward staff feel supported

Ensure that the ward consultant is notified

What additional measures may be useful in the treatment of NMS?

Monitor and correct metabolic imbalances.

Monitor temperature and cool the patient as required.

Medications such as benzodiazepines, thiamine, dextrose and/or naloxone may be needed.

Monitor kidney function and urine output.

Electro-convulsive therapy may be helpful in some patients.

What blood/laboratory tests, if any, are useful for the diagnosis and monitoring of NMS?

Possible laboratory abnormalities in NMS

Domain	Parameter	Notes
Clinical biochemistry	Blood gases	May reveal anoxia and/or metabolic acidosis
	Creatine phosphokinase	Elevated levels may be seen, reflecting myonecrosis from sustained muscle contractions (rhabdomyolysis)
	LFTs	Raised liver enzymes (LDH, ALP and AST) may be seen

⇑	U&Es	May reflect altered renal function
	Urinalysis	May reveal myoglobinuria (rhabdomyolysis)
Haematology	FBC	May reveal leucocytosis

What is the prognosis of NMS?

Mortality: Between 5% and 12% due to cardiac arrhythmia, DIC, respiratory failure, renal failure and shock.

Morbidity: Variable, better outcome in younger people and early intervention: arrhythmias, aspiration pneumonia, DIC, respiratory embarrassment, rhabdomyolysis, renal failure and seizures.

Problem solving

Remember that NMS and its differentials are potentially life-threatening conditions, and prompt action is always required. Ensure that staff are aware of the urgency of intervention, have appropriate equipment to hand and that the crash team has been alerted. There must be no delay in seeing the patient, and it is advisable to ring for an ambulance at the earliest opportunity, ensuring that the receiving hospital is also warned about the patient. A copy of the current drug chart and psychiatric notes is always helpful, as is a transfer letter.

Prior to transfer to A&E, basic interventions (airways, breathing and circulation) and basic observations should be performed, with additional input given where the doctor in charge deems this appropriate.

ADDITIONAL POINTS

In normal practice, 'heroic' interventions are not appropriate on the ward, and although you have a duty of care towards your patient, performing interventions that you are not adequately trained in or experienced with is never appropriate. Management of medical emergencies is best performed in A&E.

FURTHER READING

National Institute for Health and Care Excellence (2006) Bipolar disorder: The management of bipolar disorder in adults, children and adolescents, in primary and secondary care. http://www.nice.org.uk/nicemedia/pdf/CG38fullguideline.pdf

Schweyen, D.H., Sporka, M.C. & Burnakis, T.G. (1991) Evaluation of serum lithium concentration determinations. *American Journal of Hospital Pharmacy*, 48(7), 1536–7.

Taylor, D., Paton, C. & Kapur, S. (2015) *Maudsley Prescribing Guidelines in Psychiatry*, 12th edn. Chichester: Wiley Blackwell.

The examiners mark sheet

Domain/ percentage of marks	Essential points to pass	✓	Extra marks/comments (make notes here)
1. Communication with colleagues	Clear and professional communication		
25% of marks	Explanation of the urgency in this case		⇓

2. Recognition of the signs and symptoms of NMS

   20% of marks

Ability to synthesise the case and explain the clinical features of NMS to a colleague

3. Immediate management

   20% of marks

Basic supportive measures

4. Longer-term management

   25% of marks

Physical

Psychiatric

5. Answering other questions

   10% of marks

Appropriate responses to questions

% SCORE _____

___ **OVERALL IMPRESSION**

5 (CIRCLE ONE)

Good Pass

Pass

Borderline

Fail

Clear Fail

NOTES/Areas to improve

STATION 10: DIAGNOSIS AND MANAGEMENT OF SEROTONIN SYNDROME

INSTRUCTION TO CANDIDATE

You have been called to A&E to see Mr Richards, a 46-year-old man who has been 'medically cleared'. He was assessed by one of the PLNs, who noted that he was confused and appeared sweaty. She is concerned that he might be medically unwell and feels that a doctor's opinion is needed. The patient had apparently been taking a herbal medication, which the nurse thinks may be St John's wort. The helpful GP has confirmed that Mr Richards has a history of amphetamine abuse and had been prescribed a selective serotonin reuptake inhibitor (SSRI) due to depression, but appears to have been non-compliant. When you see him, you note that he is confused, agitated and appears to be shaking.

The PLN wonders whether he is suffering from a serotonin syndrome and would like your opinion.

ACTOR (ROLE-PLAYER) INSTRUCTIONS

You are a psychiatric liaison nurse. You have met the patient and wonder whether the symptoms are pharmacologically driven. You ask the following questions:

1. What are the possible differential diagnoses?
2. What exactly is serotonin syndrome?
3. What are the clinical signs and symptoms?
4. What immediate action needs to be taken?
5. What additional measures may be useful in the treatment of the syndrome?
6. What laboratory tests, if any, are useful for the diagnosis and monitoring of serotonin syndrome?
7. What is the prognosis of serotonin syndrome?

SUGGESTED APPROACH

Setting the scene

Introduce yourself. The current scenario should set alarm bells ringing as it implies a medical emergency that requires immediate medical input. Try to get more of a handover from the nurse and explain that you do not want to delay seeing the patient. Ask what she knows about his history, physical examination and any investigations.

Completing the tasks

What are the possible differential diagnoses?

Psychiatric:	Catatonia
Medication-related syndromes:	Malignant hyperthermia and neuroleptic malignant syndrome
Drugs/medication intoxication:	Anticholinergics, amphetamine, cocaine, lithium, MAOIs and salicylates
Drug withdrawal:	Baclofen (acute withdrawal)
Other:	Encephalitis, hyperthyroidism, meningitis, non-convulsive seizures, septicaemia and tetanus

What is serotonin syndrome?

Serotonin syndrome is a disorder that is caused by the overstimulation of serotonergic receptors following the administration of a number of medications, especially antidepressants, including SSRIs, MAOIs and TCAs. It is a rare and idiosyncratic disorder which is nearly always observed following the administration of a serotonergic agent. Clinical features are based on the triad of autonomic, cognitive/behavioural and neurological symptoms.

What are the clinical signs and symptoms?

Clinical features of serotonin syndrome	
Autonomic	Blood pressure lability
	Diaphoresis
	Dyspnoea
	Fever
	Tachycardia
Cognitive/behavioural	Changes in mental state (confusion and possible hypomania) and behaviour (agitation and insomnia) may be seen

⇩

Neurological	Akathisia
	Hyperreflexia
	Impaired coordination
	Myoclonus
	Tremor

What immediate action needs to be taken?

Severe serotonin syndrome, as appears to be the case with this patient, is a medical emergency. Thus, the medical team should be made aware immediately. Attention should be paid to airways, breathing and circulation, with supportive measures such as cooling, muscle paralysis and intubation initiated in order to prevent complications such as rhabdomyolysis, renal failure and DIC. It would be prudent to cease any putative contributory agents and, if necessary, seek advice from the local poisons unit.

What additional measures may be useful in the treatment of serotonin syndrome?

Some authorities suggest the use of serotonin antagonists, and cyproheptadine and chlorpromazine have both been used.

What laboratory tests, if any, are useful for the diagnosis and monitoring of serotonin syndrome?

Whilst the diagnosis is primarily clinical, based on the presence of autonomic, cognitive/behavioural and neurological symptoms, there are no specific diagnostic laboratory investigations. Rather, any investigations are aimed at evaluating and monitoring associated morbidity.

Possible laboratory changes in serotonin syndrome

Domain	Parameter	Notes
Clinical biochemistry	Bicarbonate	Decreased levels seen
	Creatine kinase (total)	Elevated levels seen
	Transaminases	Elevated levels seen
	Metabolic acidosis	May be seen
Haematology	Leucocytosis	May be seen
	Disseminated intravascular coagulation	

What is the prognosis of serotonin syndrome?

Although severe serotonin syndrome is a medical emergency, it is rarely life-threatening with appropriate treatment.

ADDITIONAL POINTS

In normal practice, 'heroic' interventions are not appropriate on the ward, and although you have a duty of care towards your patient, performing interventions that you are not adequately trained in or experienced with is never appropriate. Management of medical emergencies is best performed in A&E.

Two separate sets of clinical features have been proposed to assist in the diagnosis of serotonin syndrome.

The Hunter Serotonin Toxicity Criteria provide a series of 'decision rules', with spontaneous clonus in the presence of a serotonergic agent confirming the diagnosis or the presence of induced clonus with other features (agitation and sweating) or ocular clonus with other features (agitation and sweating) or tremor/hyperreflexia or hypertonia/hyperthermia/clonus (ocular or induced).

The Sternbach criteria include agitation, alteration in mental state (confusion and hypomania), diarrhoea, fever, hyperreflexia, incoordination, myoclonus, shivering, sweating and tremor.

FURTHER READING

Dunkley, E.J., Isbister, G.K., Sibbritt, D., Dawson, A.H. & Whyte, I.M. (2003) The Hunter Serotonin Toxicity Criteria: Simple and accurate diagnostic decision rules for serotonin toxicity. *QJM, 96,* 635–42.

Isbister, G.K., Buckley, N.A. & Whyte, I.M. (2007) Serotonin toxicity: A practical approach to diagnosis and treatment. *Medical Journal of Australia 187*(6), 361–5.

Sternbach, H. (1991) The serotonin syndrome. *American Journal of Psychiatry, 148*(6), 705–13.

Taylor, D., Paton, C. & Kapur, S. (2015) *Maudsley Prescribing Guidelines in Psychiatry,* 12th edn. Chichester: Wiley Blackwell.

The examiner's mark sheet

Domain/ percentage of marks	Essential points to pass	✓	Extra marks/comments (make notes here)
1. Rapport and communication 25% of marks	Clear and professional communication Explanation of the urgency in this case		
2. Recognition of the signs and symptoms of serotonin syndrome 20% of marks	Ability to synthesise the case and explain the clinical features of serotonin syndrome to a colleague		
3. Immediate management 20% of marks	Basic supportive measures		
4. Longer-term management 25% of marks	Physical Psychiatric		
5. Answering other questions 10% of marks	Appropriate responses to questions		

% SCORE _____

OVERALL IMPRESSION

5   (CIRCLE ONE)

Good Pass

Pass

Borderline

Fail

Clear Fail

NOTES/Areas to improve

STATION 11: DIAGNOSIS AND MANAGEMENT OF HYPERPROLACTINAEMIA

INSTRUCTION TO CANDIDATE

You are a new doctor in a Community Mental Health Team and have been asked to see an anxious 62-year-old man with a history of schizophrenia who is complaining of medication side effects. When you see him, he is distressed and feels that he is turning into a woman. On closer questioning, he reveals that he has been taking the same 'psycho' medications for many years. He also says that he has not been reviewed by a psychiatrist for many years. He volunteers that the medications help his mental state and that he sometimes takes one or two more of his pills on a 'stress day'. After careful questioning, he tells you that the name of the tablet is something like 'Haldone', which, on clarification, you realise is haloperidol. He says that he thinks he should be taking this at a dose of 5 mg daily.

He says that he has recently been having increasing difficulties 'down below'; he feels he is starting to grow breasts, which, embarrassingly, seem to be producing what he says is milk. He says that he never sees his GP and hates having blood tests, but says that this is stressing him out and that he is starting to get paranoid that people are paying him more attention. You see from the notes that this is a known relapse indicator for the patient. You note that he says that he has no medical problems, has never had any surgery and is not on any other medications. He says that he thinks he has a brain tumour.

You receive the results of the routine blood tests and you see that his serum prolactin level is 500 mIU/L. There are no other clinically significant results.

He has a number of questions for you:

1. What is the likely cause of the symptoms that the patient is describing?
2. What is the physiological mechanism causing these?
3. What is your explanation for the prolactin level? How would you interpret this?
4. How are you going to help him?

ACTOR (ROLE-PLAYER) INSTRUCTIONS

You are very concerned that your body is changing and worry that others see you as a woman. You are somewhat paranoid, but are not overtly psychotic – you still take regular anti-psychotic medication.

You want the doctor to help you and at the same time want to remain psychiatrically well.

You ask the doctor several times to examine your chest to see what you mean (they will not be able to do this in the examination cubicle).

You seek reassurance throughout as you worry that you have a brain tumour.

You ask the questions as indicated above.

SUGGESTED APPROACH

Setting the scene

Introduce yourself and explain that you have been asked to see this patient. Explain that some of your questions may be embarrassing, but that you will try to ask these sensitively.

Completing the tasks

What is the likely cause of the symptoms that this patient is describing?

Based on this man's history, possible differential diagnoses would include the following:

Psychiatric

Hyperprolactinaemia secondary to anti-psychotic use (thought to be less commonly associated with aripiprazole, clozapine, olanzapine, quetiapine and ziprasidone)

Anorexia nervosa

Non-psychiatric

Chronic renal failure

Ectopic secretion

Pituitary tumours

Pituitary insufficiency

Hypothalamic disease

Hypothyroidism

Liver disease

Medications (methyldopa, metoclopramide, oestrogens and reserpine)

Sarcoidosis

'Stress', including anaesthesia, insulin-induced hypoglycaemia, venepuncture and surgery

In females

Polycystic ovary syndrome

Pregnancy

Rarer causes

Argonz–Del Castillo syndrome (galactorrhoea–amenorrhoea in the absence of pregnancy associated with oestrogen deficiency and decreased urinary gonadotrophins).

Chiari–Frommel syndrome (persistent galactorrhoea and amenorrhoea postpartum).

Common symptoms in females include menstrual disturbances, galactorrhoea and infertility, while in males these include impotence, infertility and gynaecomastia.

What is the physiological mechanism causing this?

Prolactin release is inhibited by dopamine, and thus dopamine antagonists such as anti-psychotics will increase prolactin levels, likely in a dose-related manner.

How would you interpret the blood test results?

The main investigation would be serum prolactin, with levels below approximately 325 mIU/L in males considered normal and levels in females below 510 mIU/L considered abnormal. Note that different laboratories publish different reference ranges, with higher reference ranges reported for females. Levels may be affected by sampling time, as prolactin rises at night after the onset of slow-wave and cycles of rapid eye movement sleep. Where levels are markedly raised (at least twice the upper limit of normal or greater), measurement of macroprolactin, a form of prolactin bound to IgG, should be taken, as this may be found in patients with high levels of prolactin. It is not biologically active and may be a cause of apparent hyperprolactinaemia.

High levels of prolactin (in the thousands, but generally over 2,000–3,000 mIU/L) are suggestive of a prolactinoma. Measurement of other pituitary hormones should be considered where there is clinical suspicion of a pituitary tumour and high levels of prolactin have been detected.

Magnetic resonance imaging may also be helpful, and in some cases, osteoporosis may be secondary to hypogonadism and may be noted on bone density scanning.

How would you manage this patient?

This will depend on the clinical findings and the results of all investigations. This patient will require a thorough history, physical examination and appropriate investigations. A sympathetic approach is needed, given the embarrassing nature of the symptoms, and full psychiatric, medical and medication histories are especially relevant here. Physical examination should include consideration of the features of excessive hormone production, such as acromegaly and Cushing's syndrome. As some patients may present with visual symptoms, features of raised intracranial pressure or epilepsy, a full neurological examination is indicated.

Given the clinical presentation, a prolactinoma also needs to be ruled out. Medications such as bromocriptine may be used, as may quinagolide or cabergoline. In some cases, surgical intervention may be required. Where no prolactinoma is suspected, a careful history may reveal a treatable cause. It may be appropriate to discontinue and substitute his current psychotropic for a less hyper-prolactogenic agent, such as aripiprazole, clozapine, olanzapine, quetiapine or ziprasidone.

In such a case, the most likely differential is that of prolactinaemia secondary to anti-psychotic treatment. This is explained by both the clinical presentation as well as the blood results. You should reassure the patient, although you need to discuss the need for some blood tests and possibly a referral to a different specialist, depending on the results of the blood tests. You should discuss the importance of medication compliance and consider whether a dose reduction is needed or whether the medication needs to be substituted. You should discuss possible alternative medications, informing the patient that the first-choice anti-psychotic when switching from haloperidol would be one of either aripiprazole or quetiapine, but there are other alternatives should these be tolerated, such as olanzapine or ziprasidone. You should discuss the prognosis of the sexual side effects and reassure the patient that these may diminish with the new medication.

ADDITIONAL POINTS

Haloperidol is commonly associated with sexual side effects, as are all anti-psychotics to varying degrees. Such potential side effects should always be explained upon initiation of these medications, as may the finding that not all individuals who are prescribed these medications complain of sexual side effects. Taking a sexual history can be complex, and the use of a rating scale such as the Arizona Sexual Experience Scale may be helpful here.

FURTHER READING

Ajmal, A., Joffe, H. & Nachtigall, L.B. (2014) Psychotropic-induced hyperprolactinemia: A clinical review. *Psychosomatics, 55*(1), 29–36.

Foster, R. (2008) *Clinical Laboratory Investigation and Psychiatry: A Practical Handbook.* London: Informa.

Levy, A. (2014) Interpreting raised serum prolactin results. *BMJ, 348,* g3207.

Taylor, D., Paton, C. & Kapur, S. (2015) *Maudsley Prescribing Guidelines in Psychiatry,* 12th edn. Chichester: Wiley Blackwell.

The examiner's mark sheet

Domain/ percentage of marks	Essential points to pass	✓	Extra marks/comments (make notes here)
1. Rapport and communication 25% of marks	Clear communication Open and closed questions Empathy Sensitivity		
2. Recognition of clinical syndrome 25% of marks	Symptoms secondary to prolactin; likely secondary to long-term anti-psychotic use		
3. Patient education 25% of marks	Aetiology Symptoms Management plan Further investigations		
4. Answering other questions 25% of marks	Appropriate responses		

% SCORE _____

___ OVERALL IMPRESSION

4 (CIRCLE ONE)

Good Pass

Pass

Borderline

Fail

Clear Fail

NOTES/Areas to improve

O SINGLE STATIONS

STATION 1: GENDER REASSIGNMENT

INSTRUCTION TO CANDIDATE

This is Michael Green, a 28-year-old who lives with both parents. Michael is seeking comprehensive female gender reassignment and has been talking about travelling to Thailand for surgery. Michael's family are not keen on the idea and would prefer that the treatment is within the NHS.

Michael, having had feminising hormone treatment privately, is considering an NHS transgender programme and hopes to discuss this with you today. The referral notes that the patient wishes to be known as 'Charlotte'.

Speak to the patient and clarify their eligibility for gender reassignment.

Explain what a treatment programme is likely to involve.

ACTOR (ROLE-PLAYER) INSTRUCTIONS

You like to be called Charlotte and become annoyed if you are referred to as male or by the name Michael. You were born with male genitalia and brought up as male, but feel that you have always been of female gender; however, you only realised this over the past 2 years. You have been wearing women's clothes and using the name Charlotte for the last 18 months and using private feminising hormones for the past 3 months. You gain no sexual excitement from wearing women's clothes and consider yourself bisexual. You have no current symptoms of depression nor any other mental health problem.

You are seeking overseas surgery as you believe that the NHS will disregard your transsexualism and that your family would not support you through the process.

SUGGESTED APPROACH

Setting the scene

Introduce yourself and introduce the assessment. 'Hello, Charlotte, my name is Dr_____, and I am a psychiatrist. I understand you are not happy living as a man.'

Or:

'I understand that you are interested in referral to a gender reassignment programme. Can you tell me more about what led to this decision? Is it the case that you feel that the gender you were assigned at birth does not fit? When did you first notice these feelings?'

Completing the tasks

Building a rapport and being sensitive in communication is important in this task. Gender identity can be a sensitive topic so it is important that candidates understand how to use language and to appreciate the potential for discrimination and transphobia. A confident and empathic approach with careful listening will help to put the patient at ease. If you are unsure what name to use or whether to say 'he' or 'she', ask the patient their preference. 'Trans' have often experienced discrimination before and may be fearful of similar treatment in the NHS.

Diagnosing transsexualism

The ICD-10 has three diagnostic criteria (F64.0):

1. History of gender dysphoria in which the person has been subjectively uncomfortable with the gender allocated to them at birth, often accompanied by a desire to live in a way and alter their body in order to align with their internal identity.
2. They need to have a consistent and sustained desire to live as their preferred gender for at least 2 years (although they can be referred for specialist assessment prior to this).
3. Transsexualism can only be diagnosed where these beliefs and desires are not due to any other psychiatric condition (e.g. schizophrenia or the differentials outlined below) and where genitalia are unambiguous (e.g. a chromosomal disorder). Specialist assessment is needed for possible gender identity disorder in a person with intersex genitalia.

A history of gender dysphoria

Personal: take a history of the onset, duration and consistency of gender dysphoria (e.g. feeling uncomfortable with their genitalia) and secondary sexual characteristics (e.g. facial hair, voice and body shape).

Social: another component is feeling uncomfortable with others perceiving and treating them as though they were their birth-assigned gender (e.g. if male-to-female, being referred to as male or an expectation that they will dress, communicate or behave as though they were a man).

'Can you tell me when you first realised that you were transgendered? Transgender people often talk about feeling uncomfortable with their birth-assigned gender – is that the case for you? When did you first notice these feelings? How has that impacted on your life? Have there been challenges at work or with friends and family? Are there activities or places you have avoided because of this; for example, certain jobs or social occasions?'

Take a history of the onset, duration and impact of living in the desired future gender role. Behaviours specific to one gender can be subtle and differ between cultures and individuals but may include:

- Identifying as that gender to others (e.g. by a gendered name or if specifically asked)
- Changing their name by deed poll
- Dressing as that gender
- Participating in religious events in a manner appropriate to that gender where there are particular roles
- Using toilets allocated to that gender
- Indicating that gender when completing forms
- Applying for gender alteration on their passport and birth certificate via the Gender Recognition Panel

Differential diagnoses

The key differential diagnoses to exclude are dual-role transvestitism and fetishistic transvestitism.

In dual-role transvestitism, the person temporarily adopts the clothing and behavioural role of the other gender for enjoyment for a temporary period, not associated with sexual arousal and with no desire for permanent change.

In fetishistic transvestitism, clothes of the other gender are worn for sexual excitement and there is no desire to continue dressing as or any other aspect of the other gender outside of periods of sexual arousal.

'To make sure I understand your experience of your gender identity, can I ask how often you wear feminine clothes? When you do this, is there any degree of sexual excitement or is it purely an identity that you feel comfortable with? Is this something that you do or would wish to do constantly? Are there times that you don't feel a need to live as a woman?'

It is worth briefly excluding psychosis and affective disorder and enquiring into any past psychiatric history.

Management

- Referral to a specialist gender identity clinic for full assessment and guidance through the process.
- Psychological support: counselling or individual/group psychotherapy.
- Hormone therapy: this is to effect changes in the body in order to bring it in line with the person's gender identity. They can be taken indefinitely and require monitoring and clear information about side effects. Oestrogens for male-to-female reassignment require monitoring for lipids, liver function and hypertension. Give advice on the signs of thromboembolism, as this could be of increased risk. Either of the hormone treatments can reduce fertility, regardless of the birth gender, and gamete storage can be considered before commencing treatment.
- Speech and language therapy to assist with altering the voice to fit with the person's gender identity. Note that hormone treatment for female-to-male reassignment will deepen the voice, but hormone treatment for male-to-female reassignment will not raise the pitch (the larynx does not reduce in size).
- Peer support groups and support groups for the families of people going through gender reassignment.
- Hair removal treatments, particularly of facial hair in male-to-female reassignment.

Surgery

Gender reassignment surgery usually requires that the person has lived as their desired future gender role for 2 years.

For male-to-female reassignment, surgery can include phonosurgery (for voice), breast implants and the formation of a neo-vagina from existing genital tissue and autografts.

For female-to-male reassignment, surgery can include bilateral mastectomy, hysterectomy and bilateral salpingo-oophorectomy, phalloplasty/metoidioplasty, scrotoplasty and testicular implants.

It is important to ask about the intention to seek surgery overseas and to highlight the risks of not having sufficient support and preparation for surgery with major permanent effects and potential complications. Reassure them that the NHS does have specialist care for transgendered people and that they will be supported and have their rights respected throughout.

Conclusion

Having demonstrated knowledge of the diagnosis, differentials and management, it is helpful to recap the person's situation and goals. It is important to note that some hormone treatment changes and gender reassignment surgeries are permanent and the management process aims to ensure realistic expectations. Psychological and medical support continues after medical and surgical treatment.

'Thank you for talking to me today, Charlotte. From the information you have given, we can refer you to a gender reassignment clinic in order to complete the assessment and support you on the process of transitioning.'

Key considerations

A person identifying as transsexual believes that they have always had an internal gender that does not correspond to the gender they were assigned at birth on the basis of their genitalia. It is important to use the name and gender pronouns (he/him/his or she/her/hers) that they prefer.

A person's gender history prior to identifying as transsexual is confidential medical information and should not be disclosed to third parties without consent.

Persons who have a subjective gender identity that does not correspond to their bodily sex are 'transsexual' or 'transgendered', and persons who have a gender identity that does correspond to their bodily sex are often referred to as 'cissexual' or 'cisgendered'.

Patients considering gender reassignment may fear discrimination at work, from friends and family or transphobic abuse from their community.

Transsexualism occurs in both directions (i.e. male-to-female or female-to-male). This scenario concerns male-to-female reassignment, and corresponding but different hormonal treatments and surgical procedures are indicated for female-to-male reassignment.

Gender reassignment (and so transsexualism) was made a protected characteristic in Article 7 of the Equality Act 2010, making it illegal to discriminate on the basis of gender identity.

FURTHER READING

World Health Organization (1992) *The ICD-10 Classification of Mental and Behavioural Disorders. Clinical Descriptions and Diagnostic Guidelines.* Geneva: WHO Press.

Helpful explanations and advice for professionals working with transsexual patients can be found in the NHS Gender Dysphoria Guide. http://www.nhs.uk/Livewell/Transhealth/Documents/gender-dysphoria-guide-for-gps-and-other-health-care-staff.pdf

NHS Choices. Gender dysphoria (contains useful information on treatment pathways). http://www.nhs.uk/Conditions/Gender-dysphoria/Pages/Introduction.aspx

The Equality and Human Rights commission contains information on discrimination and the rights of trans people: www.equalityhumanrights.com/

The examiner's mark sheet

Domain/ percentage of marks	Essential points to pass	✓	Extra marks/comments (make notes here)
1. Rapport and communication 25% of marks	Open and closed questions Empathy Appropriate use of gendered language		
2. Takes a history of gender dysphoria 25% of marks	Makes appropriate and sensitive enquiries, taking into account onset, duration and measures already taken Explores the impact on different areas of life		
3. Excludes relevant differential diagnoses 20% of marks	Considers dual-role and fetishistic transvestitism Screens for other psychiatric disorders (e.g. psychosis, depression and substance misuse)		
4. Management 30% of marks	Explains the treatment pathway Psychological, medical and surgical interventions 2 years in preferred gender role. Notes risks and management of risks with medical/surgical management Explores reasons for seeking overseas surgery and addresses concerns		

% SCORE _____

___

4

OVERALL IMPRESSION

(CIRCLE ONE)

Good Pass

Pass

Borderline

Fail

Clear Fail

NOTES/Areas to improve

STATION 2: GRIEF REACTION

INSTRUCTION TO CANDIDATE

Mrs Smith is a 39-year-old woman who lost her husband 8 months ago due to cancer and has been attending the GP regularly with multiple non-specific complaints, and it often ends up as a counselling session. The GP has been seeing her but has not been providing any formal psychological treatment or medication. She will call the surgery often asking to speak to her doctor and has also asked him to visit her at home on a number of occasions.

The GP noticed that she continues to grieve and is unsure whether this is normal. In her medical history, she has asthma and psoriasis. There is no past psychiatric history. Her brother has an autistic spectrum disorder, but lives independently.

She is close to her mother, with whom she speaks almost every day.

Assess this woman's response to the loss of her husband.

ACTOR (ROLE-PLAYER) INSTRUCTIONS

You sleep well, have no difficulty with your daily routine and, while you cried regularly in the first few months after his death, this is now once a fortnight.

You think about your husband most days and sometimes feel sad but not pervasively low in mood; you interact normally and can see a brighter side at times.

You occasionally hear your husband call your name at home, but think this is 'all in your mind'.

You call the GP because you are afraid that minor symptoms may be early signs of cancer like your husband had and have looked this up on the Internet.

You are not delusional and accept reassurance that the bereavement may have produced some excessive worry regarding your own health.

SUGGESTED APPROACH

Setting the scene

'Hello, Mrs Smith, my name is Dr_____, and I am a psychiatrist. Your GP asked me to see you as he was concerned about how you have been feeling since you lost your husband some months ago. I'd like to ask you a bit about how you were after the bereavement, how things are now and briefly about your mental health more generally in the past. Would that be alright?'

Features of grief

The key here is whether the patient is having a normal grief reaction that may be somewhat prolonged or whether she has developed a psychiatric condition following (or even prior to) her husband's death. There are some unusual features noted by the GP for an otherwise fit 39-year-old, such as requesting home visits and multiple health complaints.

Differentials to consider are an abnormal grief (adjustment) reaction that may have led to depression with or without psychotic features, a psychotic illness, a somatoform disorder such as hypochondriasis or an anxiety disorder.

Find out a little about her husband and then her daily life before and since the bereavement.

'Losing someone close to you is always painful and I wondered how long you had known your husband for and how long you had been married. I understand from your GP that he died from cancer. Was he unwell for a long period or did his death come suddenly? Can I ask what has life been like since the loss? What do you tend to do day to day? Were you working before he passed away? What has happened with your job and social life since his death?'

Features of abnormal/complicated grief

Particular features of abnormal grief include prolonged irritability or anger relating to the death, agitation, an inability to accept the fact of the death, detachment from others who the patient was previously close to and hopelessness regarding the future.

Symptoms must be severe enough to cause a functional impairment (e.g. significant difficulty continuing with work, maintaining relationships or caring for dependents).

Six months has been suggested as the maximum duration of normal grief, but this is controversial – any time frame on normal/abnormal grieving has been removed from DSM-5.

'After we lose someone, it is of course normal to feel that loss and to take time to adjust to life without them. Sometimes this can continue for a long time and cause more difficulty for some than others. Have you found that you feel more angry or irritable since the loss? Do you ever feel agitated or restless? If you think about life a few years ago, do you still see friends and family as much? How do you feel about the future ahead of you? Do you have any plans? Of course, we never forget the death of someone we love, but do you feel as though you have been able to grieve for him and that you are gradually getting back on top of things in general?'

Exclude differentials

In normal grief, low mood and dysphoria may be intermittent and the individual is still able to reflect on happy memories of the loved one. In depression, there is more pervasive low mood and cognitive symptoms, such as feelings of worthlessness and hopelessness or guilt, particularly in relation to the death.

Clarify whether she has the core and somatic symptoms of depression and enquire about her concern over her health. Are there any nihilistic beliefs? Given her repeated calls to the GP, consider differentials of health anxiety, hypochondriasis or depression with psychotic symptoms (e.g. nihilistic delusions).

'How would you describe your mood over the past 2 weeks? Do you find that you feel sad or low all of the time or are there times when you feel better or more positive? What are your energy levels like? Do you have enough energy to go about your routine or do you feel tired most of the time? Are there things that you still enjoy doing or take your mind off things? Your GP mentioned that you have seen him quite often with general health worries. Are you concerned you may be ill? Is there anything in particular you are worried about? How do you feel after you see your GP and he has told you that he believes you are physically well? Does it reassure you?'

Screen for other delusional beliefs such as persecutory ideas, thought interference and delusions of reference.

It is normal for a bereaved person to experience brief illusions or hallucinations (whether visual or auditory) of the deceased.

'Sometimes when people have lost someone they were close to, they can seem to hear their voice or might think that they see them from time to time. Is that something you have experienced? How often does that happen? Do you ever find that you hear other people's voices talking when you are alone or that you hear anything else that others cannot hear? Is it just your husband's voice you hear or anyone else's?'

Aetiological factors

An estimated 6%–15% of bereaved people develop a complicated grief reaction and this is more likely following a sudden death or suicide, where the bereaved was dependent on the deceased, where there is a past psychiatric history or there are pressures preventing grief (e.g. dependents).

Enquire into any history of depression or other mental health problems. A history of depression increases her vulnerability to developing another episode as a result of the bereavement.

Enquire into how she has coped with any previous major losses or changes in her life.

Is there a family history of depression or other significant psychiatric disorder?

Risk

Be sure to enquire about any personal or family history of self-harm or suicide attempts.

As part of your assessment, enquire into any suicidal ideation resulting from the bereavement.

'Sometimes when people are going through a very difficult time, they think about not being alive or wanting to end it all – have thoughts like that come to you?' Be careful to distinguish any thoughts of ending her own life from a more passive wish to be with the deceased that may be common in the early stages of grief.

You should enquire about substance use.

Conclusion

Explain that you think she is having an ongoing but normal grief reaction and that this is partly being expressed as an anxiety regarding her own health, leading to repeated reliance on the GP for reassurance.

Explain that antidepressant medication is not recommended in normal grieving, but that she may benefit from bereavement counselling and that this may help with her anxiety elsewhere.

Discussing practical support (e.g. others assisting her with things that her husband may have taken a lead on in the past) and making use of her support network (e.g. her mother) are important.

Signpost that she should see her GP should she develop clear symptoms of depression or to seek urgent help if thoughts of harm to herself emerge.

FURTHER READING

Bonanno, G.A. & Kaltman, S. (2001) The varieties of grief experience. *Clinical Psychology Review, 21,* 705–34.

Hawton, K. (2007) Complicated grief after bereavement. *BMJ, 334,* 962.

Prigerson, H.G., Shear, M.K., Jacobs, S.C. et al. (1999) Consensus criteria for traumatic grief – A preliminary empirical test. *British Journal of Psychiatry, 174,* 67–73.

World Health Organization (1992) *The ICD-10 Classification of Mental and Behavioural Disorders. Clinical Descriptions and Diagnostic Guidelines.* Geneva: WHO Press.

The examiner's mark sheet

Domain/ percentage of marks	Essential points to pass	✓	Extra marks/comments (make notes here)
1. Rapport and communication 20% of marks	Clear communication Open and closed questions Empathy Demonstrating patience		
2. Explores normal grief 20% of marks	Enquires into changes to daily function Behaviours relating to the bereavement		
3. Explores abnormal grief and aetiological factors 20% of marks	Enquires into health beliefs Asks about hallucinations Evaluates severity of depressive symptoms Excludes depression, psychosis and hypochondriasis		
4. Risk 20% of marks	Assesses current and historical risk of harm to self		
5. Explains the diagnosis and management 20% of marks	No need for antidepressants Bereavement has prompted health-related anxiety Counselling and practical support		

% SCORE _____

_____

5

OVERALL IMPRESSION

(CIRCLE ONE)

Good Pass

Pass

Borderline

Fail

Clear Fail

NOTES/Areas to improve

STATION 3: SELECTIVE SEROTONIN REUPTAKE INHIBITORS AND SEXUAL DYSFUNCTION

INSTRUCTION TO CANDIDATE

This woman attends the community clinic wanting to speak to her husband's psychiatrist. She is angry that their sex life has deteriorated as a result of him taking a selective serotonin reuptake inhibitor (SSRI) antidepressant.

She has had plans to start a family. It is reported through correspondence from the GP that she may have advised her husband to stop the medication.

Speak to her and address her concerns.

ACTOR (ROLE-PLAYER) INSTRUCTIONS

You are angry with the doctor for causing the problem in your sex life, which you believe is entirely due to the antidepressant.

You are irritable and cold, but will answer questions when asked and want to know what the doctor is going to do to solve the problem – starting a family is very important to you.

Your husband became depressed 5 months ago. Loss of interest in sex was one of his symptoms. He started sertraline 100 mg OD 3 months ago and has lost even more interest in sex since then. He has not been able to have an orgasm for the past 2 months.

You think he is no longer interested in you physically and wonder whether he still loves you.

You have not felt able to talk to your husband about any of this, but did tell him he should stop the tablets 1 week ago. You do not know whether he is still taking them.

He has no other medical problems and does not take any other medication.

SUGGESTED APPROACH

Setting the scene

Introduce yourself by saying, 'Hello, my name is Dr_____, I am one of the psychiatrists. I understand you have some worries about your husband?'

She is clearly upset and may be bringing an important issue to your attention. Sexual side effects can be distressing for both partners and can damage relationships. They are also one of the main reasons for poor adherence to antidepressants in men.

Importantly, this is not your patient and you must not forget your duty of confidentiality. She can provide you with information if she wishes and you can give general information about conditions, medication effects and side effects, but you cannot give specific information about her husband's treatment.

'While I am happy to talk about general issues, I cannot give specific information about your husband's care without his permission. Have you been able to talk to him about coming here today? Please tell me about what's been happening.'

History of sexual dysfunction

What are the sexual problems? SSRIs can affect all phases of sexual behaviour: reduced libido, difficulty with arousal, erectile dysfunction and delayed or absent orgasm. This is a sensitive area, but being confident and frank will avoid making the interviewee feel more uncomfortable.

'When people talk about problems in physical intimacy, there are different things that can be affected. Some notice that they lose interest in sex; some find that it is more difficult to get aroused or have difficulty getting or keeping an erection. Some people find that it takes longer to climax or that it does not happen at all. What have you found is happening with your partner? These kinds of side effects are seen with antidepressants and this should have been explained to your husband when he started them – I'm sorry if that wasn't the case.'

It is crucial to clarify the timing of events in order to establish possible causation.

When did the symptoms of depression start?

When did the sexual problems first start?

When did the medication start and have there been any dose changes or switching?

What other medication is he on – would any of those affect sexual performance, and if so, when were they started?

Is he suffering from other side effects of SSRIs, such as dyspepsia, nausea, vomiting or insomnia? Has anything been done to address these and the sexual side effects so far?

Investigate other causes

You must ask about general medical history for other conditions that might have an impact (e.g. diabetes, cardiovascular disease, endocrine abnormalities, neurological conditions or urological procedures). Inform her that while it may be the SSRI that is causing these side effects, it is important that other possible causes are ruled out.

'We know that antidepressants can have sexual side effects, but other medical conditions can cause similar problems. Does he have any underlying conditions such as diabetes, high cholesterol, etc.? Does he smoke or drink? Does he use any recreational drugs? Has he had any injuries or operations affecting his back or genital area? It's important that we rule out other problems, and there are some blood tests that the GP can arrange to help with this, such as glucose, cholesterol and levels of a hormone called prolactin and other sex hormones.'

Exploration of broader concerns

It is important to find out why this lady is so angry and frustrated. She is hoping to start a family, but there may be other issues, such as the impact her husband's depression is having on their relationship. It is important to also clarify what kind of communication and openness she has had with the husband.

'I understand that part of why this is so upsetting is that you were hoping to become pregnant. Is that something that you and your husband have been able to have a conversation about? Depression can have a powerful impact on people's lives and on those around them. Have you found that his condition has had an impact on your relationship more generally?'

Discussion and plan

Demonstrate you are listening to her concerns and reassure her appropriately. A key part of this is acknowledging that SSRIs do cause sexual problems for some and that this can have a significant impact on both the patient and their partner.

'I am glad that you have explained what's happening and it's important to work out how we can address this. However, I cannot do anything without first getting information from your husband by also discussing what he would like to do. Do you think you can discuss this with him and ask him to see us to clarify the information and work out a plan? These medications do cause sexual side effects for some, but there may be some blood tests and examinations that the GP recommends in order to rule out other possible causes in the meantime.'

Talk through management options and also note that the aim of treatment is to remedy his depression, which can also contribute to the sexual symptoms.

'There are several things that we can do and I'll explain those now. I think it is important to bear in mind that depression itself can affect sexual feelings and behaviour and the aim of treating is to improve this in the longer term.'

Drug holidays are an option; however, her husband should be informed about discontinuation effects and the risk of a worsening of his depression or prolonging recovery.

The dose could be reduced, although this might mean less effective treatment.

Switching to another antidepressant that is less likely to cause side effects is another option. Mirtazapine is commonly used and has a lower incidence of sexual dysfunction. Bupropion (not licensed in the UK for depression) as an alternative or an adjunct and agomelatine are least likely to cause problems, although neither are first-line treatments. The uncertainty of another medication's effectiveness should be weighed against any benefit seen from sertraline.

Sex has an important psychological aspect that is relevant to sexual performance. Despite limited evidence, cognitive behavioural therapy (CBT) to address sexual dysfunction may be of benefit. Sex therapy is another option if interpersonal difficulties or performance anxiety are significant factors.

Phosphodiesterase-5 inhibitors such as sildenafil have an evidence base for improving erectile dysfunction in men and sexual dysfunction in women taking SSRIs.

Conclusion

Check whether you have addressed the problem and whether she has any questions. Emphasise again that there are things that can be done and that you take her concerns seriously, but that it is important that her husband is directly involved in anything that affects his health. Ensure that she is aware that stopping the medication risks worsening/prolonging his depression which, while impacting on sexual function independently, carries significant risks.

FURTHER READING

Balon, R. (2006) SSRI-associated sexual dysfunction. *Am J Psychiatry, 163*, 1504–9.

Taylor, D., Paton, C. & Kapur, S. (2015) *The Maudsley Prescribing Guidelines in Psychiatry*, 12th edn. Chichester: Wiley Blakwell, pp.324–7.

The examiner's mark sheet

Domain/ percentage of marks	Essential points to pass	✓	Extra marks/comments (make notes here)
1. Rapport and communication 25% of marks	Clear communication Open and closed questions Avoids confrontation Sensitive to personal issues		

2. History taking 20% of marks	Establishes the nature of the dysfunction	
	Establishes a clear timeline of depression, sexual dysfunction and medication	
	Other medication and medical conditions	
3. Explores broader concerns 20% of marks	Explores psycho-social/relationship issues	
	Addresses her concerns	
4. Discussion and management plan 25% of marks	Antidepressant alternatives	
	Psychological therapies	
	Adding medication	
	Investigation of other causes	
5. Confidentiality 10% of marks	Indicates an awareness of patient confidentiality	
	Encourages communication with the partner	

% SCORE _____

___

5

OVERALL IMPRESSION

(CIRCLE ONE)

Good Pass

Pass

Borderline

Fail

Clear Fail

NOTES/Areas to improve

STATION 4: BODY DYSMORPHIC DISORDER

INSTRUCTION TO CANDIDATE

Assess this patient who feels that his eyes are too widely spaced apart and is seeking corrective surgery.

Explain your diagnosis and how you plan to help.

ACTOR (ROLE-PLAYER) INSTRUCTIONS

You believe that since your late teens your eyes have been gradually getting further apart and this makes you unattractive.

You refuse to believe that this is not the case and think doctors are mistaken.

You have used eye makeup to minimise this and started avoiding lectures at college.

This led to you dropping out 6 months ago and you are studying a distance course with no face-to-face contact, which you enjoyed.

You have avoided seeing friends over the same time period and they call you less often – you think this is because your eyes 'look weird'.

For the past month, you have been feeling tired most of the time, anxious and low and have stopped enjoying reading for your distance course.

SUGGESTED APPROACH

Setting the scene

'Hello, Ms Smith, I am Dr_____ and I am one of the psychiatrists. I'm glad that we can meet to discuss some of your concerns. I understand you have had some concerns about your appearance and were interested in having surgery?'

History of body dysmorphia

Body dysmorphic disorder involves a preoccupation with either an imagined physical defect or a markedly excessive preoccupation with a minor physical difference to the extent of an overvalued idea (ICD-10: F5.2) or delusional belief (F22.8). A diagnosis requires a persistent preoccupation that is resistant to evidence to the contrary. Preoccupation with the defect and efforts to minimise it must cause a significant degree of distress or functional impairment.

Explore the symptoms sufficiently to reach a diagnosis and exclude differentials.

For how long have they noticed the problem? Do they think it is long-standing or new and is it progressing? Is there a history of similar concerns in the past?

Explore the impact on their behaviour and daily life.

'Do you find that this is something you can put to the back of your mind or do you end up checking your appearance quite a lot? How much time might you spend checking your reflection in a typical day? Have you tried to avoid other people noticing at all? For example, do you use makeup or clothes to hide this or do you avoid going to certain places? Is there anything this has stopped you from doing? Do you think it has had an effect on your work or social life?'

Differentials and comorbidity

This patient may be sensitive to questions around psychopathology. Asking about symptoms of depression or anxiety that might result from her distress communicates your concern for her wellbeing and is a useful place to start.

Explore other anxiety disorders including obsessive compulsive disorder (OCD) and social phobia. Substance misuse and any history of eating disorders are also relevant to the diagnosis and prognosis of body dysmorphic disorder (BDD).

Psychosis should be excluded, including features of schizophrenia (e.g. auditory hallucinations, persecutory delusions, reference and thought interference).

'It seems as though this preoccupies you a great deal and is causing you some real difficulty. How has your mood been recently?' Explore depressive symptoms in order to be able to diagnose or exclude depression.

'Do you find that you have any intrusive thoughts about other things that trouble you? For example, do you find that you repeatedly check things or worry about hygiene? Do you have any routines or rituals around these? Do you find that you feel worried or anxious a great deal of the time? What about alcohol or recreational drugs – do you find that you use anything to stop you from worrying?'

Insight

Insight is of diagnostic importance (i.e. whether their perception and preoccupation is within normal limits, whether it is an overvalued idea [with poor insight] or delusional [with no insight]). A useful way to begin is with others' perceptions of her appearance.

'Have you found other people comment on your eyes? Rather than criticise, do people ever compliment your appearance? Do you think that others notice this less than you or may have a less negative view of your appearance? Do you think there is something medically wrong with your eyes or do you think that this is normal variation and others have similar features? Have you researched anything about this on the Internet?'

Will they consider other explanations? 'It seems as though this has become an increasing worry for you and I wonder whether all of the attention that you focus on your eyes may exaggerate how badly you perceive it.'

If they think there is a medical problem or that their features are progressively changing, are they convinced by medical explanations that this is not the case?

Assess risk

What do they intend to do? A key risk issue is whether they have considered self-mutilating or surgery from unsafe sources. If so, how far have they got with planning and implementing this?

'What would you want surgery for? Have you looked at ways of altering your appearance online or thought about doing anything yourself? Do you think there could be risks associated with this?'

Is there any evidence of impulsivity or substance misuse that might impair their judgement?

You will have explored symptoms of depression. Is there any evidence of suicidal ideation, plans or intent or any history of deliberate self-harm or suicide attempts?

'It is clear that this has been causing you a great deal of distress and worry. When people are going through a difficult time, they sometimes have thoughts about wanting to harm themselves or about dying. Have any thoughts like this come to you?'

Management

Explain the diagnosis and what you would recommend as a management plan. NICE recommends a choice of either CBT or SSRIs, and a combination if more severe.

'I understand that you are worried about your eyes appearing too far apart, but my concern is that this preoccupies you so much that it exaggerates the problem and leads you to take dramatic steps that could make things worse. That could be avoiding other people who are important to you or thinking about surgery. I believe you have developed a condition called body dysmorphic disorder, which affects how you perceive a part of your body and can be very distressing. We would recommend you consider two treatments that may be helpful: cognitive behavioural therapy or medication. Cognitive behavioural therapy or "CBT" is a talking therapy usually over ten or more weekly sessions that look at the way you think about your appearance, your day-to-day behaviours relating to it and the emotional states that come up with those thoughts and behaviours. You learn to recognise how your emotions, behaviours and thoughts interact to compound the problem. You then introduce different ways of thinking and acting that reduce the distress it causes you; for example, training yourself to divert attention away from your appearance or how you believe others will respond.'

If their problems are more severe, you would offer them a SSRI alone or in combination with CBT.

'These medications are often used for depression and anxiety, but have been shown to help in other conditions. Benefits in depression tend to appear within 2 weeks, but in conditions such as BDD, this can take up to 12 weeks.'

Describe the common side effects; explain that the SSRIs are not addictive, but that discontinuation effects can occur if stopped quickly. As for OCD, higher doses of SSRIs are used.

Explain that there can be increased anxiety or agitation in the initiation period. It is recommended to continue the medication for up to 12 months after any improvement.

If there is time, you could go on to discuss a second medication, clomipramine, which can be used if there is no benefit from one or more SSRIs.

There are also self-help materials and support groups available and it would be very useful to involve a trusted friend or family member that they could confide in to support their treatment.

Rapport and communication

A particular challenge here is that this concerns something of great importance to the person (their appearance and everything that they think this will have an impact on in their life) and that they lack insight into their perceptual distortions. In particular, they may be annoyed at seeing a psychiatrist for what they see as a cosmetic or surgical issue.

You will need to balance empathy with their distress and not colluding with their beliefs. One approach is to acknowledge the very real distress they are suffering and openly explore the nature, duration and extent of their beliefs before challenging them.

It is not advised to offer your own opinion on their appearance. Ideally, draw from their objective experience of how others respond to their appearance.

> **FURTHER READING**
>
> NICE guidance for BDD is included in their guidance for OCD. https://www.nice.org.uk/guidance/cg31
>
> Veale, D. (2001) Cognitive–behavioural therapy for body dysmorphic disorder. *Advances in Psychiatric Treatment*, 7, 125–32.

The examiner's mark sheet

Domain/ percentage of marks	Essential points to pass	✓	Extra marks/comments (make notes here)
1. Rapport and communication 25% of marks	Clear communication Open and closed questions Empathy Demonstrating patience		

⬆ 2. Diagnosis of BDD and insight 30% of marks	Preoccupation with feature of appearance	
	Checking behaviours	
	Concealing/avoidance behaviours	
	Severity and frequency	
	Considers comorbid conditions	
3. Assessment of risk 20% of marks	Comorbid depression	
	Suicidal ideation/plans/intent	
	Self-mutilation/risky surgical intentions	
4. Management plan 25% of marks	CBT and/or SSRI	
	Combination treatment	
	Involving friends/family members	

% SCORE _____

___

4

OVERALL IMPRESSION

(CIRCLE ONE)

Good Pass

Pass

Borderline

Fail

Clear Fail

NOTES/Areas to improve

STATION 5: SEASONAL AFFECTIVE DISORDER

INSTRUCTION TO CANDIDATE

You have been asked to assess this 32-year-old gentleman. He has been to his GP on and off for 5 years complaining of changes in his sleeping pattern and mood. Whilst working abroad for a year during the winter, he did not complain of low mood.

The GP informs you that he is noticeably more depressed between October and April, during which he will sleep excessively and put on weight. As spring arrives, he can become mildly elated and irritable. His partner is finding his unpredictability difficult to manage.

The GP referred him for psychotherapy, but this did not help. He wonders whether excessive travelling is responsible for his unstable mental state.

What is the differential diagnosis? Explain your rationale for each.

Give him advice on what can be done to help.

ACTOR (ROLE-PLAYER) INSTRUCTIONS

You have felt low and irritable every winter from about November through to April for the past 5 years, except for 1 year ago in which you spent the majority of your time in the tropics with work from November through to February.

During the winter, you have often taken several weeks off with 'stress', and last winter, you had a poor appraisal that further damaged your confidence, prompting this referral from the GP.

In the spring and early summer, you find that you need far less sleep, are at times irritable and get slightly 'hyper' in a way that frustrates your partner. You have never done anything risky or irresponsible during these periods.

You drink alcohol rarely, are an ex-smoker and take no illicit drugs. You have no medical problems other than mild asthma.

You have never had any thoughts of suicide and have never attempted to end your life.

SUGGESTED APPROACH

Setting the scene

'Hello, my name is Dr_____, thank you for coming. I am a psychiatrist and your GP has written to me explaining that you have problems with low mood and sleep and these seem to happen at particular times of the year, is that right?'

Seasonal affective disorder

To reach a diagnosis, there must have been at least 2 years with a pattern of depression in the winter months that remits in the spring and summer. There should not be a conflicting year where depression occurred in the summer.

'Can you describe the problems with your mood and sleep that you have been seeing your GP for?'

Take care to elicit as full a set of depressive symptoms as possible, particularly atypical symptoms, with increased appetite, weight gain, anergia and increased sleep duration – these are characteristic in seasonal affective disorder (SAD).

'The letter implied that these seem to happen at certain times of the year. What time does your low mood usually start? When do you begin to feel better? So by spring and moving into summer, perhaps May to June, do you find that you have any difficulties with your mood and energy or are you back to your normal self? And has this pattern in which you develop low mood, increased sleep and appetite and reduced energy and little enjoyment in things ever happened during the spring or summer? Are there any winters where this has not happened? Was there anything different about that time?'

Remember in any station related to depressive symptoms to ask about suicidal ideation.

Differential diagnoses

You have considered recurrent depressive disorder in asking about non-seasonal episodes of depression.

It is important to exclude adjustment reactions to stressors that might occur at particular times in the year and confound the diagnosis (e.g. changes in work pattern).

'Are there other changes in your life – perhaps the nature of your job or things in your personal life – which change significantly because of the time of year? Are these things that cause you a great deal of concern or worry?'

As with any station involving depression, ask for a history of mania or hypomania that may point to bipolar affective disorder.

'Do you ever have periods lasting days to weeks or longer with unusually good mood and increased energy or talkativeness? Does this ever become problematic, perhaps leading to not completing tasks or being so talkative that others find it difficult to be around you?'

Ask about a lifelong history of prolonged cyclical changes in mood that may not have adhered to a seasonal pattern. Another differential is cyclothymia, although in such a case you would not expect these periods of low mood to last for the full duration of winter.

Remember also to ask about substance use, particularly alcohol, which may explain the mood symptoms. Think about whether this is prior to the onset of symptoms or whether it may be a form of self-medication.

It is also important to mention physical health and to check their thyroid function.

Management strategy

Start by saying that there are various options you can consider, but it might be useful to ask his partner's perspective on his symptoms in winter and particularly the change during spring if he is agreeable to your speaking to them.

The leading diagnosis is SAD. The NICE guidelines recommend approaching SAD in the same manner as depression with CBT and/or SSRIs as the first line depending on the severity and duration of symptoms and patient preference.

NICE advises against using bright light therapy as an alternative, but this can be used to supplement the treatment, as there is some evidence of a benefit. The patient would need to be exposed to 10,000 lux of white fluorescent light using a light box for at least 30 minutes every day during early morning or on rising. They need to stay awake during this with their eyes open. They could read or do any other light activity that allows them to stay by the light source. Benefit may be felt after several days, although it usually takes up to 2 weeks to reach full effect. Ideally, treatment should be started in late summer or early autumn.

Conclusion

The symptoms of irritability and becoming 'hyper' in the summer may point towards a bipolar affective disorder, but this requires a more in-depth interview and you can suggest meeting for further assessment, as well as obtaining collateral from his partner. Recurrent depressive disorder is another differential if there are episodes that do not fit the SAD pattern. The clear leading diagnosis, however, is of seasonal affective disorder.

Be sure to clarify time courses and confounders, summarise the symptoms reported in order to make it clear that you have reached a diagnosis and always cover risk to self.

FURTHER READING

Eagles, J.M. (2003) Seasonal affective disorder. *British Journal of Psychiatry*, 182, 174–6.

NICE Clinical Guidance CG90 1.6.1.2 (2009) Advises against using light therapy as an alternative instead of antidepressants or CBT. https://www.nice.org.uk/guidance/cg90

The examiner's mark sheet

Domain/percentage of marks	Essential points to pass	✓	Extra marks/comments (make notes here)
1. Rapport and communication 25% of marks	Clear communication Open and closed questions Empathy Demonstrating patience		
2. History of seasonal affective disorder 20% of marks	Depression in winter months Atypical features Remission in the summer 2 years and no conflicting patterns or confounders		
3. Differential diagnoses 30% of marks	Recurrent depressive disorder Bipolar affective disorder Annual stressor/adjustment reactions Medical conditions and blood tests Substance use		
4. Management 25% of marks	Explains the differentials Offers further assessment/collateral history SSRI and/or CBT Additional option of bright light therapy Risk of self-harm		

% SCORE _____

OVERALL IMPRESSION

4 (CIRCLE ONE)

Good Pass

Pass

Borderline

Fail

Clear Fail

NOTES/Areas to improve

STATION 6: URINE DRUG SCREEN

INSTRUCTION TO CANDIDATE

You are the junior doctor on call and have been asked to see this 23-year-old male patient who came back late from Section 17 leave and is behaving strangely. He has a diagnosis of paranoid schizophrenia with a history of relapse secondary to poor compliance in the context of substance misuse. He has been improving with anti-psychotics and abstinence. Nursing staff have suspended their leave and asked for a urine drug screen, which he/she has refused.

Talk to the patient and manage the situation. Do NOT conduct a full mental state examination.

ACTOR (ROLE-PLAYER) INSTRUCTIONS

You have been on leave and overstayed into the evening after taking cannabis and some cocaine at a friend's flat, where you talked and played computer games.

You are feeling slightly paranoid but do not have any delusions, and the 'voices' you hear are quieter and vague.

You believe that the anti-psychotics make you feel calmer and help you sleep, but do not have an understanding of the psychotic symptoms you experienced earlier in the admission.

You refused the urine drug screen because you have been arrested in the past for possession of drugs and believe the ward will call the police to punish you.

You think that the ward would punish you because you were told on a previous admission that you would be discharged if you broke any of the ward rules – you think they may also discharge you home if the urine drug screen shows you have taken recreational drugs.

You do not want to be sent home to your flat as you owe money to a drug dealer that lives in the same building and are afraid that they may hurt you.

SUGGESTED APPROACH

Setting the scene

Introduce yourself as the doctor on call and explain why you have been asked to see him.

'Hello, _____, my name is Dr_____, and the nurses asked me to see you because you came back from leave late and we are concerned about what may have happened. Is it alright if I talk to you for a while? The nurses also said that they asked for a urine sample for a drugs test but you weren't happy to do one, is that correct?'

This station is largely about building rapport and trust so that you can take a history regarding a sensitive issue from a vulnerable patient. You will need to explain to him/her why you are concerned and the reasons for a urine sample and ascertain his expectations and concerns.

Ascertain what happened during the leave, whether he/she used any illicit substances and whether there was any risk of him/her coming to harm. This is a good opportunity to reassure him/her and show an interest in his wellbeing.

'How was your leave? Did you enjoy it? Did you see any friends or family? How did that go? Sometimes when people have been unwell in hospital, others may try to take advantage of them – did you meet anyone that made you uncomfortable or did anything bad happen to you? Did anybody try to attack you or try to take money from you?'

Explore his/her concerns about giving the sample

'It sounds like you're worried about what might happen if a test shows up drugs in your urine. Can I ask why you are not happy to give a urine sample? Have you given samples to the ward before? What happened? Sometimes people worry that we are going to punish them or call the police, but we don't think that would be helpful for patients.'

Explain the reason for asking for a urine sample

'It might help if I explain why we think it's useful. The team thinks that one of the reasons that you became unwell was because some recreational drugs you took brought the mental illness back on. They also seem to interfere with the tablets you usually take. The nurses felt that you were not your usual self when you came back from leave and we are wondering whether that might be because of something you may have taken or if it is a sign that we are not treating the schizophrenia well enough. A urine sample would show us whether any difference in your mental wellbeing might be because of drugs, rather than the medication not working for you. Another concern we have is that the drugs tend to act against the medication and may mean that you end up spending longer in hospital. The reason why the nurses have stopped your leave for the present is the concern that more drugs may set you back and stop you from being well enough to go home.'

Rapport and communication

It is important to demonstrate to the patient that you have their interests at heart and encourage them to voice their concerns or anxieties.

Asking after their wellbeing and their view on their illness, medication, the admission and drug use is important to understanding why they have refused. A motivational interviewing approach where you 'roll with resistance' and avoid telling the patient what they should and should not do, but rather encourage reflection on harms and benefits, is more likely to work.

Conclusion

Ask again whether they would allow a urine sample to be taken and offer to come back and talk to them about it later. If there is time, you can ask whether they understand the reason for their leave being stopped and the behavioural contract with the staff. Acknowledge again that stopping recreational drug use is difficult and there can be great pressure to buy and use substances in the community. Emphasise the expectation that they will get better faster and get out of hospital sooner if they do not use drugs which both affect their mental state and interact with their medication. The hope is to develop a relationship of trust regarding leave and to enable staff to reduce restrictions on liberty while being confident that the patient's mental health will not suffer. Be mindful throughout that the patient may well experience their leave being stopped as punitive and feel mistrustful towards the team.

The examiner's mark sheet

Domain/ percentage of marks	Essential points to pass	✓	Extra marks/comments (make notes here)
1. Rapport and communication 20% of marks	Clear communication		
	Open and closed questions		
	Empathy		
	Demonstrating patience		

⇧ 2. Takes a history about events during leave

30% of marks

What happened, why was he late?

Any risk events to self/others

Any vulnerable adult issues – financial abuse or assault?

Any drug taking divulged

3. Explores the patient's concerns

30% of marks

What are his expectations?

What has happened previously?

Delusional beliefs?

Forensic history?

Owes money to drug dealers?

4. Explains the rationale and addresses concerns

20% of marks

Explains the need to tell whether the symptoms observed may be due to drugs versus illness

Reassures the patient

Explains the importance of abstinence in working towards discharge

% SCORE _____

___

4

OVERALL IMPRESSION

(CIRCLE ONE)

Good Pass

Pass

Borderline

Fail

Clear Fail

NOTES/Areas to improve

STATION 7: PSYCHOTIC DEPRESSION IN AN OLDER ADULT

INSTRUCTION TO CANDIDATE

You are asked to see Mrs Oswald, a 77-year-old woman who presented to the local police station in her nightie stating that she had committed a crime. The police have brought her to accident and emergency (A&E), where you are assessing her as the duty psychiatrist.

Take a history and perform a mental state examination in order to arrive at a diagnosis.

ACTOR (ROLE-PLAYER) INSTRUCTIONS

You are terrified that you have committed a crime and are giving yourself up so that you can be put in jail. You believe that you stole from the hospital where your son was born as you took him home in the blankets used by the maternity ward.

You are convinced that this means you stole from the government and should be punished. You cannot be convinced that you are not in serious trouble.

You were depressed 20 years ago after your son died in a car crash, but did not have any treatment. You do not want any treatment now and would refuse to go into hospital.

You are agitated and restless, with low mood, anxiety, reduced sleep and appetite for 6 months since your husband died. You have not slept for the past 3 nights at all.

You occasionally hear your husband's voice call your name, but have no other hallucinations. You do not have any other psychotic symptoms.

You have thought about throwing yourself from your third floor balcony where you live alone.

SUGGESTED APPROACH

Setting the scene

Introduce yourself: 'Hello, my name is Dr_____, and I am a psychiatrist. I understand that you came to the police station because you are worried you have done something wrong. You seem very distressed – would you mind telling me what has happened?'

This is a distressed and agitated patient – remaining calm, speaking clearly and repeating where needful will help to hold her attention.

Symptoms of psychotic depression

Ask her to explain her concerns and offer reassurance. Explore her responses: 'So you are worried that you may have stolen linens from the NHS many years ago. Can I ask why this is something that you have become worried about now? Why do you think the hospital and the police would be concerned about one blanket going missing? It sounds like it was an honest mistake – do you think the police would want to charge you for taking a blanket by accident? I am sure that many mothers must have made the same mistake over the years. Do you think that the police are trying to find everyone that might have taken a blanket?'

It is important to establish whether there are symptoms of depression. Ensure you ask about mood, anhedonia, anergia and biological symptoms.

Differentials

Late-onset schizophrenia-like psychoses, delirium and behavioural and psychological symptoms in dementia are key differentials.

Delirium is a medical emergency and would require full medical assessment – asking about past medical history and any symptoms of urinary tract infection (UTI) or chest infection indicates that you are thinking about this.

There is not enough time to conduct a complete cognitive screen, but asking about orientation to time and place is useful and demonstrates that you are aware that this may be a presentation related to cognitive impairment or confusion. A brief test of attention is serial sevens or digit span test would be useful.

Given that she is presenting with delusional beliefs, other forms of psychosis should be excluded. Screen for symptoms of schizophrenia (e.g. auditory hallucinations, persecutory delusions, ideas of reference, passivity and thought interference). Is there any evidence of racing thoughts, pressured speech or grandiosity?

You could also consider post-traumatic stress disorder by inquiring about traumatic events (e.g. the two family bereavements) and intrusive imagery, nightmares or avoidance.

Ask about past psychiatric history. Previous episodes of depression support a recurrent episode in the present.

Risk

'When people are going through a very distressing time, they sometimes think about harming themselves or ending their lives. Have you had any thoughts like that? Have you thought about any particular way that you would try to kill yourself?'

Ask who is at home with her and what supports there may be.

Is she using alcohol and is there any evidence of impulsivity?

Has she every tried to end her life in the past?

Is there a family history of suicide?

Has she been eating and drinking? What is her hydration status?

Does this patient drive?

Does she ever look after any minors (e.g. grandchildren)?

Has she had any falls?

Immediate management

This lady is presenting with psychotic depression (delusional beliefs) in the context of a recent bereavement and previous depressive episodes. Given her suicidal ideation in the context of agitation and without supports at home, she is potentially high risk and needs to be fully assessed in an in-patient setting.

'Mrs Oswald, you seem to be very upset and worried and I am thinking about what may be the best way to help you. In particular, I am concerned that you may be suffering from a form of depression at the moment. How would you feel about coming into hospital for a period of time where you would have people to support you and we could address what treatment may help?'

If the patient refuses to consider admission, with clear evidence of risks and mental disorder, you will need to discuss a Mental Health Act assessment.

'From the things you have told me about how you have been feeling, I am concerned that you may have developed a severe depression. I am quite concerned and I think it may be important for your safety to come into hospital and to have a full assessment and treatment, even if you are not happy to do so. Sometimes this happens under a part of the law called the Mental Health Act if people are very unwell and their condition is putting them at risk of harm. I will ask for two doctors and an approved mental health professional who is not a doctor to meet with you in order to talk about your worries and why you came to the police station. They will see you for a Mental Health Act assessment, which means that they will consider whether you are unwell and require being in hospital under the Mental Health Act. This is sometimes called being placed under a Section and would mean that you go from A&E to a mental health hospital for a period of time in order to work out what is wrong and try to get you better.'

If there is time, you can explain Section 2 for assessment and treatment and that this lasts for a maximum of 28 days.

A patient with severe depression and delusional beliefs is unlikely to be able to engage with psychological therapies.

The first line will be antidepressants augmented with an anti-psychotic either at initiation or if there is no response to antidepressant monotherapy. Doses should take into account the patient's age.

Tricyclic antidepressants may be more effective in psychotic depression, although they are not tolerated as well as SSRIs.

If she does not respond to treatment at an appropriate dose, switching and augmenting strategies should be used.

If she is not responsive to sufficient trials on pharmacotherapy or if rapid response is needed (e.g. poor dietary intake), electro-convulsive therapy has a good evidence base in psychotic depression.

Conclusion

This is severe depression with psychotic features and suicidal ideation, agitation, no carers in the community and easy access to a potentially lethal method (jumping from her balcony). Given the level of risk, she should be managed in hospital. Explaining that you feel an admission is needed and discussing a Mental Health Act if she refuses demonstrates your awareness of the severity of risk.

The hallucinations of her husband's voice may or may not be relevant to the diagnosis – these could be a normal experience in uncomplicated grief and may have predated the depression. However, there is sufficient evidence for the diagnosis of severe depression with psychotic features due to her nihilistic delusions of guilt.

FURTHER READING

Taylor, D., Paton, C. & Kapur, S. (2015) *The Maudsley Prescribing Guidelines in Psychiatry*, 12th edn. Chichester: Wiley Blackwell, pp.266–8.

The examiner's mark sheet

Domain/ percentage of marks	Essential points to pass	✓	Extra marks/comments (make notes here)
1. Rapport and communication 20% of marks	Clear communication Open and closed questions Empathy Remains calm despite agitated patient		
2. Symptoms of psychotic depression 20% of marks	Symptoms of depression Psychotic symptoms Duration of symptoms Trigger factors		

⇧ 3. Differential diagnoses Delirium
   15% of marks   Cognitive impairment
                           Paranoid psychosis
                           Substance misuse

4. Risk assessment   Suicidal ideation, method
   20% of marks   and intent
                           Social support
                           Eating and drinking
                           Driving
                           Minors
                           Falls

5. Immediate management   Admission
   25% of marks   Mental Health Act (MHA)
                           assessment if patient
                           refuses
                           Antidepressant with or
                           without anti-psychotic

% SCORE _____

___

5

OVERALL IMPRESSION

(CIRCLE ONE)

Good Pass

Pass

Borderline

Fail

Clear Fail

NOTES/Areas to improve

INDEX